Editorial Board Members' Collection Series: Biomaterials Design

Editorial Board Members' Collection Series: Biomaterials Design

Editors

Richard Drevet
Hicham Benhayoune

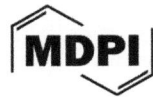

Basel • Beijing • Wuhan • Barcelona • Belgrade • Novi Sad • Cluj • Manchester

Editors

Richard Drevet
Department of Physical Electronics
Masaryk University
Brno
Czech Republic

Hicham Benhayoune
Institut de Thermique Mécanique et Matériaux (ITheMM)
Université de Reims Champagne-Ardenne (URCA)
Reims
France

Editorial Office
MDPI AG
Grosspeteranlage 5
4052 Basel, Switzerland

This is a reprint of articles from the Topical Collection published online in the open access journal *Designs* (ISSN 2411-9660) (available at: https://www.mdpi.com/journal/designs/topical_collections/Q5P5XA1Y8U).

For citation purposes, cite each article independently as indicated on the article page online and as indicated below:

Lastname, A.A.; Lastname, B.B. Article Title. *Journal Name* **Year**, *Volume Number*, Page Range.

ISBN 978-3-7258-1691-0 (Hbk)
ISBN 978-3-7258-1692-7 (PDF)
doi.org/10.3390/books978-3-7258-1692-7

© 2024 by the authors. Articles in this book are Open Access and distributed under the Creative Commons Attribution (CC BY) license. The book as a whole is distributed by MDPI under the terms and conditions of the Creative Commons Attribution-NonCommercial-NoDerivs (CC BY-NC-ND) license.

Contents

Richard Drevet and Hicham Benhayoune
Biomaterials Design for Human Body Repair
Reprinted from: *Designs* **2024**, *8*, 65, doi:10.3390/designs8040065 1

Nuzul Ficky Nuswantoro, Muhammad Adly Rahandi Lubis, Dian Juliadmi, Efri Mardawati, Petar Antov, Lubos Kristak and Lee Seng Hua
Bio-Based Adhesives for Orthopedic Applications: Sources, Preparation, Characterization, Challenges, and Future Perspectives
Reprinted from: *Designs* **2022**, *6*, 96, doi:10.3390/designs6050096 5

Carlos Aurelio Andreucci, Elza M. M. Fonseca and Renato N. Jorge
Bio-Lubricant Properties Analysis of Drilling an Innovative Design of Bioactive Kinetic Screw into Bone
Reprinted from: *Designs* **2023**, *7*, 21, doi:10.3390/designs7010021 29

Elisa Bertrand, Sergej Zankovic, Johannes Vinke, Hagen Schmal and Michael Seidenstuecker
About the Mechanical Strength of Calcium Phosphate Cement Scaffolds
Reprinted from: *Designs* **2023**, *7*, 87, doi:10.3390/designs7040087 40

Alexandros Efstathiadis, Ioanna Symeonidou, Konstantinos Tsongas, Emmanouil K. Tzimtzimis and Dimitrios Tzetzis
3D Printed Voronoi Structures Inspired by *Paracentrotus lividus* Shells
Reprinted from: *Designs* **2023**, *7*, 113, doi:10.3390/designs7050113 58

Rumana Islam and Mohammed Tarique
Investigating the Performance of Gammatone Filters and Their Applicability to Design Cochlear Implant Processing System
Reprinted from: *Designs* **2024**, *8*, 16, doi:10.3390/designs8010016 76

Jia Uddin
Attention-Based DenseNet for Lung Cancer Classification Using CT Scan and Histopathological Images
Reprinted from: *Designs* **2024**, *8*, 27, doi:10.3390/designs8020027 97

Ana Pais, Catarina Moreira and Jorge Belinha
The Biomechanical Analysis of Tibial Implants Using Meshless Methods: Stress and Bone Tissue Remodeling Analysis
Reprinted from: *Designs* **2024**, *8*, 28, doi:10.3390/designs8020028 115

Manuel Mejía Rodríguez, Octavio Andrés González-Estrada and Diego Fernando Villegas-Bermúdez
Finite Element Analysis of Patient-Specific Cranial Implants under Different Design Parameters for Material Selection
Reprinted from: *Designs* **2024**, *8*, 31, doi:10.3390/designs8020031 133

Paweł Turek, Wojciech Bezłada, Klaudia Cierpisz, Karol Dubiel, Adrian Frydrych and Jacek Misiura
Analysis of the Accuracy of CAD Modeling in Engineering and Medical Industries Based on Measurement Data Using Reverse Engineering Methods
Reprinted from: *Designs* **2024**, *8*, 50, doi:10.3390/designs8030050 146

Konstantinos Chatzipapas, Anastasia Nika and Agathoklis A. Krimpenis
Introduction of Hybrid Additive Manufacturing for Producing Multi-Material Artificial Organs for Education and In Vitro Testing
Reprinted from: *Designs* **2024**, *8*, 51, doi:10.3390/designs8030051 . . . . **168**

Carlos Aurelio Andreucci, Elza M. M. Fonseca and Renato N. Jorge
Biomechanics of a Novel 3D Mandibular Osteotomy Design
Reprinted from: *Designs* **2024**, *8*, 57, doi:10.3390/designs8030057 . . . . **179**

Luis Miguel Pires and José Martins
Design and Implementation of a Low-Power Device for Non-Invasive Blood Glucose
Reprinted from: *Designs* **2024**, *8*, 63, doi:10.3390/designs8040063 . . . . **190**

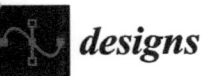 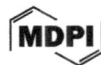

Editorial

Biomaterials Design for Human Body Repair

Richard Drevet [1,*] and Hicham Benhayoune [2]

1 Department of Plasma Physics and Technology, Masaryk University, Kotlářská 2, CZ-61137 Brno, Czech Republic
2 Institut de Thermique, Mécanique et Matériaux (ITheMM), EA 7548, Université de Reims Champagne-Ardenne (URCA), Bât.6, Moulin de la Housse, BP 1039, 51687 Reims CEDEX 2. France; hicham.benhayoune@univ-reims.fr
* Correspondence: drevet@mail.muni.cz or richarddrevet@yahoo.fr

The global clinical demand for biomaterials is constantly increasing due to the aging population [1,2]. Biomaterials are biocompatible materials made of metal [3–5], polymer [6–8], bioactive glass [9–11], ceramic [12–17] or a composite of these materials. The International Union of Pure and Applied Chemistry (IUPAC) defines biocompatibility as the *ability of a material to be in contact with a biological system without producing an adverse effect* [18–23]. Academic and industrial research permanently develops new biomaterials with extended lifespans and improved properties to repair or replace tissue functions of the body. Implanted materials need specific biological, physical, chemical, and mechanical properties to interact appropriately with the physiological environment. The biomedical applications of biomaterials include, but are not limited to, joint replacements, bone implants, intraocular lenses, artificial organs, artificial ligaments and tendons, dental implants, blood vessel prostheses, heart valves, skin repair, cochlear implants, drug delivery systems, stents, nerve conduits, surgical sutures, pins and screws for fracture stabilization, and surgical mesh.

This topical collection gathers feature articles and reviews presenting the latest achievements in the field and the next challenges for future investigations of the design and applications of biomaterials (Figure 1).

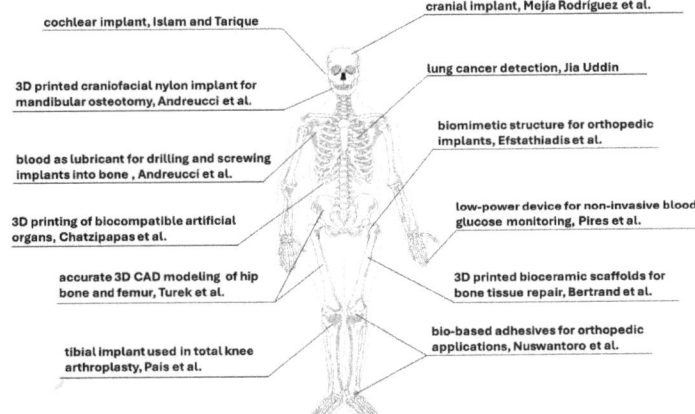

Figure 1. Biomaterials studied in the articles of this topical collection: Pires et al. [24], Andreucci et al. [25], Chatzipapas et al. [26], Turek et al. [27], Mejía Rodríguez et al. [28], Pais et al. [29], Jia Uddin [30], Islam and Tarique [31], Efstathiadis et al. [32], Bertrand et al. [33], Andreucci et al. [34], Nuswantoro et al. [35].

In their article, Pires et al. designed a low-power device for non-invasive blood glucose monitoring [24]. The blood glucose concentration is measured with a near-infrared sensor integrated into a small box placed on the tip of the patient's finger. This innovative device provides high-precision measurements.

In another article, Andreucci et al. describe the use of 3D images from CT scans of patients and 3D printing (also known as additive manufacturing) for mandibular osteotomy [25]. This method of maxillofacial surgery aims to readjust the position of the lower jaw (mandible). The material used to produce the 3D-printed craniofacial implant is nylon, a bioactive polymer material with properties close to bone.

The article by Chatzipapas et al. describes an innovative 3D printing method to produce a biocompatible artificial liver including veins and arteries [26]. Polylactic acid (PLA) is used to create a mold of a liver that is filled with biocompatible light-bodied silicone (polysiloxane). Molds of the veins and arteries are printed using polyvinyl alcohol (PVA). The method is relevant in producing artificial livers with expected applications in medical training, personalized medicine, and organ transplantation.

In another article, Turek et al. describe a reverse engineering (RE) method to accurately reconstruct the geometry of three-dimensional computer-aided designed (3D CAD) models [27]. They show the influence of the measurement parameters, the accuracy of the data fitting, and the parameterization method on the precision of the model. Their innovative method produces accurate bone models (hip bone and femur) with a ± 0.1 mm deviation.

Mejía Rodríguez et al. use finite element analysis (FEA) to study polymeric cranial implants under different design parameters [28]. They describe the mechanical behavior of poly(methyl methacrylate) (PMMA) and polyether ether ketone (PEEK) and discuss the impact of thickness and perforations used in surgical procedures. They conclude that both PMMA and PEEK biomaterials are suitable for producing cranial implants because they withstand deformation in the normal direction.

Another article by Pais et al. reports a computational analysis of the mechanical behavior of tibial implants used in total knee arthroplasty (TKA) [29]. They describe the influence of the knee joint implant properties on the bone remodeling process of the tibia after implantation. The results show the impact of the length of the tibial stem on the maximum stress and displacement distributions in the proximal tibia.

Jia Uddin's article describes a new method using CT scans and histopathological images to improve lung cancer detection and classification [30]. Deep learning technologies are used to improve the precision and reliability of lung cancer diagnostics for early detection and treatment.

In their article, Islam and Tarique studied the performance and optimization of gammatone filters used to design cochlear implants [31]. This theoretical research evaluates the impact of several parameters such as the filter bandwidth, signal frequency, and interferences on the cochlear implant performance.

Efstathiadis et al. investigate the mechanical behavior of polylactic acid (PLA) specimens made by using a 3D printing process called fused filament fabrication (FFF) [32]. The specimens are printed in a biomimetic Voronoi structure inspired by the microstructure of the shell of the sea urchin *Paracentrotus lividus*. The experimental results of this biomimetic design strategy are compared with computational results obtained by finite element analysis.

The research proposed by Bertrand et al. focuses on the mechanical strength of calcium phosphate cement scaffolds produced by 3D printing [33]. This biomaterial is expected to be used for bone tissue repair. The authors describe the influence of the number of printed layers and the influence of the needle's inner diameter on the compressive strength of the 3D-printed bioceramic scaffolds.

The tribological study by Andreucci et al. describes the use of blood as a biological lubricant for drilling and screwing implants into bone [34]. The viscosity of the blood plasma combined with the elastic properties provided by the red blood cells improves the sliding and frictional interfaces between the bone and implant surfaces.

Nuswantoro et al. comprehensively review various types of bio-based adhesives used in orthopedic applications [35]. They are polymer materials with powerful properties for bone fracture healing. In addition to strong adhesion characteristics, bio-based adhesives exhibit biocompatibility, biodegradability, large molecular weight, excellent resorbability, ease of use, and low immunoreactivity.

Author Contributions: Conceptualization, R.D. and H.B.; validation, R.D. and H.B.; resources, R.D. and H.B.; writing—original draft preparation, R.D. and H.B.; writing—review and editing, R.D. and H.B. All authors have read and agreed to the published version of the manuscript.

Funding: This research received no external funding.

Data Availability Statement: The original contributions presented in the study are included in the article.

Conflicts of Interest: The authors declare no conflicts of interest.

References

1. Gheno, R.; Cepparo, J.M.; Rosca, C.E.; Cotton, A. Musculoskeletal Disorders in the Elderly. *J. Clin. Imaging Sci.* **2012**, *2*, 39. [CrossRef]
2. Li, G.; Thabane, L.; Papaioannou, A.; Ioannidis, G.; Levine, M.A.H.; Adachi, J.D. An overview of osteoporosis and frailty in the elderly. *BMC Musculoskelet. Disord.* **2017**, *18*, 46. [CrossRef]
3. Geetha, M.; Singh, A.K.; Asokamani, R.; Gogia, A.K. Ti based biomaterials, the ultimate choice for orthopaedic implants—A review. *Prog. Mater. Sci.* **2009**, *54*, 397–425. [CrossRef]
4. Chen, Q.; Thouas, G.A. Metallic implant biomaterials. *Mater. Sci. Eng. R* **2015**, *87*, 1–57. [CrossRef]
5. Tchana Nkonta, D.V.; Drevet, R.; Fauré, J.; Benhayoune, H. Effect of surface mechanical attrition treatment on the microstructure of cobalt–chromium–molybdenum biomedical alloy. *Microsc. Res. Tech.* **2021**, *84*, 238–245. [CrossRef]
6. Bartmański, M.; Ronowska, A.; Mania, S.; Banach-Kopeć, A.; Kozłowska, J. Biological and antibacterial properties of chitosan-based coatings with AgNPs and CuNPs obtained on oxidized Ti13Zr13Nb titanium alloy. *Mater. Lett.* **2024**, *360*, 135997. [CrossRef]
7. Ferroni, L.; Gardin, C.; Rigoni, F.; Balliana, E.; Zanotti, F.; Scatto, M.; Riello, P.; Zavan, B. The Impact of Graphene Oxide on Polycaprolactone PCL Surfaces: Antimicrobial Activity and Osteogenic Differentiation of Mesenchymal Stem Cell. *Coatings* **2022**, *12*, 799. [CrossRef]
8. Kalirajan, C.; Dukle, A.; Nathanael, A.J.; Oh, T.H.; Manivasagam, G. A Critical Review on Polymeric Biomaterials for Biomedical Applications. *Polymers* **2021**, *13*, 3015. [CrossRef]
9. Sergi, R.; Bellucci, D.; Cannillo, V. A Comprehensive Review of Bioactive Glass Coatings: State of the Art, Challenges and Future Perspectives. *Coatings* **2020**, *10*, 757. [CrossRef]
10. Drevet, R.; Fauré, J.; Benhayoune, H. Calcium Phosphates and Bioactive Glasses for Bone Implant Applications. *Coatings* **2023**, *13*, 1217. [CrossRef]
11. Shaikh, M.S.; Fareed, M.A.; Zafar, M.S. Bioactive Glass Applications in Different Periodontal Lesions: A Narrative Review. *Coatings* **2023**, *13*, 716. [CrossRef]
12. Ginebra, M.P.; Montufar, E.B. Injectable biomedical foams for bone regeneration. In *Biomedical Foams for Tissue Engineering Applications*, 1st ed.; Netti, P.A., Ed.; Woodhead Publishing: Sawston, UK, 2014; Part 2; pp. 281–312. [CrossRef]
13. Dorozhkin, S.V. Calcium Orthophosphate (CaPO$_4$)-Based Bioceramics: Preparation, Properties, and Applications. *Coatings* **2022**, *12*, 1380. [CrossRef]
14. Heimann, R.B. Structural Changes of Hydroxylapatite during Plasma Spraying: Raman and NMR Spectroscopy Results. *Coatings* **2021**, *11*, 987. [CrossRef]
15. Furko, M.; Balázsi, C. Calcium Phosphate Based Bioactive Ceramic Layers on Implant Materials Preparation, Properties, and Biological Performance. *Coatings* **2020**, *10*, 823. [CrossRef]
16. Drevet, R.; Faure, J.; Benhayoune, H. Bioactive Calcium Phosphate Coatings for Bone Implant Applications: A Review. *Coatings* **2023**, *13*, 1091. [CrossRef]
17. Paital, S.R.; Dahotre, N.B. Calcium phosphate coatings for bio-implant applications: Materials, performance factors, and methodologies. *Mater. Sci. Eng. R* **2009**, *66*, 1–70. [CrossRef]
18. Williams, D.F. On the mechanisms of biocompatibility. *Biomaterials* **2008**, *29*, 2941–2953. [CrossRef]
19. Gao, C.; Peng, S.; Feng, P.; Shuai, C. Bone biomaterials and interactions with stem cells. *Bone Res.* **2017**, *5*, 17059. [CrossRef]
20. Williams, D.F. On the nature of biomaterials. *Biomaterials* **2009**, *30*, 5897–5909. [CrossRef]
21. Williams, D.F. Biocompatibility pathways and mechanisms for bioactive materials: The bioactivity zone. *Bioact. Mater.* **2022**, *10*, 306–322. [CrossRef]
22. Albrektsson, T.; Johansson, C. Osteoinduction, osteoconduction and osseointegration. *Eur. Spine J.* **2001**, *10*, S96–S101. [CrossRef]

23. Drevet, R.; Viteaux, A.; Maurin, J.C.; Benhayoune, H. Human osteoblast-like cells response to pulsed electrodeposited calcium phosphate coatings. *RSC Adv.* **2013**, *28*, 11148–11154. [CrossRef]
24. Pires, L.M.; Martins, J. Design and Implementation Low-Power Device for Non-Invasive Blood Glucose. *Designs* **2024**, *8*, 63. [CrossRef]
25. Andreucci, C.A.; Fonseca, E.M.M.; Jorge, R.N. Biomechanics of a Novel 3D Mandibular Osteotomy Design. *Designs* **2024**, *8*, 57. [CrossRef]
26. Chatzipapas, K.; Nika, A.; Krimpenis, A.A. Introduction of Hybrid Additive Manufacturing for producing multi-material artificial organs for education and in-vitro testing. *Designs* **2024**, *8*, 51. [CrossRef]
27. Turek, P.; Bezłada, W.; Cierpisz, K.; Dubiel, K.; Frydrych, A.; Misiura, J. Analysis of the accuracy of CAD modeling in engineering and medical industries based on measurement data using reverse engineering methods. *Designs* **2024**, *8*, 50. [CrossRef]
28. Mejía Rodríguez, M.; González-Estrada, O.A.; Villegas-Bermúdez, D.F. Finite Element Analysis of Patient-Specific Cranial Implants under Different Design Parameters for Material Selection. *Designs* **2024**, *8*, 31. [CrossRef]
29. Pais, A.; Moreira, C.; Belinha, J. The Biomechanical Analysis of Tibial Implants Using Meshless Methods: Stress and Bone Tissue Remodeling Analysis. *Designs* **2024**, *8*, 28. [CrossRef]
30. Uddin, J. Attention-Based DenseNet for Lung Cancer Classification Using CT Scan and Histopathological Images. *Designs* **2024**, *8*, 27. [CrossRef]
31. Islam, R.; Tarique, M. Investigating the Performance of Gammatone Filters and Their Applicability to Design Cochlear Implant Processing System. *Designs* **2024**, *8*, 16. [CrossRef]
32. Efstathiadis, A.; Symeonidou, I.; Tsongas, K.; Tzimtzimis, E.K.; Tzetzis, D. 3D Printed Voronoi Structures Inspired by *Paracentrotus lividus* Shells. *Designs* **2023**, *7*, 113. [CrossRef]
33. Bertrand, E.; Zankovic, S.; Vinke, J.; Schmal, H.; Seidenstuecker, M. About the Mechanical Strength of Calcium Phosphate Cement Scaffolds. *Designs* **2023**, *7*, 87. [CrossRef]
34. Andreucci, C.A.; Fonseca, E.M.M.; Jorge, R.N. Bio-lubricant Properties Analysis of Drilling an Innovative Design of Bioactive Kinetic Screw into Bone. *Designs* **2023**, *7*, 21. [CrossRef]
35. Nuswantoro, N.F.; Rahandi Lubis, M.A.; Juliadmi, D.; Mardawati, E.; Antov, P.; Kristak, L.; Lee, S.H. Bio-Based Adhesives for Orthopedic Applications: Sources, Preparation, Characterization, Challenges, and Future Perspectives. *Designs* **2022**, *6*, 96. [CrossRef]

Disclaimer/Publisher's Note: The statements, opinions and data contained in all publications are solely those of the individual author(s) and contributor(s) and not of MDPI and/or the editor(s). MDPI and/or the editor(s) disclaim responsibility for any injury to people or property resulting from any ideas, methods, instructions or products referred to in the content.

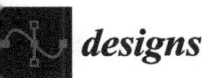

Review

Bio-Based Adhesives for Orthopedic Applications: Sources, Preparation, Characterization, Challenges, and Future Perspectives

Nuzul Ficky Nuswantoro [1,2,*], Muhammad Adly Rahandi Lubis [1,3,*], Dian Juliadmi [1,2], Efri Mardawati [3,4], Petar Antov [5,*], Lubos Kristak [6] and Lee Seng Hua [7]

1. Research Center for Biomass and Bioproducts, National Research and Innovation Agency, Cibinong 16911, Indonesia
2. Research Collaboration Center for Biomedical Scaffold between BRIN and Fakultas Kedokteran Gigi Universitas Gadjah Mada, Yogyakarta 55281, Indonesia
3. Research Collaboration Center for Biomass and Biorefinery between BRIN and Universitas Padjadjaran, Jatinangor 40600, Indonesia
4. Department of Agro-industrial Technology, Universitas Padjadjaran, Jatinangor 40600, Indonesia
5. Faculty of Forest Industry, University of Forestry, 1797 Sofia, Bulgaria
6. Faculty of Wood Sciences and Technology, Technical University in Zvolen, 96001 Zvolen, Slovakia
7. Laboratory of Biopolymer and Derivatives, Institute of Tropical Forestry and Forest Product, Universiti Putra Malaysia, Serdang 43400, Malaysia
* Correspondence: nuzul.ficky.nuswantoro@brin.go.id (N.F.N.); marl@biomaterial.lipi.go.id (M.A.R.L.); p.antov@ltu.bg (P.A.)

Abstract: Bone fracture healing involves complex physiological processes that require biological events that are well coordinated. In recent decades, the process of fracture healing has been upheld through various treatments, including bone implants and bio-adhesive utilization. Bio-adhesion can be interpreted as the process in which synthetic or natural materials adhere to body surfaces. Bio-based adhesives have superiority in many value-added applications because of their biocompatibility, biodegradability, and large molecular weight. The increased variety and utilization of bio-based materials with strong adhesion characteristics provide new possibilities in the field of orthopedics in terms of using bio-based adhesives with excellent resorbability, biocompatibility, ease of use, and low immunoreactivity. The aim of this review is to provide comprehensive information and evaluation of the various types of bio-based adhesives used clinically with a specific focus on their application in orthopedics. The main properties of bio-based adhesives, their benefits, and challenges compared with the traditional bio-based materials in orthopedics, as well as the future perspectives in the field, have also been outlined and discussed.

Keywords: adhesion; bio-based adhesives; bio-polymers; ceramics; orthopedic; biomaterials

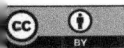

1. Introduction

1.1. Bone Fracture Healing

Bone fracture healing involves complex physiological processes that require biological events that are well coordinated. The knowledge of this process has significantly increased since the expansion of comprehension of the various factors and biological pathways involved. In the near future, advanced developments in bone fracture healing are expected. It is already known that numerous bone diseases can lead to secondary trauma, aging, and metabolic disorders, but a new treatment protocol can solve these problems effectively. Bone fracture healing can be distinguished into direct (primary) and indirect (secondary) healing according to histological perspective. When inflexible internal fixation anatomically diminishes the fracture sections, subsequently, it can lead to direct fracture healing and reducing inter-fragmentary strain. A direct endeavor by the cortex to establish new

Haversian systems by shaping different remodeling aggregations known as cutting cones is involved in this process; the purpose of this process is to reestablish mechanical continuity. The osteoblasts that are required for bone remodeling are differentiated from osteoprogenitor cells that are produced by vascular endothelial cells and perivascular mesenchymal cells. During this process, there are no periosteal or only a few reactions recorded (there is no callus formation) [1,2].

Usually, bone fracture healing is conducted by indirect fracture healing. This process involves callus formation that is produced by the combination of intra-membranous and endochondral ossification. Micro-motion can upgrade this process, which is also hindered by rigid fixation. New bone tissue can be formed straightforwardly through intra-membranous ossification without forming cartilage from committed osteoprogenitor cells in the first place and mesenchymal cells which, not yet differentiated, dwell within the periosteum arranged away from the fracture location. Callus formation is produced from this process, which is known as a hard callus. In this process of bone fracture healing, bone marrow is contributed to bone healing at the early phase of bone healing where endothelial cells are changed into polymorphic cells which have an osteoblastic phenotype. After that, the process is continued by recruitment, proliferation, and differentiation of mesenchymal cells into cartilage, which gets to be calcified and eventually replaced by bone. This process is known as endochondral ossification. The bone healing process requires a few stages, i.e., an initial stage of hematoma formation and inflammation, subsequent angiogenesis and formation of cartilage, cartilage calcification, cartilage removal, bone formation, and ultimately bone remodeling. In this type of fracture, healing the adjacent periosteum and the external soft tissues forms an early callus as a bridge, known as soft callus, and the fracture fragments in the location will stabilized by this callus. The ongoing investigations aimed at better understanding of bone regeneration have provided advanced knowledge of the cellular and molecular processes that oversee these occasions [1–5]. The process of fracture healing is upheld through various treatments, including bone implants and bio-adhesive utilization.

1.2. Bio-Adhesion and Bio-Based Adhesives

Bio-adhesion can be interpreted as the process in which synthetic or natural materials adhere to body surfaces. Bio-based adhesives have found increased utilization in a wide variety of value-added applications due to their sustainability, renewability, biocompatibility, biodegradability, and large molecular weight [6,7]. Bio-adhesion has been extensively used in various biomedical applications, such as orthopedics, orthodontics, surgery, drug administration systems, etc. [8–10]. The constituent utilized for bio-adhesives can be derived from natural resources or be synthesized. In its application, the bio-adhesive must have some capability including the reduction of surgery time, seals strengthening, ease to remove materials, user friendly, enhanced quality of sealing air leaks, etc. Bio-based adhesives, used in biomedical applications, should meet certain criteria such as excellent biocompatibility, resorbability, ease of handling, good strength with effectiveness in biological conditions, and typically low immunogenicity [11]. Bio-based adhesives have found increased application in surgery as sealants and hemostats. Bio-based adhesives have an objective to bond the tissues during the healing period of injuries and maintain a strategic distance from the foreign body reaction at the injury location. In addition, bio-based adhesives ought to work at a particular site and progress along with the healing process with the most extreme safety, i.e., they should not impair the surrounding tissues. The challenging assessment of bio-adhesion is in the wet surfaces, but marine organisms like mussels, fungi, and other bacteria have provided a natural solution to this problem. The bio-based adhesive proteins produced by marine mussels provided them with the ability to adhere to extremely wet surfaces. The adhesive proteins produced by mussels, called mussel foot prints (MFP), are characterized by excellent adhesion characteristics. The MFP is mainly consisted of 3, 4 Dihydroxyphenylalanine (DOPA), derived from tyrocine. The binding and solidifying properties of MFP obtained from catechol side chain of DOPA are cross-linked with the surface of the substrate by chemical reactions. The MFP inspired the development of novel bio-based adhesives materials to fulfill the demands of satisfactory adhesive ability to wet surfaces by utilizing the advantages provided by adhesive proteins [11–13].

The inspiration for developing sustainable bio-based adhesives are based on plants and animals that have inherent bio-adhesion to substrates and tissues. Character similarity with nature is the main factor for the efficient utilization of high-performance, bio-based adhesives in various applications. Bio-based adhesives based on proteins or polysaccharides can imitate the process of blood coagulation. Typical examples of protein-based bio-based adhesives are fibrin sealants, gelatin, and collagen, while examples of polysaccharide-based bio-adhesives include alginate, chondroitin, and chitosan [14–16]. In addition, bio-adhesion construct can be utilized for drug delivery system (DDS) via drug carriers into specific sites [17,18]. Bio-based adhesives can also be utilized to hold mucous or epithelial tissues. Bio-based adhesives that adhere to mucosal tissue surfaces are called mucoadhesives. Mucoadhesives are characterized by easy administration and enhanced adhesion which provides extended contact time and active agent protection, resulting in better patient adherence to the treatment. Ocular cavities, rectal, vaginal, oesophageal, oral, and nasal bio-based adhesives are typical examples of tissue location that provide muco-adhesion [12,19,20].

In spite of the various advantages of the bio-adhesion, it also can cause adverse effect such as bio-fouling. Bacterial bio-film can cause an infection or inflammation like cystic fibrosis and endocarditis that is more often to have prominent resistance against antibiotics. It is considered that there are over 500 type of bacteria which can be found on teeth and gums [12,19,21,22]. The aim of this review is to provide comprehensive information and critical evaluation on the various types of bio-based adhesives used clinically with a specific focus on their application in orthopedics. The main properties of bio-based adhesives, their benefits and challenges compared with the traditional bio-based materials in orthopedics, as well as the future perspectives in the field, have also been outlined and discussed.

2. Sources and Types of Bio-Based Adhesives

Bio-based adhesives can be classified into internal and external ones in accordance with their function and application conditions. Internal bio-based adhesives are largely used in intracorporal conditions with direct contact to organs, tissues, and body fluids. Internal bio-based adhesives have two specific characteristics, i.e., the bio-based adhesives should be able to dissolve in a liquid solution without adding the organic solvent to the primary constituents. Moreover, the primary constituents of bio-based adhesives must be capable to conduct cross linkage. Internal bio-based adhesives are developed to be in contact with internal organs and fluids frequently, so bio-based adhesive must have minimum toxic content along with aqueous solutions. Bio-based adhesives have special characteristics that can set up their adhesive function as it were when it is conducting cross-linking with the substrate in a wet environment just like the internal organs that have liquid circulation with rich blood supply. Toxicities due to long-term application and adverse effects may happen in the patient's body, in case the bio-based adhesives applied inside the body are unable to dissolve and degrade in body fluids which are excrete by excretion system. In general, external bio-based adhesives are applied in topical medications, e.g., epidermal grafting and wound closure [11,19,23,24].

Cyanoacrylate-based tissue adhesive is the most broadly utilized type of external bio-based adhesive. The application of this material can be found at wound dressings treatment, plastic surgeries, and skin transplantations. Some examples of cyanoacrylate-based bio-adhesive are Trufill n-BCA and Dermabond. USA Food and Drug Association (FDA) have approved these types of bio-based adhesives. Cyanoacrylates are distinguished by points of interest, such as their short time for bio-adhesion and improved bonding strength. Nevertheless, in application at tropical zones formaldehyde and respective alkyl compound of cyanoacrylates can be harmful to the human body. This toxic component can also act as carcinogenic agent that can cause tumor or cancer if used for long time period separated from the common complications like necrosis, thrombo-embolic, and septic complications. Cyanoacrylates could see expanded utilization in numerous applications in case the optimum brittleness and adhesion strength of the material can be optimized by adjusting the length of alkyl groups [25].

Other common synthetic polymers, used in bone adhesive applications are polyurethanes, poly(methyl methacrylate)s (PMMAs) (Figure 1), and polycyanoacrylates. Polyurethanes can be synthesized from polyisocyanates and polyols using ultraviolet light orcatalyst. Shifting the orientation of the molecule, chemical groups, cross-linking, and crystallinity of polyurethanes makes this material degrade optimally when utilized as bio-adhesive. If the composition of the molecule, degree of cross-linking, and stiffness of polyurethanes are tuned, these polymers can show diverse properties, suitable for a wide variety of applications, such as bio-based adhesives, wound dressing treatment, tube of catheter, and bone fillers. Since polyurethanes have been widely utilized as bio-based adhesives for soft tissue and sealants, they have found a recent application as bone adhesives. The mechanism that occurs when these polymers physically adhere to bone is through hydrogen bonding, but also through chemical process that involve the arrangement of urea bonds through reaction of the amine at mineralized collagenous extracellular matrix of bone with carbamate group of polyurethanes. In any case, the biomedical environment stability of this material in long-term utilization is still questionable, whereas degradation of this polymer through hydrolysis and enzymatic process is reported by several studies concluding that the degradation caused by in vivo utilization is negligible [26].

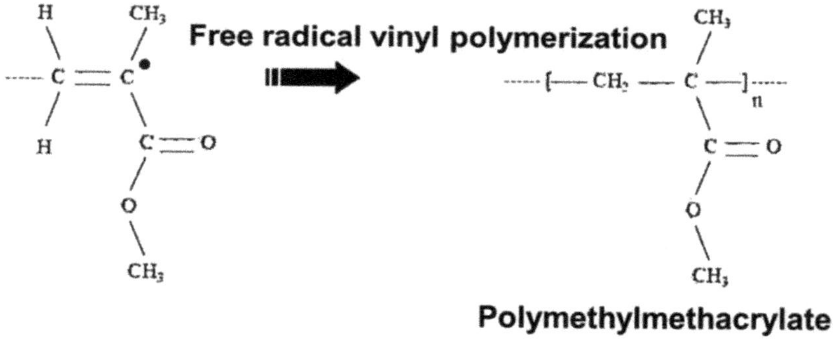

Figure 1. Formation of a polymer chain of PMMA cement. Reused from an Open Access article [27].

Kryptonite is a polyurethane-based polymer used as bone adhesive. Recent studied have reported its successful functional adherence to bone tissue in order to get vertebral augmentation, cranial reconstruction, and sterna closure. Kryptonite covers calcium carbonate powder, castor oil-based polyol, and a reactive isocyanate. However, for utilization as bone cement the formulation of this polymer still should be optimized. In addition, a novel adhesive which has foam-like form consisted of 4,4-methylene diphenyl diisocyanate (MDI)M which was polyurethane-based polymer, a polycaprolactone-based polyol with biodegradable properties and hydroxyapatite particles reinforcement was developed in order to achieve applications of bone-to-bone bonding. Based on the mechanical testing, it can be concluded that a four-fold improved adhesion yields a better result compared to conventional PMMA cement. However, this four-fold improved bio-adhesion is still not considered adequate to attain optimal bone healing since bio-adhesion of PMMA adhesives to bone tissue is slightly low. The cytocompatibility of this adhesive is firstly assessed in vitro which affirmed the good result. At that point, the healing of broken frog hind limb tarsus bone was conducted as the in vivo response. The tissue immunological response of the adhesive material is found based on histological results that comparable to control specimens of bone tissue. However, the estimate impediments of the animal species hold the appropriate evaluation of adhesive to bone bonding strength. In this manner, in order to convincingly as certain the biocompatibility of this material, long-term in vivo studies are required [26].

Actually, PMMA cements show weak bio-adhesion to bone in damp conditions because of hydrophobic properties of this material. Mechanical interlocks with the porous bone are formed when PPMA adhesive is placed. In common, PMMA is encapsulated by fibrous instead of hard tissue, but unfavorable tissue reactions have been reported for bio-adhesives from PMMA-based. In spite of the fact mutagenesis has been reported in bacteria related to utilization of PMMA but carcinogenesis still unknown to be associated with these biomaterials. During application of the PMMA, heat can be released to the surrounding bone tissue caused by an exothermic polymerization reaction that eventually might lead to thermal necrosis. Numerous endeavors have been reported to improve the adhesion of PMMAs to bone, such as bone pre-treatment, intermediate bonding agent application, and PMMA cement chemical modification [11,23,28,29].

In the first place, cyanoacrylates were developed for household, automotive, and construction industries. Dermabond®, Indermil®, Glubran®, and Histoacryl® are examples of cyanoacrylate-based soft tissue bio-based adhesives that are already commercially available. Although this biomaterial has been utilized in clinics as bone glue, cyanoacrylates have not been purposed particularly for application as bone bio-based adhesive. Cyacrin was a cyanoacrylate adhesive, used for the first time in 1963 for bone adhesive, but this material was characterized by high infection rate, no adhesion after the placement, formation of fistula, and several local reactions. Furthermore, Biobond is an ethyl cyanoacrylate which, mixed with polyisocyanate and nitrile rubber, yields better initial results based on in vivo testing. Carcinogenicity is associated with cyanoacrylates that have short alkyl chains due to the releasing of formaldehyde and cyanoacetate caused by erosion of the polymers that happen through hydrolysis reaction. Because of that, American Food and Drug Administration banned methyl cyanoacrylate-based adhesives for human use. Cyanoacrylates that have longer alkyl chain showed a gentler reaction in bone tissue based on further studies, due to steric hindrance and hydrophobicity that makes this material degrade slower. A cyanoacrylate-based adhesive called butyl 2-cyanoacrylate, known as Histoacryl® is already recognized for utilization in surgery to conduct wound closure because of its biocompatibility. Besides, several potential bone adhesives for fractures healing are also tested, such as butyl, isobutyl and octyl 2-cyanoacrylates. However, inadequate bonding strength for stabilization at fracture location after six weeks, cytotoxicity, and inflammatory responses in undiluted form are reported in some cases, although cytotoxicity was appropriate when diluted with culture medium for ten times. For general, cyanoacrylates-based bio-based adhesives need more biocompatibility studies in order to better determine their utilization as bone adhesives [11,25,28,30].

There are numerous natural polymers that function as bone bio-based adhesives, mostly polymers consisted of animal-inspired bio-based adhesives, such as frog, sandcastle, mussel, polysaccharides, and fibrin glue [31–38]. The most broadly utilized material for soft tissue bio-based adhesives, sealants, and hemostatic agents is fibrin. Fibrin is a fibrous non-globular protein involved in the blood clotting mechanism. However, there are numerous factors that affect the fibrin gel architecture, such as thrombin and fibrinogen concentration, temperature of preparation process, pH, ionic strength, and concentration of calcium ion can affect the materials mechanical properties. The gel mechanical strength will be affected by the presence of Factor XIII covalently cross-linking with the polymer chains. Moreover, the adhesive strength of the fibrin-based adhesive can be affected by water, fat, and collagen contents. However, the adhesive strength of fibrin-based bio-adhesive against bone tissue is still low when compared to synthetic bio-adhesives (0.17 MPa), which can also be assumed due to the poor cohesive strength of the fibrin itself, although the fibrin-based bio-adhesive adhere to bone tissues through the formation of covalent bonds between carboxylic acid groups within the collagenous matrix of bone tissue with amino groups of fibrin or fibronectin. Based on the excellent biocompatibility, biodegradability, and cost-effectiveness, fibrin-based bio-adhesive prove to be more superior to synthetic bio-adhesives such as cyanoacrylates. Therefore, these materials proved to be extensively utilized in orthopedic surgery. Currently, the fibrin-based adhesives are utilized for treatment to osteochondral defects. Accelerated revascularization of the osteochondral fragment can be achieved by using fibrin sealant in a thin layer form, this process also confidently followed by union and healing of bone fracture [11,39–41].

There are several important groups of polysaccharides utilized as soft tissue adhesives and hemostatic materials, such as chitin, chitosan, dextran or chondroitin. These materials yield biocompatible and biodegradable adhesives that are composed of natural sugar building blocks that are easy to prepare and apply [21,42–45]. A study reported the successful developed of novel biocompatible and degradable biopolymers based on a two-component bio-adhesive system (chitosan and starch). Based on biomechanical studies, it is known that these bio-adhesive polymers have better strength of bio-adhesion when compared to fibrin glue, but they also have a poorer strength of bio-adhesion than cyanoacrylates on bovine cortical bone specimens. Excellent biocompatibility was also demonstrated in *in vitro* cell testing, so this bio-based adhesive can be a promising candidate for clinical utilization [21,42,46–48].

A cellulose polysaccharides-based scaffold with good mechanical properties and suitability for load-bearing bone healing applications has been reported. Plant cell walls have a linear polysaccharide of D-glucose units linked by $\beta(1\rightarrow4)$ glycosidic bonds that are called cellulose. These materials have a particular strength and provide water-insoluble properties despite their hydrophilic nature because of the highly cohesive hydrogen-bonded structure that composed the cellulose fibers. The character of the cellulose made the scaffolds provide a good compressive strength, which is similar to the mid-range of human trabecular bone. Esterification reaction between the carboxylic acid groups within the bone tissue organic matrix and hydroxyl groups within cellulose was the main mechanism that provides the bio-adhesion of this material. However, in 24 h this adhesive exhibited a weight loss about 10–15% because of degradation under in vitro conditions. In order to decrease the degradation of this scaffold, its chemical structure should be modified for better tissue engineering applications [7,11,23,46,49].

In order to anchor themselves to in water or wet environment, saltwater animals, as well as marine worms, limpets, mussels, and oysters, produce bio-based adhesive proteins. In an environment that has various levels of salinity and humidity there is an organism like *Mytlius edulis* (blue mussel) that has the capability to adhere itself to a substrate, either inorganic or organic. Furthermore, a non-sticky material such as polytetrafluoroethylene (PTFE) can also adhere to this organism. However, there are some technical difficulties due to extraction and high production cost that hold this bio-adhesive to utilize widely in many practical applications. Moreover, large exogenous proteins produced from mussel adhesive utilization can trigger an allergic reaction based on in vivo examination. Because of that, there are many bio-mimetic polymers that have been developed in order to assess the characters and examine the constituents that provide mussels with substantial adhesive capability. Based on the research, it is known that a high concentration of compound at the interface of adhesive substrate of mussels endow this animal with strong adhesive ability. This compound belongs to the so called DOPA groups. Furthermore, it was found that $Fe(DOPA)_3$ was formed from cross-linking reaction between high concentration iron on mussel adhesive with cathecolic hydroxyl group of DOPA. The concentration of iron in mussel bio-adhesives is actually higher (100,000 times) than its concentration in the peripheral water. Ultimately, the bonding between protein and protein or bonding of protein and surface for adhesion actually occurs when iron induces the oxidation of DOPA to produce an organic radical [10–12,50,51].

Because bone is made up of both organic and inorganic components, the type of bio-adhesion that bone has, either to organic or inorganic chemicals, has become the most important factor to take into account in the process of developing bone bio-based adhesives. Because the carboxylic acid and the hydroxyl groups from the catechol of DOPA can establish ionic bonding with calcium, there is a presumption that DOPA could adhere to bone tissue. The process of in vivo maturation of new bones takes place when DOPA stimulates the formation of bone tissue. Additionally, the newly growing bones have a density that is comparable to that of normal bone, as well as in vitro osteogenic differentiation of osteoblast cells. The creation of adhesives modeled after mussels is also being carried out by mixing DOPA, also known as 3,4-dihydroxyphenethylamine (dopamine), with synthetic polymers and hydrogels such as PEG, Pluronic®, and PMMA co-polymers recently. Because of the development that was carried out, a wide variety of tissue bio-based adhesives and hydrogels are now manufactured. However, their potential use as bone bio-based adhesives has been the subject of intensive research [13,47,52–56].

Phragmatopoma calafornica is another marine animal that has inspired researchers in developing bio-based adhesives. This animal produces a bio-based adhesive, commonly known as sandcastle glue. This bio-based adhesive is made of polyphenolic proteins that function as shield for the animal by pasting sea shell, sand, and grains together. These proteins are oppositely charged polyelectrolytes which coagulate due to pH changes. The protein produced by this animal can be a promising bone bio-based adhesive material since the presence of phosphate and amine side groups. The Australian frog *Notaden bennetti* is known to secrete a protein-based material which can produce a sticky elastic hydrogel rapidly. This protein is considered as frog glue. It is known that there are proteins (55–60% of dry weight) rich in glycine (15–16 mol %), proline (8–9 mol %), glutamic acid/glutamine (14–15 mol %), and 4-hydroxyproline (4–5 mol %) which compose this frog glue. Research indicated that this frog glue can solidify spontaneously and function well as a bio-based adhesive in wet environments by creating a proteinaceous pressure-sensitive adhesive. This frog glue can conduct covalent bonding with amines which consist in collagen matrix of bone because the main proteins contain carboxylic acid groups. It is reported that the glue performed significantly better than fibrin glues, although this bio-based adhesive did not perform better as cyanoacrylate in a repair model of ovine meniscal cartilage. This frog glue also enhanced bone-tendon fixation in an ovine model of rotator cuff repair. However, further research must be performed to examine its utilization as a bio-based adhesive for orthopedic applications; even this material has a good in vivo biocompatibility and resorbability. Overall, the distinctive characters of the frog bio-adhesive suggest that a bio-mimetic co-polymer can have a substantial potency for utilization as bone bio-based adhesive [11,12,19,49,53,56–58].

Another material that can be considered for utilization as a bio-based adhesive is from the ceramics group. It is already know that there are various ceramics materials that can be utilize in orthopedic application including calcium phosphate and hydroxyapatite [59–61]. Hydroxyapatite can actually be synthesized chemically from the precipitate of calcium and phosphate. However, this material can also be synthesized from natural resources included clam shells, egg shells, or animal bones like bovine bone [62–68]. Hydroxyapatite was chosen as bio-based adhesive material in orthopedic application because of its biocompatibility and bio-activity, since hydroxyapatite is actually a natural matrix of human bone which constructs the bone tissue along with protein and other organic compound [69–73].

Hydroxyapatite has been used widely for numerous applications in orthopedics, such as metal implants coating, bone graft, bone cement, bone adhesive, and bone scaffold. There are many studies that have been conducted in order to examine the ability of hydroxyapatite to perform a good bone healing either as used as implants coating, bone graft, bone cement, bone adhesive, or bone scaffold. The result of these study demonstrated that hydroxyapatite can enhance the adhesive bonding (osseointegration) between metal implant and bone tissue. As bone graft and bone cement, hydroxyapatite also shows a good result. Furthermore, as a scaffold, hydroxyapatite demonstrated a good performance since this material can promote new bone remodeling without any serious negative effect. Ultimately, hydroxyapatite can be a good candidate as bone bio-adhesive for utilization in orthopedic applications [69,71,74–83]. Summarized information on different bio-based adhesive materials, preparation, and applications is given in Table 1.

Table 1. Summary of Bio-Adhesive Source, Materials, Preparation, and Applications.

No.	Materials	Mechanical Properties	Preparation	Applications	Reference
1.	1. Dopamine methacrylamide (DMA) 2. Methacrylic anhydride (MPC)	1. Surface Roughness (Ra) = 14.5 nm 2. Shear strength 54.6 MPa	Polymerization	1. Implant coating 2. Self-lubrication	[84]
2.	1. Hidroksiapatit (HA) 2. Polyvinyl Alcohol/K-carrageenan (PVACar)	1. Cumulative Release (CR) 200% in 200 h (pH 7.4) and 60% in 250 h (pH 3.0)	Polymerization	Bone Scaffold	[85]
3.	1. Poly(dopamine) (DP) 2. Nitrodopamine (NDP) 3. Titanium oxide nanotubes (NT-TiO$_2$/Ti)	1. Surface Roughness 128 nm (Poly(dopamine)) and 220 nm (Nitrodopamine) 2. Surface Energy 56.98 mJ/mm^2 (Poly(dopamine) and 69.05 mJ/mm^2 (Nitrodopamine) 3. Bending resistance 8.64 MPa (Poly(dopamine)) and 5.32 MPa (Nitrodopamine)	Polymerization	Implant Coating	[86]
4.	1. Albumin/genipinbioglue 2. Bovine serum albumin (BSA) 3. Genipin (GP)	1. Adhesion strength 0.98 N	Polymerization	Tissue glue	[87]
5.	1. Chitosan	1. Tensile bond strength up to 0.024 ± 0.0036 MPa 2. Shear bond strength up to 0.031 ± 0.0069 MPa 3. Fracture toughness of 2.38 ± 0.54 J/m^2	Cross-linking	Bone glue	[88]
6.	1. Chitosan-graft-polypeptide 2. N-carboxyanhydrides (NCAs)—3,4-di-hydroxyphenylalanine-N-carboxyanhydride (DOPA-NCA) 3. Cysteine-NCA (Cys-NCA) 4. Aginine-NCA (Arg-NCA)	1. Lap-shear adhesion strength 195.97 ± 21.1 kPa and 3080 ± 320 kPa 2. Tensile adhesion strength 642.70 ± 61.1 kPa	Ring opening polymerization	Bone glue	[89]
7.	1. Chitosan	1. Tensile strength 0.082 ± 0.03 MPa 2. Elasticity 19.42 ± 6.9% elongation	Cross-linking	Bone Glue	[90]
8.	1. Tris(trimethylsiloxy)silyl (M3T) 2. Trimethoxysilane propyl methacrylate (TMOSPMA) 3. Propyl methacrylate (PMA) 4. Terpolymer (M3T-co-PMA-co-TMOSPMA)	1. Water Contact Angle 98 +/− 0.4° 2. Pencil hardness B	Polymerization	Anti-bacterial implant coating	[91]
9.	1. Tantalum 2. Magnesium 3. Polydopamine (Ta-PDA-Mg)	1. Compression strength 116.46 ± 1.01 MPa 2. Elastic modulus 4.85 ± 0.11 GPa	3D Printing	Scaffold and drug release	[92]

Table 1. Cont.

No.	Materials	Mechanical Properties	Preparation	Applications	Reference
10.	1. Polydimethylsiloxane and poly(ether) ether ketone (PDMS-PEEK)	1. Elastic modulus 3.68 MPa 2. Ultimate tensile strength 1.57 MPa 3. Elongation at break 180.74%	Polymerization	1. Orthodontic prosthetic 2. Artificial vein 3. Cartilage Scaffold	[93]
11.	1. Sodium alginate hydrogel	1. Elastic modulus 4–21 kPa	Cross-linking	Tissue engineering	[94]
12.	1. Visible-light-activated naturally derived polymer (gelatin) 2. Antimicrobial peptide (AMP)	1. Adhesive strength 55.3 G 6.7 kPa 2. Lap shear strength 60 kPa 3. Burst pressure 37.7 G 6.5 kPa	Cross-linking	Scaffold for teeth	[95]
13.	1. Poly(2-oxazoline)	1. Tensile strength 1–4 MPa 2. Tensile Modulus 20–80 MPa	Polymerization	Bone implant	[96]
14.	1. Poly(octamethylene maleate (anhydride) citrate) (POMaC) 2. Poly(ethylene glycol) diacrylate (PEGDA)	1. Young's modulus 1.22 ± 0.01 MPa 2. Tensile strength 0.163 ± 0.010 MPa 3. Elongation 15.44 ± 0.05 4. adhesive strengths 190 g.cm^{-2}	1. 3D Printing 2. Polymerization	Scaffold	[97]
15.	1. Soybean 2. Porcine Bone 3. Xanthan Gum 4. Calcium Chloride 5. Phosphate buffer saline (PBS) 6. Ethyl ether	1. Adhesion strength 361 kPa	Polymerization	Bone adhesive	[98]
16.	1. Bovine serum albumin (BSA) 2. Electro-oxidized alginate-dopa 3. Polyacrylic acid (PAA)	1. Shear strength on vessel 80 kPa, stomach 30 kPa, liver 30 kPa, intestine 32 kPa, and heart 40 kPa. 2. Adhesion strength on vessel 0.25 MPa, stomach 0.13 MPa, liver 0.15 MPa, intestine 0.1 MPa, and heart 0.15 MPa	Cross-linking	1. Closing wound in surgeries 2. Fixing implantable devices 3. Haemostasis	[99]
17.	1. Hydrogel system (MGC-g-CD-ic-TCS) composed by triclosan (TCS)-complexed beta-cyclodextrin (β-CD)-conjugated methacrylated glycol chitosan (MGC)	1. Lap shear strength 40 kPa	Photo-cross-linking via Visible Light Irradiation	Tissue bio-adhesive and anti-bacterial	[100]
18.	1. TiO$_2$ nanotube (TNT) 2. Icariin (Ica) 3. Polydopamine (DP)	1. Surface roughness 159 nm 2. Surface Energy 59.27 mJ/m^2	Electrochemical Anodization	Bone implant osseointegration	[101]

Table 1. *Cont.*

No.	Materials	Mechanical Properties	Preparation	Applications	Reference
19.	1. Sulfate-Catechol Biopolymer	1. Compresive strength 7.8 ± 1.0 kPa	Carbodiimide coupling reaction	Soft tissue engineering	[102]
20.	1. Bio-adhesive polysaccharide-based hydrogels 2. Carboxymethyl chitosan 3. Modified sodium alginate 4. Tannic acid	1. Adhesion strength 162.6 kPa	1. Dynamic covalent bonds 2. Photo-triggered covalent bonds 3. Hydrogen bonds 4. Multi-cross-linking	1. Wound healing 2. Hemostatic 3. Anti-bacterial	[103]
21.	1. Polymerization N-acryloyl aspartic acid (PAASP)	1. Adhesion strength 120 kPa	Polymerization	1. Tissue and organ repair 2. Wound healing	[104]
22.	1. Nitrodopamine (NDP) 2. Poly-Dopamine (DP)	1. Surface roughness 220 ± 9 nm 2. Surface energy 56.98 mJ/m^2 3. Elongation 60 N 4. Adhesive strength 8.64 MPa	Melt grafting	Implant Coating	[86]
23.	1. Polycaprolactane (PCL, Mw 45,000) 2. Beta-tricalcium phosphate (βTCP)	1. Shear strength 157.6 ± 25.1 kDa	Cross-linking	Bone scaffold	[105]
24.	1. Multifunctional injectable temperature-sensitive gelatin-based adhesive double-network hydrogel (DNGel)	1. Adhesive strength 3.75 MPa	1. Cross-linking 2. Facile dual-syringe methodology	Wound healing	[106]
25.	1. PMMA 2. CaP 3. BG 4. Collagen 5. ECM 6. BcP 7. Alginate 8. Chitosan 9. HA	1. Compressive strength 15 MPa	1. Polimerization 2. Cross-linking 3. 3D Printing	1. Bone Adhesive 2. Bone Scaffold 3. Bone Graft 4. Bone Cement	[107]
26.	1. Isocyanate-terminated urethane methacrylate precursors (UMP)	1. Tensile strength 34 ± 4 MPa	Polymerization	Orthodontic	[108]
27.	1. Polycatechol (PC) 2. Pyrocatechol (PC), lithium chloride (LiCl), sodium chloride (NaCl), potassium chloride (KCl), tetramethylammonium chloride (NMe4Cl), potassium nitrate (KNO3) and N, N-bis(2-hydroxyethyl) glycine (bicine)	1. Adhesion Fad/R ~ 27.36 mN/m	Polymerization	1. Implant coating 2. Tissue engineering	[56]

Table 1. Cont.

No.	Materials	Mechanical Properties	Preparation	Applications	Reference
28.	1. Poly(γ-glutamicacid) (γ-PGA)-dopamine (PGADA)	1. Adhesive strength 260 kPa	Cross-linking	Tissue adhesive	[109]
29.	1. Dopamine modified chondroitin sulfate (CSD) 2. N-(3-dimethylaminopropyl)-N′-ethylcarbodiimide hydrochloride/N-hydroxysuccinimide(EDC/NHS)	1. Lap shear strength 163.3 ± 9.1 kPa	Coupling reaction	1. Bone graft 2. Implant coating	[110]
30.	1. Semiflexible biopolymers (modeling)	1. Adhesive strength range ($\varepsilon A \geq 2.5$ kBT)	1. Cross-linking	1. Tissue engineering	[111]
31.	1. Ethylene propylene diene monomer rubber (EPDM)	1. Tensile strength 378 ± 17 MPa	Polymerization	Tissue engineering	[112]
32.	1. Dopamine-conjugated dialdehyde−HA (DAHA) hydrogels	1. Adhesive strength of 90.0 ± 6.7 kPa	Cross-linking	Wound healing	[55]
33.	1. Silk fibroin (SF) 2. Poly(ethylene glycol) (PEG)	1. Tensile strength 503.32 ? 16.54 kPa	Cross-linking	Wound healing	[113]
34.	1. 3,4-dihydroxyphenyalanine (DOPA) 2. dopamine (DA) 3. 3,4-dihydroxybenzaldehyde(DBA) 4. 3-(3,4-dihydroxyphenyl) propionic acid (DPPA)	1. Adhesive strength 57 kPa	1. Polymerization 2. Cross-linking	Tissue adhesive	[52]
35.	1. IPAM 2. BPAM 3. SAM	1. Adhesive strength 5.7 kPa	Genetic engineering	Tissue adhesive	[51]
36.	1. P-D-C/A/W hydrogel	1. Adhesive strength 5.5 kPa	Cross-linking	1. Biomedicine 2. Flexible electronic	[114]
37.	1. Novel gelatin-based hydrogel system crosslinked using a carbodiimide 2. Chlorhexidine (CHX)	1. Burst strength (sealing ability) 233–357 mmHg 2. Tensile modulus 47–69 kPa 3. Compressive modulus 58–104 kPa 4. Tensile strain 42–113%	Cross-linking	1. Local treatment for periodontal infections	[115]
38.	1. Chitosan-based Adhesive	1. Tensile strength 0.024 ± 0.0036 MPa, 2. Shear strength 0.031 ± 0.0069 MPa 3. Fracture toughness 2.38 ± 0.54 J/m2	Cross-linking	Bone Bio-Adhesive	[88]
39.	1. Catechol-conjugated chitosan (CCs)	1. Adhesive shear strength 64.8 ± 5.7 kPa	1. Chemical Conjugation 2. Chemical Oxidation	Surgical Adhesive	[54]

Table 1. Cont.

No.	Materials	Mechanical Properties	Preparation	Applications	Reference
40.	1. 3,4-dihydroxyphenyl propionic acid (DPA) 2. Dopamine (DA) 3. Chitosan (CS) 4. y-polyglutamic acid yPGA)	1. Adhesive strength 150 kPa	Cross-linking	1. Bone adhesive 2. Wound healing	[53]
41.	1. 3,4-dihydroxyphenylalanine (DOPA) 2. l-3,4-dihydroxyphenylalanine methyl ester (l-DOPAME) 3. Candida antartica fraction B (CAL-B) lipase	1. Covalent adhesion 100% after 90 min	1. Direct conjugation of DOPA at the C-terminus on the surface of the protein 2. Protein conjugation with tailor-made glycopolymers (DOPA-hyaluronic acid (HA) polymers) at the N-terminus	Tissue adhesive	[47]
42.	1. Polypetide-based adhesive	1. Covalent cross-linked adhesives 110 mN with $F \cdot w^{-1} = 22$ $N \cdot m^{-1}$	1. Recombinant protein fusion 2. DOPA modified polymers or peptide 3. Polymerization 4. Cross-linking	1. Tissue adhesive	[49]
43.	1. Coldwater fish skin "type A" gelatin (G7041) 2. Alginic acid sodium salt (A1112) 3. Crosslinking agent: N-(3-dimethy laminopropyl)-N-ethylcarbodiimide hydrochloride (EDC, E7750) 4. Fillers: Sodium montmorillonite (Cloisite Na+) 5. Kaolin (K1512) 6. Cellulose fibers TECHNOCEL® 300 (fiber length 500 μm)	1. Bonding strength 400 and 485 KPa 2. Burst strength 605 and 562 3. Tensile strength 90 kPa 4. Young's Modulus 150 kPa	Cross-linking	Wound healing	[116]
44.	1. PEGDMA 2. Poly(ethylene glycol)	1. Adhesion strength 150 kPa	Cross-linking	Tissue engineering	[117]
45.	1. Magnesium oxide (MgO) 2. Poly(ethylene glycol)-block-poly(propylene glycol)-block-poly(ethylene glycol) (PEG-PPG-PEG, Pluronic® L-31) 3. Dopamine	1. Tensile strength $\leq$ 4.5 MPa 2. Adhesion strength 125 kPa	Cross-linking	Tissue engineering	[118]
46.	1. Acrylamide 2. Acrylic acid 3. N, N'-Methylenebis (acrylamide) 4. 3-(trimethoxysilyl) propyl methacrylate (TMSPMA, Aladdin, S111153) 5. Hydrogel ini- tiators include α-Ketoglutaric acid (Aladdin, K105571) and α, α'-Azodiisobutyramidinedihydrochloride (V50, ShangHaiD&B Biological Science and Technology Co. Ltd., Shanghai, China)	1. Work of debonding 129 J/m^2	Cross-linking	Tissue engineering	[119]

Table 1. Cont.

No.		Materials		Mechanical Properties	Preparation	Applications	Reference
47.	1.	Polycaprolactane (PCL, Mw 45,000), and beta-tricalcium phosphate (βTCP)	1.	Shear strength 157.6 kDa ± 25.1	3D printing	1. Scaffold 2. Tissue engineering	[105]
48.	1. 2. 3. 4. 5. 6.	Cellulose-reinforced catechol-modified polyacrylic acid-Zn2+ PAA, N,N0- dicyclohexylcarbodiimide (DCC) and sodium tetraborate ($Na_2B_4O_7$) Cellulose fibers Dopamine hydrochloride (DOPA HCl), N-hydroxysuccinimide (NHS)and zinc chloride (ZnCl2) Cellulose nanocrystals Polyvinyl alcohol glue, polyurethane glue, epoxy glue and cyanoacrylate glue	1.	Bonding strength 10 MPa	Amidation reaction	Implant coating	[120]
49.	1. 2. 3. 4. 5. 6. 7.	(L)-Lactic acid, anhydrous glycerol, and methacrylic anhydride p-Toluenesulfonic acid (≥99.0%; Merck) Toluene (≥99.8%; Merck) 2-Hydroxyethylmethacrylate (HEMA) MMA (≥99.0%, Merck) Benzoylperoxide (BP) (A75%; Merck) ASA and N,N,N′,N′- tetramethylethylenediamine	1.	Thermal−mechanical properties (LSS: 8.62 MPa, Tdeg: 370 °C)	Condensation reaction of glycerin and LA	Biomedical application	[121]
50.	1. 2. 3.	PEG crosslinked by trilysine amine Polyethylene glycol (PEG)—polyethylenimine (PEI) copolymer Polyurethane polymer	1. 2.	Ultimate Tensile Strength 21.6 ± 8.4 MPa Elastic Modulus 83.3 ± 34.9 MPa	Cross-linking	Spinal sealant	[30]
51.	1. 2. 3.	Dopamine (DA) Sodium carboxymethyl cellulose (CMC) Catechol-modified CMC–DA	1.	Adhesion strength 11.37 ± 2.62 kPa	1. Carbodiimide chemistry method 2. Cross-linking	Wound healing	[46]
52.	1. 2.	Chitosan Protocatechuic acid (PCA)	1.	Adhesion strength of 4.56 ± 0.54 MPa	Michael-type addition	Bio-glue	[58]
53.	1. 2.	Poly (ethylene glycol) (PEG) based sealants Albumin and glutaraldehyde	1.	Adhesion strength 0.31 MPa	Cross-linking	1. Sealing graft 2. Bone graft	[50]
54.	1.	TGI/HA-CS (tilapia type I gelatin/hyaluronic acid-chondroitin sulfate)	1.	Compressive strength 11.34 ± 1.18 MPa	Cross-linking	temporomandibular joint disc	[122]
55.	1.	CAG@PLys@PDA-Cu^{2+}	1. 2. 3.	Tensile stress 5.5 MPa (Strain 400%) Tensile zzzstrangth 5.3 MPa Young's Modulus 1 Mpa	step-wise modification of parallel-microgroove-patterned	Endothelial healing	[123]

3. Preparation of Bio-Based Adhesives

Based on the numerous studies that have been conducted in order to examine the bio-adhesive synthesis and preparation, it can be concluded that there are two major process used to produce a bio-adhesive, i.e., polymerization and cross-linking [12,21,23,28,124–126]. The cross-linking process usually utilizes some type of bonding that can happen in the reaction, including hydrogen bonding, ionic bonding, host–guest interaction, hydrophobic bonds, imine bonds, disulfide bond, Acylhydrazone bonds, Diels-Alder reaction, boronate bonds, and oxime bonds [125]. In orthopedic surgery and orthodontics, poly(methyl methacrylate)s (PMMA) has been widely used. The polymerization of methyl methacrylate (MMA) via a free radical process utilizing an azo compound or peroxide as an initiator is a method to produce PMMA. Commercially, polymerization can be conducted, i.e., in bulk, solution, suspension, or emulsion. A viscous paste will be formed after blending these constituents which solidify via monomer radicals or anionic polymerization [11,26].

Alkyl 2-cyanoacrylates are now the most researched and most widely used group of bone adhesives. By altering the length of the alkyl chain, it is possible to produce a wide range of different 2-cyanoacrylates esters. The structure of poly (alkyl cyanoacrylate) (PACA), which was investigated for potential use in bone bio-based adhesives, is presented in Figure 2 [127]. The polymerization process can be carried out at room temperature without the need of a heating step, the addition of a catalyst, or the application of pressure thanks to the profound reactivity of these materials. The reaction that must take place in order to generate these materials begins with the anionic polymerization of the monomers, which is triggered by water. The acrylate bond can be broken by a nucleophilic attack carried out by weak bases such as water or amines. In order to accomplish bio-adhesion to bone, an electron-withdrawing nitrile group polarizes the acrylate bond. Because of this, the acrylate bond is susceptible to nucleophilic attack by weak bases, such as the amines that are found in the collagenous matrix of bone tissues. Increasing the length of the alkyl chain can, in general, result in greater polymerization rates, stronger bonding strengths in bone tissues, and can form more flexible chains [25].

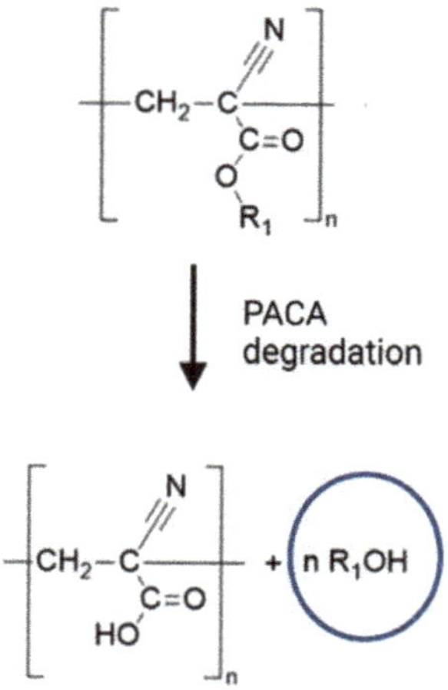

Figure 2. Structure of Poly (alkyl cyanoacrylate) (PACA). Reused from an open access article [127].

Mixing a solution that contains a fibrinogen source (from plasma, platelet-rich plasma), or heterologous/autologous cryoprecipitate) and factor XIII with another separate solution consisting of thrombin source (bovine, human, or recombinant), anti-fibrinolytic agent, and calcium to prevent rapid fibrinolysis is the most common method that is used to produce fibrin-based adhesive systems. When brought together, these substances cause the formation of a clot that is devoid of cells. During this process, thrombin cleaves fibrinogen, which results in the production of soluble fibrin monomers. These monomers then self-assemble into loosely aggregated fibrils via hydrogen bonding, and then into a more robust cross-linked fibrin polymer via covalent bonding. Thrombin also activates factor XIII, which, in the presence of calcium, provides for the formation of covalent bonds between fibrin polymer chains. However, a considerable amount of preparation is required before employing this adhesive made from biomaterials [11,39].

Starch was oxidized with periodic acid in order to produce aldehyde side groups, and chitosan was used as the amino-group carrier throughout this process. In the bio-based adhesives system, amino groups that are present in the surrounding tissues will react with aldehyde groups in a manner analogous to that of chitosan. After being mixed together in water, the two components produce a Schiff's base, which results in a covalent cross-linking that allows for a strong adhesion to tissue. This is accomplished by the production of covalent bonds. The bio-based glue had the potential to form bonds with any other exposed amino groups, such as those that are present in shattered bone for example. In addition, increasing the bio-adhesion strength to bone can be accomplished by conjugating starch or dextran compounds with 3,4-dihydroxy—phenylalanine (DOPA) [21,42,46–48]. A study reported that free radical copolymerization of monoacryloxyethyl phosphate (MAEP), dopamine methacrylate (DMA), and acrylamide (Aam) are used to produce bio-mimetic adhesive complex. This bio-based adhesive has the capability to bond wet bones together either in vitro and in vivo, demonstrating suitability for utilizing in the reconstruction of craniofacial fractures, and showed good degradability and osteoconductivity [11].

Biocompatible in situ-gelling Schiff's base reaction and ionic interactions was conducted to produce carboxymethyl cellulose (CMC)-glycol chitosan (GC) hydrogel, a potential three-dimensional (3D) printing biomaterial ink for tissue engineering applications, the probable reaction is shown at Figure 3 [15]. A successful strategy to address cell-behavior on biomaterials was also presented by the plasma enhanced–chemical vapor deposition (PE-CVD) of polyethylene oxide-like (PEO)-like coatings [128]. Moreover, Tris(trimethylsiloxy)silyl (M3T) containing methacrylate copolymers with low surface energy were designed and synthesized [91].

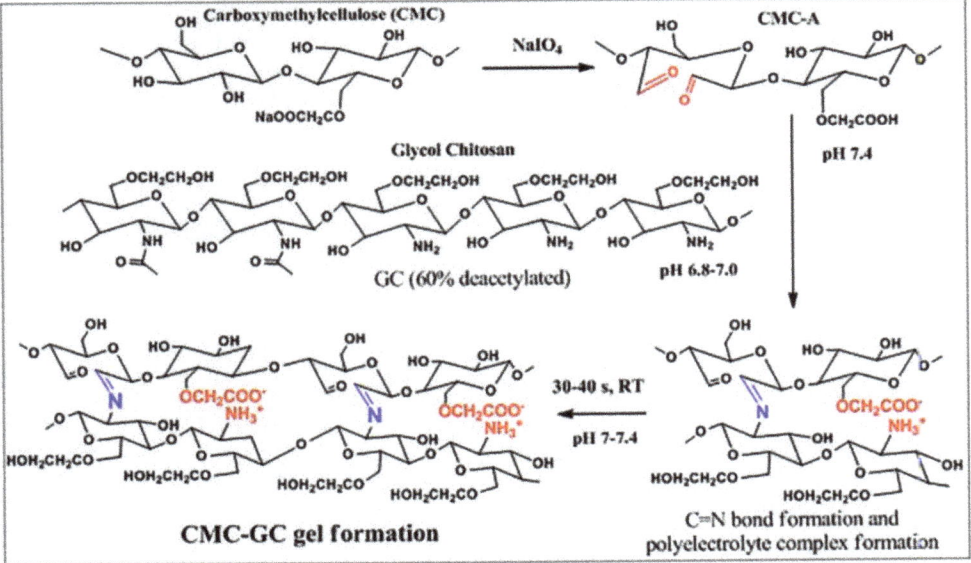

Figure 3. Probable mechanism of gel formation using Schiff's base reaction method. Reused/adapted with permission from Ref. [15]. 2020, Elsevier, License Number 5401720806257.

Chitosan thiomer derivatives are utilized in order to produce a novel three-dimensional (3D) scaffold with potential soft tissue repair applications. A covalent coupling reaction was conducted to synthesize amino acid-grafted chitosan (cysteine, CHICys) and N-acylated chitosan (11- mercaptoundecanoic acid, CHIMerc) derivatives, and hydrogel scaffolds were produced by freeze-drying process. They were comprehensively characterized by swelling and degradation behaviors, NMR, FTIR, and Raman spectroscopy, SEM, and X-ray microcomputed tomography [14]. A series of chitosan-graft- polypeptides were synthesized by ring-opening polymerization of three N-carboxyanhydrides (NCAs)—3,4-dihydroxyphenylalanine-N-carboxyanhydride (DOPA-NCA), cysteine-NCA (Cys-NCA) and arginine-NCA (Arg- NCA)—using partial-NH2-protected chitosan as an initiator since inspired by the mussel foot protein and chitosan-based macromolecular adhesives. Based on the result, these copolymers demonstrated good biodegradability and low cytotoxicity for application in orthopedic implant and scaffold [89].

A research also reported utilizing the 3,4-dihydroxyphenylalanine (DOPA), l-3,4-dihydroxyphenylalanine methyl ester (l-DOPAME), and Candida antartica fraction B (CAL-B) lipase in order to produce bio-based tissue adhesive by conducting direct conjugation of DOPA at the C-terminus on the surface of the protein and protein conjugation with tailor-made glycopolymers (DOPA-hyaluronic acid (HA) polymers) at the N-terminus [47]. The above are some examples of preparation process of bio-based adhesive production.

4. Characterization of Bio-Adhesives

4.1. In Vitro Methods

4.1.1. Shear Strength Measurement

The strength of bio-adhesion is commonly characterized by using mechanical testing, including crack growth assessment, peel test, and shear strength test. In the case of mucoadhesive assessment, shear strength measurements are commonly utilized to measure the forces within the mucus layer that slides each other in a parallel direction to the contact plane. Another method that can be utilized to measure the mucoadhesive strength is the flow channel method. The method assesses the shear strength by measuring the force needed to get the particle of adhesive from the mucin gel surface using forced humid air via flow cell. Furthermore, in order to assess the development of crack yielding from the dental implant, the bending tests were also conducted in the application of bio-based adhesive in orthodontic. The cracks are usually produced as a result of polymerization due to the shrinkage of the composite materials used in the implant. Characterization and interpretation of the bending test results is conducted using Griffith's energy balance model. For example, the teeth elastic energy (usually the average elastic energy of tooth and the dental implant material) and the crack surface energy is set up using this balancing model. The experimental crack development assessment will decide the strain energy release rate or the stress intensity while the Poisson's ration and modulus of the implant material will calculate the fracture energy [9,11,12,19,23].

4.1.2. Peel Strength Evaluation

Fractographic techniques, e.g., transmission electron microscopy (TEM) or scanning electron microscopy (SEM), are used in order to assess the quality of the dental implants-surface after performing the tensile test. American Standards for Testing and Materials (ASTM) with various tests are conducted on the interface of adhesion and the substrates. In order to obtain better shear strength, peel strength, and adhesion failure temperature, a pressure-sensitive adhesive (PSA) is formed as a composite material by supplementing it with montmorillonite, an organo-clay based element [14].

4.1.3. Flow through Experiment and Plate Method

The flow through channel method, which is the macro-scale measure of flow rate that can yield the depletion of bio-adhesive coated over the substrate sphere, is conducted to measure the mucoadhesion of DDS. The biophysical assessment method is conducted to measure the fluctuation in sedimentation coefficient that emerges due to the molecular weight change through an analytical centrifuge. The Wilhelm plate method is used for surface tension evaluation by utilizing natural or synthetic mucus rather than a conventional water medium. This method is known for use as macro-scale bio-adhesion assessment method. This method is conducted by coating a plate with any polymer material before the changes in interfacial properties and the bio-adhesion property are measured with respect to time [11,19].

4.2. Ex Vitro Methods

4.2.1. Adhesion Weight Method

A specific test method is developed in order to determine the weight of adherent particles that emerged in the interior mucous layers of guinea pig digestive tract due to the ion exchange. The particle size effect and adhesion charge after 5 min of time with the pig's digestive tract was determined using this method. Based on the result it is recommended that the weight of the digestive tract increased due to bio-adhesion. However, when a larger change within the biological tissue emerged due to regeneration or degeneration of the digestive tract tissues, this method will posture a diminished reproducibility of the data [11,19].

4.2.2. Fluorescent Probe Methods

Fluorescent probe methods could determine the relationship between the polymer molecules and epithelial cell membranes. The formulation of an orally utilized bio-based adhesive polymer can actually be improved by knowing its structural requirements. The investigated bio-based adhesives can be tagged on to the cell membrane which consists of proteins and the lipid bi-layer membranes and the variations in fluorescent spectrum are noted. Excimer and monomer bands are two different Pyrene bands shown by these materials, and environmental viscosity will administer the ratio of these bands. Because of that, by assessing the bands ratio, the viscosity changes can be noted. Based on this result, it can be concluded that the adhesion strength is directly related to the viscosity change. The bond between polymer and protein membrane can be observed using a quantitative method (fluorescence depolarization), while the interactions of soluble polymers can be compared with that of peel of the cell [11,19].

5. Challenges

Based on the findings, presented in numerous research articles, it can be seen that bio-based adhesives have demonstrated their superiority in various medical applications. At present, the application of bio-based adhesives in the medical sector, including orthopedics, is an area of great scientific interest due to the recent advances in their formulations.

Bio-based adhesives consist of synthetic materials and natural materials. A number of studies have shown that synthetic materials have advantages from several aspects, especially with regards to mechanical properties [129]. Synthetic materials have adhesive strength, shear strength, and tensile strength which are much higher than natural materials, but these synthetic materials have major weaknesses in terms of biocompatibility and cytotoxicity, as it is known that synthetic materials have elements that are toxic to the human body. Meanwhile, natural materials have advantages in terms of biocompatibility and cytotoxicity because they are acceptable for use in the human body, but these materials still have weaknesses in terms of mechanical properties. Several studies have shown that the adhesive strength produced from bio-based adhesives derived from natural raw materials is still very low and is only sufficient to meet the need for adhesives for soft tissue or surgical sutures. Therefore, it is necessary to conduct future research to optimize the material properties of bio-based adhesives in order to obtain materials that have both satisfactory mechanical properties and good biocompatibility properties.

Bio-based adhesives for orthopedic applications, which are produced from utilization of natural resource polymers, are less studied. The main challenge in using bio-based adhesives for orthopedic applications is meeting the stringent requirements for high bond strength in a demanding clinical environment [116]. Markedly, bio-based adhesives have better biodegradability and biocompatibility properties, although bio-based adhesives from synthetic or chemical preparation have higher adhesion strength to bone. Polymers known as hydrogels are more suitable to be used in bio-based adhesive applications for soft tissue than bio-based adhesives for bone adhesive due to the low cohesive strength produced by these materials. A more rational design should be executed to develop bio-based adhesive materials with particular bonding strength to bone tissue. Bone type, age of the patients, fracture location, samples storage, and treatment can affect the physicochemical properties of bone, so a particular method is required to characterize the properties of bio-based bone adhesives. Various distinctive assessment methods have been conducted, including the foremost common butt tensile strength tests, which compromise coordinate comparison between various tests. In this respect, the establishment of standardized and reproducible assessment protocols for the adhesion strength of bio-based adhesives to bone is of utmost importance.

Another obstacle in this field is lowering the cost of bio-based adhesive materials [117]. Several researchers have emphasized the growing need to convert available agricultural wastes into biocompatible and biodegradable products [118,119]. Nonetheless, research on the subject is still lacking, necessitating ongoing investigations.

6. Future Perspectives

Polymers with biodegradability properties, prepared using synthetic or chemical methods, can be designed by tuning the chemical groups, the degree of cross-linking, viscosity, and surface tension. They represent a promising approach for bone fracture healing. The chemical composition of bone must be the main consideration for future bone adhesive design. A matrix consisting of organic collagen ($\approx$30 wt.%), reinforced by nanocrystals of calcium phosphate mineral ($\approx$70 wt.%), is the main constituent of bone tissue. Biodegradable polymers, such as PEG or alginate, can be outlined to connect firmly to bone tissue through functionalization with the addition of chemical groups, which have high bonding strength with bone components. N-hydroxysuccinimide esters (NHS esters) are known to build solid covalent amide bonds with primary amines found within the collagenous extracellular bone matrix. On the other hand, a few functional groups are known to bind to Ca^{2+} as present within the mineral phase of bone tissue, i.e., hydroxyapatite. Bisphosphonates (BP) are anti-osteoporotic particles that are known for their uncommonly strong affinity for hydroxyapatite. Moreover, in this manner, BP-functionalized polymers might strongly adhere to bone by forming ionic bonds between pendant BP groups and Ca^{2+}. Organic compounds, consisting of carboxyl groups with strong adhesion for Ca^{2+}, generally include proteins, sequences of peptide, amino acids in single form, and carboxyl groups, such as sulfate groups, hydroxyl, and catechol. Moreover, the adhesion to bone can be improved by expanding the amount of functional (side) groups with high affinity to bone in the polymer.

The use of bio-based adhesives can reduce the complicated invasive techniques currently used in orthopedics, which in turn will result in improved patient treatment protocols and quality of life. It can be expected that, in the future, the bio-based bone adhesive materials with more judicious design will permit bone fracture fixation utilizing internal fixation.

Future research should be focused on comprehensive studies of the suitability of various bio-based adhesives for bone tissue scaffolds, development of innovative injectable adhesives for fracture treatment, and mechanical testing of bio-based adhesives intended for orthopedic applications. The existing studies in the field remain rather limited, and the results will be of great importance for the development of bio-based adhesives for orthopedic applications with optimal performance.

Author Contributions: Conceptualization, N.F.N.,M.A.R.L. and P.A.; methodology, N.F.N. and M.A.R.L.; validation, N.F.N., M.A.R.L. and P.A.; investigation, N.F.N. and M.A.R.L.; resources, N.F.N.,M.A.R.L., D.J., E.M., P.A., L.K. and L.S.H.; data curation, N.F.N.; writing—original draft preparation, N.F.N.; writing—review and editing, N.F.N.,M.A.R.L., P.A., L.K. and L.S.H.; visualization, D.J. and E.M.; supervision, M.A.R.L. and P.A.; project administration, M.A.R.L., D.J. and P.A. All authors have read and agreed to the published version of the manuscript.

Funding: This research received no external funding.

Institutional Review Board Statement: The study did not require ethical approval.

Informed Consent Statement: Not applicable.

Data Availability Statement: Not applicable.

Acknowledgments: This study was supported by Research Collaboration Center for Biomass and Biorefinery between BRIN and Universitas Padjadjaran, and Research Collaboration Center for Biomedical Scaffold between BRIN and Universitas Gadjah Mada.

Conflicts of Interest: The authors declare no conflict of interest.

References

1. Tsiridis, E.; Upadhyay, N.; Giannoudis, P. Molecular Aspects of Fracture Healing: Which Are the Important Molecules? *Int. J. Care Inj.* **2007**, *38S1*, S11–S25. [CrossRef] [PubMed]
2. Dimitriou, R.; Tsiridis, E.; Giannoudis, P.V. Current Concepts of Molecular Aspects of Bone Healing. *Injury* **2005**, *36*, 1392–1404. [CrossRef] [PubMed]
3. Marsell, R.; Einhorn, T.A. The Biology of Fracture Healing. *Injury* **2011**, *42*, 551–555. [CrossRef] [PubMed]
4. Barnes, G.L.; Kostenuik, P.J.; Gerstenfeld, L.C.; Einhorn, T.A. Growth Factor Regulation of Fracture Repair. *J. Bone Miner. Res.* **1999**, *14*, 1805–1815. [CrossRef]
5. Al-Aql, Z.S.; Alagl, A.S.; Graves, D.T.; Gerstenfeld, L.C.; Einhorn, T.A. Molecular Mechanisms Controlling Bone Formation During Fracture Healing and Distraction Osteogenesis. *J. Dent. Res.* **2008**, *87*, 107–118. [CrossRef] [PubMed]
6. Yu, Y.; Brió Pérez, M.; Cao, C.; de Beer, S. Switching (Bio-) Adhesion and Friction in Liquid by Stimulus Responsive Polymer Coatings. *Eur. Polym. J.* **2021**, *147*, 110298. [CrossRef]
7. Kumar, M.; Tomar, M.; Punia, S.; Dhakane-Lad, J.; Dhumal, S.; Changan, S.; Senapathy, M.; Berwal, M.K.; Sampathrajan, V.; Sayed, A.A.S.; et al. Plant-Based Proteins and Their Multifaceted Industrial Applications. *Lwt* **2022**, *154*, 112620. [CrossRef]
8. Sardella, E.; Gristina, R.; Fanelli, F.; Veronico, V.; Da Ponte, G.; Kroth, J.; Fracassi, F.; Favia, P. How to Confer a Permanent Bio-Repelling and Bio-Adhesive Character to Biomedical Materials through Cold Plasmas. *Appl. Sci.* **2020**, *10*, 9101. [CrossRef]
9. Majeed, H.; Rehman, K.; Ali, A.; Khalid, M.F.; Akash, M.S.H. Wound Healing Adhesives. In *Green Adhesives*; John Wiley & Sons, Inc.: Hoboken, NJ, USA, 2020; pp. 181–204.
10. Xiang, L. *Molecular Interaction and Adhesion Mechanisms of Mussel-Inspired Adhesive Coatings*; University of Alberta: Alberta, Canada, 2020.
11. Ramesh, M.; Kumar, L.R. Bioadhesives. In *Green Adhesives: Preparation, Properties and Applications*; John Wiley & Sons: Inc Hoboken, NJ, USA, 2020; pp. 145–163.
12. Rathi, S.; Saka, R.; Domb, A.J.; Khan, W. Protein-Based Bioadhesives and Bioglues. *Polym. Adv. Technol.* **2019**, *30*, 217–234. [CrossRef]
13. Bolghari, N.; Shahsavarani, H.; Anvari, M.; Habibollahi, H. A Novel Recombinant Chimeric Bio-Adhesive Protein Consisting of Mussel Foot Protein 3, 5, Gas Vesicle Protein A, and CsgA Curli Protein Expressed in Pichia Pastoris. *AMB Express* **2022**, *12*, 1–19. [CrossRef]
14. Medeiros Borsagli, F.G.L.; Carvalho, I.C.; Mansur, H.S. Amino Acid-Grafted and N-Acylated Chitosan Thiomers: Construction of 3D Bio-Scaffolds for Potential Cartilage Repair Applications. *Int. J. Biol. Macromol.* **2018**, *114*, 270–282. [CrossRef] [PubMed]
15. Janarthanan, G.; Tran, H.N.; Cha, E.; Lee, C.; Das, D.; Noh, I. 3D Printable and Injectable Lactoferrin-Loaded Carboxymethyl Cellulose-Glycol Chitosan Hydrogels for Tissue Engineering Applications. *Mater. Sci. Eng. C* **2020**, *113*, 111008. [CrossRef] [PubMed]
16. Shahryarimorad, K.; Alipour, A.; Honar, Y.S.; Abtahi, B. In Silico Prediction and in Vitro Validation of the Effect of pH on Adhesive Behaviour of the Fused CsgA - MFP3 Protein. *AMB Express* **2022**, *12*, 1–13. [CrossRef] [PubMed]
17. Kazemi, S.; Pourmadadi, M.; Yazdian, F.; Ghadami, A. The Synthesis and Characterization of Targeted Delivery Curcumin Using Chitosan-Magnetite-Reduced Graphene Oxide as Nano-Carrier. *Int. J. Biol. Macromol.* **2021**, *186*, 554–562. [CrossRef] [PubMed]
18. Alqosaibi, A.I. Nanocarriers for Anticancer Drugs: Challenges and Perspectives. *Saudi J. Biol. Sci.* **2022**, *29*, 103298. [CrossRef] [PubMed]
19. Chopra, H.; Kumar, S.; Singh, I. Bioadhesive Hydrogels and Their Applications. In *Bioadhesives in Drug Delivery*; John Wiley & Sons: Inc Hoboken, NJ, USA, 2020; pp. 147–170. ISBN 9781119640240.

20. Lyu, Q.; Peng, L.; Hong, X.; Fan, T.; Li, J.; Cui, Y.; Zhang, H.; Zhao, J. Smart Nano-Micro Platforms for Ophthalmological Applications: The State-of-the-Art and Future Perspectives. *Biomaterials* **2021**, *270*, 120682. [CrossRef] [PubMed]
21. Li, D.; Chen, J.; Wang, X.; Zhang, M.; Li, C.; Zhou, J. Recent Advances on Synthetic and Polysaccharide Adhesives for Biological Hemostatic Applications. *Front. Bioeng. Biotechnol.* **2020**, *8*, 926. [CrossRef] [PubMed]
22. Guo, Q.; Chen, J.; Wang, J.; Zeng, H.; Yu, J. Recent Progress in Synthesis and Application of Mussel-Inspired Adhesives. *Nanoscale* **2020**, *12*, 1307–1324. [CrossRef]
23. Bu, Y.; Pandit, A. Cohesion Mechanisms for Bioadhesives. *Bioact. Mater.* **2022**, *13*, 105–118. [CrossRef]
24. Patil, N.A.; Kandasubramanian, B. Functionalized Polylysine Biomaterials for Advanced Medical Applications: A Review. *Eur. Polym. J.* **2021**, *146*, 110248. [CrossRef]
25. Korde, J.M.; Kandasubramanian, B. Biocompatible Alkyl Cyanoacrylates and Their Derivatives as Bio-Adhesives. *Biomater. Sci.* **2018**, *6*, 1691–1711. [CrossRef] [PubMed]
26. Al-Abassi, A.; Papini, M.; Towler, M. Review of Biomechanical Studies and Finite Element Modeling of Sternal Closure Using Bio-Active Adhesives. *Bioengineering* **2022**, *9*, 198. [CrossRef] [PubMed]
27. Yousefi, A.M. A Review of Calcium Phosphate Cements and Acrylic Bone Cements as Injectable Materials for Bone Repair and Implant Fixation. *J. Appl. Biomater. Funct. Mater.* **2019**, *17*, 2280800019872594. [CrossRef]
28. Chen, S.; Gil, C.J.; Ning, L.; Jin, L.; Perez, L.; Kabboul, G.; Tomov, M.L.; Serpooshan, V. Adhesive Tissue Engineered Scaffolds: Mechanisms and Applications. *Front. Bioeng. Biotechnol.* **2021**, *9*, 683079. [CrossRef] [PubMed]
29. Venturella, F. *Development of Nontoxic Bio–Adhesives for Wet Environments*; Università degli Studi di Palermo: Palermo, Italy, 2021.
30. Gillman, N.; Lloyd, D.; Bindra, R.; Ruan, R.; Zheng, M. Surgical Applications of Intracorporal Tissue Adhesive Agents: Current Evidence and Future Development. *Expert Rev. Med. Devices* **2020**, *17*, 443–460. [CrossRef]
31. Park, K.; Kim, S.; Jo, Y.; Park, J.; Kim, I.; Hwang, S.; Lee, Y.; Kim, S.Y.; Seo, J. Lubricant Skin on Diverse Biomaterials with Complex Shapes via Polydopamine-Mediated Surface Functionalization for Biomedical Applications. *Bioact. Mater.* **2022**. [CrossRef]
32. Zheng, D.; Ruan, H.; Chen, W.; Zhang, Y.; Cui, W.; Chen, H.; Shen, H. Advances in Extracellular Vesicle Functionalization Strategies for Tissue Regeneration. *Bioact. Mater.* **2022**. [CrossRef]
33. Liu, C.; Yu, Q.; Yuan, Z.; Guo, Q.; Liao, X.; Han, F.; Feng, T.; Liu, G.; Zhao, R.; Zhu, Z.; et al. Engineering the Viscoelasticity of Gelatin Methacryloyl (GelMA) Hydrogels via Small "Dynamic Bridges" to Regulate BMSC Behaviors for Osteochondral Regeneration. *Bioact. Mater.* **2022**. [CrossRef]
34. Shokri, M.; Dalili, F.; Kharaziha, M.; Baghaban Eslaminejad, M.; Ahmadi Tafti, H. Strong and Bioactive Bioinspired Biomaterials, next Generation of Bone Adhesives. *Adv. Colloid Interface Sci.* **2022**, *305*, 102706. [CrossRef]
35. Wang, X.; Fang, X.; Gao, X.; Wang, H.; Li, S.; Li, C.; Qing, Y.; Qin, Y. Strong Adhesive and Drug-Loaded Hydrogels for Enhancing Bone–Implant Interface Fixation and Anti-Infection Properties. *Colloids Surf. B Biointerfaces* **2022**, *219*, 112817. [CrossRef]
36. Du, J.; Zhou, Y.; Bao, X.; Kang, Z.; Huang, J.; Xu, G.; Yi, C.; Li, D. Surface Polydopamine Modification of Bone Defect Repair Materials: Characteristics and Applications. *Front. Bioeng. Biotechnol.* **2022**, *10*, 1–18. [CrossRef] [PubMed]
37. Abourehab, M.A.S.; Rajendran, R.R.; Singh, A.; Pramanik, S.; Shrivastav, P.; Ansari, M.J.; Manne, R.; Amaral, L.S.; Deepak, A. Alginate as a Promising Biopolymer in Drug Delivery and Wound Healing: A Review of the State-of-the-Art. *Int. J. Mol. Sci.* **2022**, *23*, 9035. [CrossRef] [PubMed]
38. Bohara, S.; Suthakorn, J. Surface Coating of Orthopedic Implant to Enhance the Osseointegration and Reduction of Bacterial Colonization: A Review. *Biomater. Res.* **2022**, *26*, 1–17. [CrossRef] [PubMed]
39. Pei, X.; Wang, J.; Cong, Y.; Fu, J. Recent Progress in Polymer Hydrogel Bioadhesives. *J. Polym. Sci.* **2021**, *59*, 1312–1337. [CrossRef]
40. Espinoza-Ramirez, A.; Fuentes-Rodriguez, H.; Hernandez-Herrera, E.; Mora-Sandi, A.; Vega-Baudrit, J.R. Nanobiodiversity and Biomimetic Adhesives Development: From Nature to Production and Application. *J. Biomater. Nanobiotechnol.* **2019**, *10*, 78–101. [CrossRef]
41. Zheng, G.; Cui, Y.; Lu, L.; Guo, M.; Hu, X.; Wang, L.; Yu, S.; Sun, S.; Li, Y.; Zhang, X.; et al. Microfluidic Chemostatic Bioreactor for High-Throughput Screening and Sustainable Co-Harvesting of Biomass and Biodiesel in Microalgae. *Bioact. Mater.* **2022**, 1–11. [CrossRef]
42. Samyn, P. A Platform for Functionalization of Cellulose, Chitin/Chitosan, Alginate with Polydopamine: A Review on Fundamentals and Technical Applications. *Int. J. Biol. Macromol.* **2021**, *178*, 71–93. [CrossRef]
43. Dongre, R.S. *Marine Polysaccharides in Pharmaceutical Uses*; Springer: Berlin/Heidelberg, Germany, 2022; ISBN 9783030357344.
44. Bashir, S.M.; Rather, G.A.; Patrício, A.; Haq, Z.; Sheikh, A.A.; Zahoor, M.; Singh, H.; Khan, A.A.; Imtiyaz, S.; Ahmad, S.B. Chitosan Nanoparticles: A Versatile Platform for Biomedical Applications. *Materials* **2022**, *15*, 6521. [CrossRef]
45. Abourehab, M.A.S.; Pramanik, S.; Abdelgawad, M.A.; Abualsoud, B.M.; Kadi, A.; Ansari, M.J.; Deepak, A. Recent Advances of Chitosan Formulations in Biomedical Applications. *Int. J. Mol. Sci.* **2022**, *23*, 10975. [CrossRef] [PubMed]
46. Chen, Y.; Cui, G.; Dan, N.; Huang, Y.; Bai, Z.; Yang, C.; Dan, W. Preparation and Characterization of Dopamine–Sodium Carboxymethyl Cellulose Hydrogel. *SN Appl. Sci.* **2019**, *1*, 1–10. [CrossRef]
47. Jaramillo, J.; Rodriguez-Oliva, I.; Abian, O.; Palomo, J.M. Specific Chemical Incorporation of L-DOPA and Functionalized l-DOPA-Hyaluronic Acid in Candida Antarctica Lipase: Creating Potential Mussel-Inspired Bioadhesives. *SN Appl. Sci.* **2020**, *2*, 1–12. [CrossRef]
48. Lutz, T.M.; Kimna, C.; Casini, A.; Lieleg, O. Bio-Based and Bio-Inspired Adhesives from Animals and Plants for Biomedical Applications. *Mater. Today Bio.* **2022**, *13*, 100203. [CrossRef] [PubMed]

49. Sun, J. *Fabrication and Mechanical Properties of Supercharged Polypeptides Based Biomaterials: From Adhesives to Fibers*; University of Groningen: The Netherlands, 2020.
50. Pandey, N.; Soto-Garcia, L.F.; Liao, J.; Zimmern, P.; Nguyen, K.T.; Hong, Y. Mussel-Inspired Bioadhesives in Healthcare: Design Parameters, Current Trends, and Future Perspectives. *Biomater. Sci.* **2020**, *8*, 1240–1255. [CrossRef] [PubMed]
51. Kang, V.; Lengerer, B.; Wattiez, R.; Flammang, P. Molecular Insights into the Powerful Mucus-Based Adhesion of Limpets (*Patella Vulgata* L.): Molecular Insights into Limpets Adhesion. *Open Biol.* **2020**, *10*, 200019. [CrossRef]
52. Wang, H.; Wang, L.; Zhang, S.; Zhang, W.; Li, J.; Han, Y. Mussel-Inspired Polymer Materials Derived from Nonphytogenic and Phytogenic Catechol Derivatives and Their Applications. *Polym. Int.* **2021**, *70*, 1209–1224. [CrossRef]
53. Shi, C.; Chen, X.; Zhang, Z.; Chen, Q.; Shi, D.; Kaneko, D. Mussel Inspired Bio-Adhesive with Multi-Interactions for Tissue Repair. *J. Biomater. Sci. Polym. Ed.* **2020**, *31*, 491–503. [CrossRef]
54. Park, M.K.; Li, M.X.; Yeo, I.; Jung, J.; Yoon, B.I.L.; Joung, Y.K. Balanced Adhesion and Cohesion of Chitosan Matrices by Conjugation and Oxidation of Catechol for High-Performance Surgical Adhesives. *Carbohydr. Polym.* **2020**, *248*, 116760. [CrossRef] [PubMed]
55. Zhou, D.; Li, S.; Pei, M.; Yang, H.; Gu, S.; Tao, Y.; Ye, D.; Zhou, Y.; Xu, W.; Xiao, P. Dopamine-Modified Hyaluronic Acid Hydrogel Adhesives with Fast-Forming and High Tissue Adhesion. *ACS Appl. Mater. Interfaces* **2020**, *12*, 18225–18234. [CrossRef] [PubMed]
56. Xiang, L.; Zhang, J.; Wang, W.; Gong, L.; Zhang, L.; Yan, B.; Zeng, H. Nanomechanics of π-Cation-π Interaction with Implications for Bio-Inspired Wet Adhesion. *Acta Biomater.* **2020**, *117*, 294–301. [CrossRef] [PubMed]
57. Ventura, I.V.P. *Characterization of Glycoproteins Involved in Sea Urchin Adhesion*; University of Coimbra: Portugal, 2020.
58. Capitain, C.; Wagner, S.; Hummel, J.; Tippkötter, N. Investigation of C–N Formation Between Catechols and Chitosan for the Formation of a Strong, Novel Adhesive Mimicking Mussel Adhesion. *Waste Biomass Valorization* **2021**, *12*, 1761–1779. [CrossRef]
59. Kwon, Y.; Yang, D.H.; Lee, D. A Titanium Surface-Modified with Nano-Sized Hydroxyapatite and Simvastatin Enhances Bone Formation and Osseointegration. *J. Biomed. Nanotechnol.* **2015**, *11*, 1007–1015. [CrossRef] [PubMed]
60. Cheng, Z.; Guo, C.; Dong, W.; He, F.; Zhao, S.; Yang, G. Effect of Thin Nano-Hydroxyapatite Coating on Implant Osseointegration in Ovariectomized Rats. *Oral Maxillofac. Surg.* **2012**, *113*, 48–53. [CrossRef]
61. Pang, K.-M.; Lee, J.-K.; Seo, Y.-K.; Kim, S.-M.; Kim, M.-J.; Lee, J.-H. Biologic Properties of Nano-Hydroxyapatite: An in Vivo Study of Calvarial Defects, Ectopic Bone Formation and Bone Implantation. *Biomed. Mater. Eng.* **2015**, *25*, 25–38. [CrossRef] [PubMed]
62. Juliadmi, D.; Nuswantoro, N.F.; Fajri, H.; Indriyani, I.Y.; Affi, J.; Manjas, M.; Tjong, D.H.; Gunawarman. The Coating of Bovine-Source Hydroxyapatite on Titanium Alloy (Ti-6Al-4V ELI) Using Electrophoretic Deposition for Biomedical Application. *Mater. Sci. Forum* **2020**, *1000*, 97–106. [CrossRef]
63. Kusrini, E.; Sontang, M. Characterization of X-Ray Diffraction and Electron Spin Resonance: Effects of Sintering Time and Temperature on Bovine Hydroxyapatite. *Radiat. Phys. Chem.* **2012**, *81*, 118–125. [CrossRef]
64. Khandan, A.; Abdellahi, M.; Ozada, N.; Ghayour, H. Study of the Bioactivity, Wettability and Hardness Behaviour of the Bovine Hydroxyapatite-Diopside Bio-Nanocomposite Coating. *J. Taiwan Inst. Chem. Eng.* **2016**, *60*, 538–546. [CrossRef]
65. Mihailescu, N.; Stan, G.E.; Duta, L.; Chifiriuc, C.M.; Bleotu, C.; Sopronyi, M.; Luculescu, C.; Oktar, F.N.; Mihailescu, I.N. Structural, Compositional, Mechanical Characterization and Biological Assessment of Bovine-Derived Hydroxyapatite Coatings Reinforced with MgF2 or MgO for Implants Functionalization. *Mater. Sci. Eng. C* **2016**, *59*, 863–874. [CrossRef]
66. Gunawarman; Mulyadi, I.H.; Arif, Z.; Nuswantoro, N.F.; Affi, J.; Niinomi, M. Effect of Particle Size on Adhesion Strength of Bovine Hydroxyapatite Layer on Ti-12Cr Coated by Using Electrophoretic Deposition (EPD) Method. In Proceedings of the 2nd Conference on Innovation in Technology (CITES 2020), Padang, Indonesia, 4–5 November 2020; pp. 1–8.
67. Fajri, H.; Ramadhan, F.; Nuswantoro, N.F.; Juliadmi, D.; Tjong, D.H.; Manjas, M.; Affi, J.; Yetri, Y.; Gunawarman. Electrophoretic Deposition (EPD) of Natural Hydroxyapatite Coatings on Titanium Ti-29Nb-13Ta-4.6Zr Substrates for Implant Material. *Mater. Sci. Forum* **2020**, *1000*, 123–131. [CrossRef]
68. Gunawarman; Affi, J.; Yetri, Y.; Ilhamdi; Juliadmi, D.; Nuswantoro, N.F.; Fajri, H.; Ahli, A.; Gundini, R.; Nur, H. Synthesis and Characterization of Calcium Precursor for Hydroxyapatite Synthesis from Blood Clam Shell (Anadara Antiquata) Using Planetary Ball Mill Process. In Proceedings of the IOP Conference Series: Materials Science and Engineering, Padang, Indonesia, 8–9 November 2018; pp. 1–6.
69. Khalili, V.; Khalil-allafi, J.; Xia, W.; Parsa, A.B.; Frenzel, J.; Somsen, C.; Eggeler, G. Preparing Hydroxyapatite-Silicon Composite Suspensions with Homogeneous Distribution of Multi-Walled Carbon Nano-Tubes for Electrophoretic Coating of NiTi Bone Implant and Their Effect on the Surface Morphology. *Appl. Surf. Sci.* **2016**, *366*, 158–165. [CrossRef]
70. Gunawarman; Nuswantoro, N.F.; Juliadmi, D.; Fajri, H.; Budiman, A.; Djong, H.T.; Manjas, M. Hydroxyapatite Coatings on Titanium Alloy TNTZ Using Electrophoretic Deposition. In Proceedings of the IOP Conference Series: Materials Science and Engineering, Padang, Indonesia, 8–9 November 2018; pp. 1–11.
71. Juliadmi, D.; Fauzi, V.R.; Gunawarman; Nur, H.; Idris, M.H. Hydroxyapatite Coating on Titanium Alloy Ti-6Al-4V with Electrophoretic Deposition (EPD) for Dental Root Application. *Int. J. Adv. Sci. Eng. Informational Technol.* **2017**, *7*, 2152–2158. [CrossRef]
72. Łukaszewska-Kuska, M.; Krawczyk, P.; Martyla, A.; Hędzelek, W.; Dorocka-bobkowska, B.; Dorocka-bobkowska, B. Hydroxyapatite Coating on Titanium Endosseous Implants for Improved Osseointegration: Physical and Chemical Considerations Address for Correspondence. *Adv. Clin. Exper. Med.* **2018**, *27*, 1055–1059. [CrossRef] [PubMed]

73. Liang, H.; Xu, X.; Feng, X.; Deng, X.; Wu, S.; Liu, X.; Yang, C. Gold Nanoparticles-Loaded Hydroxyapatite Composites Guide Osteogenic Differentiation of Human Mesenchymal Stem Cells through Wnt/β–Catenin Signaling Pathway. *Int. J. Nanomed.* **2019**, *14*, 6151–6163. [CrossRef] [PubMed]
74. Nuswantoro, N.F.; Juliadmi, D.; Fajri, H.; Manjas, M.; Suharti, N.; Tjong, D.H.; Affi, J.; Gunawarman. Electrophoretic Deposition Performance of Hydroxyapatite Coating on Titanium Alloys for Orthopedic Implant Application. *Mater. Sci. Forum* **2020**, *1000*, 69–81. [CrossRef]
75. Nuswantoro, N.F.; Manjas, M.; Suharti, N.; Juliadmi, D.; Fajri, H.; Tjong, D.H.; Affi, J.; Niinomi, M.; Gunawarman. Hydroxyapatite Coating on Titanium Alloy TNTZ for Increasing Osseointegration and Reducing Inflammatory Response in Vivo on Rattus Norvegicus Wistar Rats. *Ceram. Int.* **2021**, *47*, 16094–16100. [CrossRef]
76. Nuswantoro, N.F.; Gunawarman; Saputra, M.R.; Nanda, I.P.; Idris, M.H.; Arafat, A. Microstructure Analysis of Hydroxyapatite Coating on Stainless Steel 316L Using Investment Casting Technique for Implant Application. *Int. J. Adv. Sci. Eng. Inform. Technol.* **2018**, *8*, 2168–2174. [CrossRef]
77. Beig, B.; Liaqat, U.; Niazi, M.F.K.; Douna, I.; Zahoor, M.; Niazi, M.B.K. Current Challenges and Innovative Developments in Hydroxyapatite-Based Coatings on Metallic Materials for Bone Implantation: A Review. *Coatings* **2020**, *10*, 1249. [CrossRef]
78. Bose, S.; Tarafder, S.; Bandyopadhyay, A. Hydroxyapatite Coatings for Metallic Implants. In Hydroxyapatite (HAP) for Biomedical Applications. Elsevier Ltd.: Amsterdam, The Netherlands, 2015; Volume 7, pp. 143–157. ISBN 9781782420330.
79. Nuswantoro, N.F.; Maulana, I.; Djong, H.T.; Manjas, M.; Gunawarman. Hydroxyapatite Coating on New Type Titanium, TNTZ, Using Electrophoretic Deposition. *J. Ocean. Mech. Aerosp.* **2018**, *56*, 1–4.
80. Gunawarman; Affi, J.; Sutanto, A.; Putri, D.M.; Juliadmi, D.; Nuswantoro, N.F.; Fajri, H.; Tjong, D.H.; Manjas, M. Adhesion Strength of Hydroxyapatite Coating on Titanium Alloy (Ti-6Al- 4V ELI) for Biomedical Application. In Proceedings of the International Colloquium on Computational and Experimental Mechanics (ICCEM 2020), Selangor, Malaysia, 25–26 June 2020; pp. 1–9.
81. Araghi, A.; Hadianfard, M.J. Fabrication and Characterization of Functionally Graded Hydroxyapatite/TiO2 Multilayer Coating on Ti-6Al-4V Titanium Alloy for Biomedical Applications. *Ceram. Int.* **2015**, *41*, 12668–12679. [CrossRef]
82. Nuswantoro, N.F.; Budiman, I.; Septiawarman, A.; Djong, H.T.; Manjas, M.; Gunawarman. Effect of Applied Voltage and Coating Time on Nano Hydroxyapatite Coating on Titanium Alloy Ti6Al4V Using Electrophoretic Deposition for Orthopaedic Implant Application. In Proceedings of the IOP Conference Series: Materials Science and Engineering, Bandung, Indonesia, 6–7 September 2018; Volume 547, pp. 1–11.
83. Bovand, D.; Allazadeh, M.R.; Rasouli, S.; Khodadad, E.; Borhani, E. Studying the Effect of Hydroxyapatite Particles in Osteoconductivity of Ti-HA Bioceramic. *J. Aust. Ceram. Soc.* **2019**, *55*, 395–403. [CrossRef]
84. Han, Y.; Zhao, W.; Zheng, Y.; Wang, H.; Sun, Y.; Zhang, Y.; Luo, J.; Zhang, H. Self-Adhesive Lubricated Coating for Enhanced Bacterial Resistance. *Bioact. Mater.* **2021**, *6*, 2535–2545. [CrossRef] [PubMed]
85. Alinavaz, S.; Mahdavinia, G.R.; Jafari, H.; Hazrati, M.; Akbari, A. Hydroxyapatite (HA)-Based Hybrid Bionanocomposite Hydrogels: Ciprofloxacin Delivery, Release Kinetics and Antibacterial Activity. *J. Mol. Struct.* **2021**, *1225*, 129095. [CrossRef]
86. Albu, A.M.; Draghicescu, W.; Munteanu, T.; Ion, R.; Mitran, V.; Cimpean, A.; Popescu, S.; Pirvu, C. Nitrodopamine vs Dopamine as an Intermediate Layer for Bone Regeneration Applications. *Mater. Sci. Eng. C* **2019**, *98*, 461–471. [CrossRef]
87. Wang, Y.; Guo, J.; Li, B.; Li, D.; Meng, Z.; Sun, S.K. Biocompatible Therapeutic Albumin/Genipin Bioglue for Postoperative Wound Adhesion and Residual Tumor Ablation. *Biomaterials* **2021**, *279*, 121179. [CrossRef] [PubMed]
88. Vargas Villanueva, J.G.; Sarmiento Huertas, P.A.; Galan, F.S.; Esteban Rueda, R.J.; Briceño Triana, J.C.; Casas Rodriguez, J.P. Bio-Adhesion Evaluation of a Chitosan-Based Bone Bio-Adhesive. *Int. J. Adhes. Adhes.* **2019**, *92*, 80–88. [CrossRef]
89. Lu, D.; Wang, H.; Wang, X.; Li, Y.; Guo, H.; Sun, S.; Zhao, X.; Yang, Z.; Lei, Z. Biomimetic Chitosan-Graft-Polypeptides for Improved Adhesion in Tissue and Metal. *Carbohydr. Polym.* **2019**, *215*, 20–28. [CrossRef] [PubMed]
90. Singh, G.; Nayal, A.; Malhotra, S.; Koul, V. Dual Functionalized Chitosan Based Composite Hydrogel for Haemostatic Efficacy and Adhesive Property. *Carbohydr. Polym.* **2020**, *247*, 116757. [CrossRef]
91. Lei, H.; Xiong, M.; Xiao, J.; Zheng, L.; Zhuang, Q. Fluorine-Free Coating with Low Surface Energy and Anti-Biofouling Properties. *Prog. Org. Coatings* **2018**, *124*, 158–164. [CrossRef]
92. Ma, L.; Cheng, S.; Ji, X.; Zhou, Y.; Zhang, Y.; Li, Q.; Tan, C.; Peng, F.; Zhang, Y.; Huang, W. Immobilizing Magnesium Ions on 3D Printed Porous Tantalum Scaffolds with Polydopamine for Improved Vascularization and Osteogenesis. *Mater. Sci. Eng. C* **2020**, *117*, 111303. [CrossRef]
93. Smith, J.A.; Mele, E.; Rimington, R.P.; Capel, A.J.; Lewis, M.P.; Silberschmidt, V.V.; Li, S. Polydimethylsiloxane and Poly(Ether) Ether Ketone Functionally Graded Composites for Biomedical Applications. *J. Mech. Behav. Biomed. Mater.* **2019**, *93*, 130–142. [CrossRef]
94. Kazi, G.A.S.; Yamamoto, O. Effectiveness of the Sodium Alginate as Surgical Sealant Materials. *Wound Med.* **2019**, *24*, 18–23. [CrossRef]
95. Shirzaei Sani, E.; Portillo Lara, R.; Aldawood, Z.; Bassir, S.H.; Nguyen, D.; Kantarci, A.; Intini, G.; Annabi, N. An Antimicrobial Dental Light Curable Bioadhesive Hydrogel for Treatment of Peri-Implant Diseases. *Matter* **2019**, *1*, 926–944. [CrossRef] [PubMed]
96. Fernandez, M.J.S. Development of Poly (2-Oxazoline) -Based Bone-Adhesive Biomaterials. *J. Biomed. Mater. Res. Part B Appl. Biomater.* **2021**.

97. Wales, D.J.; Keshavarz, M.; Howe, C.; Yeatman, E. 3D Printability Assessment of Poly(Octamethylene Maleate (Anhydride) Citrate) and Poly(Ethylene Glycol) Diacrylate Copolymers for Biomedical Applications. *Appl. Polym. Mater.* **2022**. [CrossRef]
98. Feng, C.; Wang, F.; Xu, Z.; Sui, H.; Fang, Y.; Tang, X.; Shen, X. Characterization of Soybean Protein Adhesives Modified by Xanthan Gum. *Coatings* **2018**, *8*, 342. [CrossRef]
99. Xue, B.; Gu, J.; Li, L.; Yu, W.; Yin, S.; Qin, M.; Jiang, Q.; Wang, W.; Cao, Y. Hydrogel Tapes for Fault-Tolerant Strong Wet Adhesion. *Nat. Commun.* **2021**, *12*, 1–12. [CrossRef] [PubMed]
100. Moon, Y.J.; Yoon, S.J.; Koo, J.H.; Yoon, Y.; Byun, H.J.; Kim, H.S.; Khang, G.; Chun, H.J.; Yang, D.H. β-Cyclodextrin/Triclosan Complex-Grafted Methacrylated Glycol Chitosan Hydrogel by Photocrosslinking via Visible Light Irradiation for a Tissue Bio-Adhesive. *Int. J. Mol. Sci.* **2021**, *22*, 700. [CrossRef]
101. Negrescu, A.M.; Mitran, V.; Draghicescu, W.; Popescu, S.; Pirvu, C.; Ionascu, I.; Soare, T.; Uzun, S.; Croitoru, S.M.; Cimpean, A. TiO2 Nanotubes Functionalized with Icariin for an Attenuated In Vitro Immune Response and Improved In Vivo Osseointegration. *J. Funct. Biomater.* **2022**, *13*, 43. [CrossRef]
102. Scalzone, A.; Bonifacio, M.A.; Cometa, S.; Cucinotta, F.; De Giglio, E.; Ferreira, A.M.; Gentile, P. PH-Triggered Adhesiveness and Cohesiveness of Chondroitin Sulfate-Catechol Biopolymer for Biomedical Applications. *Front. Bioeng. Biotechnol.* **2020**, *8*, 1–14. [CrossRef]
103. Zou, C.Y.; Lei, X.X.; Hu, J.J.; Jiang, Y.L.; Li, Q.J.; Song, Y.T.; Zhang, Q.Y.; Li-Ling, J.; Xie, H.Q. Multi-Crosslinking Hydrogels with Robust Bio-Adhesion and pro-Coagulant Activity for First-Aid Hemostasis and Infected Wound Healing. *Bioact. Mater.* **2022**, *16*, 388–402. [CrossRef]
104. Yu, J.; Qin, Y.; Yang, Y.; Zhao, X.; Zhang, Z.; Zhang, Q.; Su, Y.; Zhang, Y.; Cheng, Y. Robust Hydrogel Adhesives for Emergency Rescue and Gastric Perforation Repair. *Bioact. Mater.* **2022**, *19*, 703–716. [CrossRef]
105. Tabatabaei, F.; Rasoulianboroujeni, M.; Yadegari, A.; Tajik, S.; Moharamzadeh, K.; Tayebi, L. Osteo-Mucosal Engineered Construct: In Situ Adhesion of Hard-Soft Tissues. *Mater. Sci. Eng. C* **2021**, *128*, 112255. [CrossRef] [PubMed]
106. Hou, M.; Wang, X.; Yue, O.; Zheng, M.; Zhang, H.; Liu, X. Development of a Multifunctional Injectable Temperature-Sensitive Gelatin-Based Adhesive Double-Network Hydrogel. *Mater. Sci. Eng. C* **2021**, *134*, 112556. [CrossRef] [PubMed]
107. Zhou, H.; Liang, C.; Wei, Z.; Bai, Y.; Bhaduri, S.B.; Webster, T.J.; Bian, L.; Yang, L. Injectable Biomaterials for Translational Medicine. *Mater. Today* **2019**, *28*, 81–97. [CrossRef]
108. Xu, R.; Yu, F.; Huang, L.; Zhou, W.; Wang, Y.; Wang, F.; Sun, X.; Chang, G.; Fang, M.; Zhang, L.; et al. Isocyanate-Terminated Urethane-Based Dental Adhesive Bridges Dentinal Matrix Collagen with Adhesive Resin. *Acta Biomater.* **2019**, *83*, 140–152. [CrossRef]
109. Kim, M.H.; Lee, J.N.; Lee, J.; Lee, H.; Park, W.H. Enzymatically Cross-Linked Poly(γ-Glutamic Acid) Hydrogel with Enhanced Tissue Adhesive Property. *ACS Biomater. Sci. Eng.* **2020**, *6*, 3103–3113. [CrossRef]
110. Tao, C.; Jin, M.; Yao, H.; Wang, D.A. Dopamine Based Adhesive Nano-Coatings on Extracellular Matrix (ECM) Based Grafts for Enhanced Host-Graft Interfacing Affinity. *Nanoscale* **2021**, *13*, 18148–18159. [CrossRef]
111. Zhang, Y.; Debenedictis, E.P.; Keten, S. Cohesive and Adhesive Properties of Crosslinked Semiflexible Biopolymer Networks. *Soft Matter* **2019**, *15*, 3807–3816. [CrossRef]
112. Wang, A. Molecular Mechanisms Governing the Mechanics of Polymeric and Protein-Based Materials. *Adv. Drug Del. Rev.* **2021**.
113. Liu, H.; Yuan, M.; Sonamuthu, J.; Yan, S.; Huang, W.; Cai, Y.; Yao, J. A Dopamine-Functionalized Aqueous-Based Silk Protein Hydrogel Bioadhesive for Biomedical Wound Closure. *New J. Chem.* **2020**, *44*, 884–891. [CrossRef]
114. Wang, H.; Su, X.; Chai, Z.; Tian, Z.; Xie, W.; Wang, Y.; Wan, Z.; Deng, M.; Yuan, Z.; Huang, J. A Hydra Tentacle-Inspired Hydrogel with Underwater Ultra-Stretchability for Adhering Adipose Surfaces. *Chem. Eng. J.* **2022**, *428*, 131049. [CrossRef]
115. Zussma, M.; Giladi, S.; Zilberman, M. In Vitro Characterization of Injectable Chlorhexidine-Eluting Gelatin Hydrogels for Local Treatment of Periodontal Infections. *Polym. Adv. Technol.* **2022**, 1–12.
116. Eshkol-Yogev, I.; Tobias, T.; Keren, A.; Gilhar, A.; Gilboa, E.; Furer, A.; Ullman, Y.; Zilberman, M. Dual Composite Bioadhesives for Wound Closure Applications: An in Vitro and in Vivo Study. *Polym. Adv. Technol.* **2022**, 1–16. [CrossRef]
117. Karami, P. Design and Development of Injectable, Tough and Intrinsically-Adhesive Hydrogels for Biomedical Applications. *EPFL* **2021**.
118. Lu, X.; Shi, S.; Li, H.; Gerhard, E.; Lu, Z.; Tan, X.; Li, W.; Rahn, K.M.; Xie, D.; Xu, G.; et al. Magnesium Oxide-Crosslinked Low-Swelling Citrate-Based Mussel-Inspired Tissue Adhesives. *Biomaterials* **2020**, *232*, 119719. [CrossRef]
119. Li, Q.; Zhang, P.; Yang, C.; Duan, H.; Hong, W. Switchable Adhesion between Hydrogels by Wrinkling. *Extrem. Mech. Lett.* **2021**, *43*, 101193. [CrossRef]
120. Li, A.; Xu, Z.; Sun, N.; Si, Z.; Xu, Y.; Guo, X. Cellulose-Reinforced Catechol-Modified Polyacrylic Acid-Zn2+ Coacervate as Strong Composite Adhesive. *J. Appl. Polym. Sci.* **2019**, *136*, 3–9. [CrossRef]
121. Moini, N.; Khaghanipour, M.; Kabiri, K.; Salimi, A.; Zohuriaan-Mehr, M.J.; Jahandideh, A. Engineered Green Adhesives Based on Demands: Star-Shaped Glycerol-Lactic Acid Oligomers in Anaerobic Adhesives. *ACS Sustain. Chem. Eng.* **2019**, *7*, 16247–16256. [CrossRef]
122. Xu, X.; Sui, B.; Liu, X.; Sun, J. A Bioinspired and High-Strengthed Hydrogel for Regeneration of Perforated Temporomandibular Joint Disc: Construction and Pleiotropic Immunomodulatory Effects. *Bioact. Mater.* **2022**. [CrossRef]
123. Yi, B.; Zhou, B.; Song, Z.; Yu, L.; Wang, W.; Liu, W. Step-Wise CAG@PLys@PDA-Cu2+ Modification on Micropatterned Nanofibers for Programmed Endothelial Healing. *Bioact. Mater.* **2022**. [CrossRef]

124. Chávez-Villarreal, A.; de los Ángeles Andrea Carvajal-Montes de Oca, M.; Garza-Enríquez, M.; Elizondo-Cantú, O. The Use of Cyanoacrylate in Surgical Procedure in Periodontics: A Literature Review. *Int. J. Appl. Dent. Sci.* **2019**, *5*, 330–332.
125. Anupama Devi, V.K.; Shyam, R.; Palaniappan, A.; Jaiswal, A.K.; Oh, T.H.; Nathanael, A.J. Self-Healing Hydrogels: Preparation, Mechanism and Advancement in Biomedical Applications. *Polymers* **2021**, *13*, 3782. [CrossRef] [PubMed]
126. Khadem, E.; Kharaziha, M.; Bakhsheshi-Rad, H.R.; Das, O.; Berto, F. Cutting-Edge Progress in Stimuli-Responsive Bioadhesives: From Synthesis to Clinical Applications . *Polymers* **2022**, *14*, 1709. [CrossRef] [PubMed]
127. Hyldbakk, A.; Mørch, Y.; Snipstad, S.; Åslund, A.K.O.; Klinkenberg, G.; Nakstad, V.T.; Wågbø, A.M.; Schmid, R.; Molesworth, P.P. Identification of Novel Cyanoacrylate Monomers for Use in Nanoparticle Drug Delivery Systems Prepared by Miniemulsion Polymerisation—A Multistep Screening Approach. *Int. J. Pharm. X* **2022**, *4*, 100124. [CrossRef] [PubMed]
128. Li, D.; Zhuang, B.; Wang, X.; Wu, Z.; Wei, W.; Aladejana, J.T.; Hou, X.; Yves, K.G.; Xie, Y.; Liu, J. Chitosan Used as a Specific Coupling Agent to Modify Starch in Preparation of Adhesive Film. *J. Clean. Prod.* **2020**, *277*, 123210. [CrossRef]
129. Salama, A.H.; Abdelkhalek, A.A.; Elkasabgy, N.A. Etoricoxib-Loaded Bio-Adhesive Hybridized Polylactic Acid-Based Nanoparticles as an Intra-Articular Injection for the Treatment of Osteoarthritis. *Int. J. Pharm.* **2020**, *578*, 119081. [CrossRef] [PubMed]

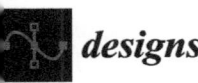

Article

Bio-Lubricant Properties Analysis of Drilling an Innovative Design of Bioactive Kinetic Screw into Bone

Carlos Aurelio Andreucci [1], Elza M. M. Fonseca [2,*] and Renato N. Jorge [3]

1. Mechanical Engineering Department, Faculty of Engineering, University of Porto, Rua Dr. Roberto Frias, 712, 4200-465 Porto, Portugal
2. LAETA, INEGI, ISEP, Instituto Politécnico do Porto, R. Dr. António Bernardino de Almeida, 4249-015 Porto, Portugal
3. LAETA, INEGI, Mechanical Engineering Department, Faculty of Engineering, University of Porto, Rua Dr. Roberto Frias, 712, 4200-465 Porto, Portugal
* Correspondence: elz@isep.ipp.pt

Citation: Andreucci, C.A.; Fonseca, E.M.M.; Jorge, R.N. Bio-Lubricant Properties Analysis of Drilling an Innovative Design of Bioactive Kinetic Screw into Bone. *Designs* 2023, 7, 21. https://doi.org/10.3390/designs7010021

Academic Editors: Richard Drevet and Hicham Benhayoune

Received: 18 December 2022
Revised: 18 January 2023
Accepted: 29 January 2023
Published: 1 February 2023

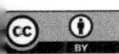

Copyright: © 2023 by the authors. Licensee MDPI, Basel, Switzerland. This article is an open access article distributed under the terms and conditions of the Creative Commons Attribution (CC BY) license (https://creativecommons.org/licenses/by/4.0/).

Abstract: Biotribology is applied to study the friction, wear, and lubrication of biological systems or natural phenomena under relative motion in the human body. It is a multidisciplinary field and tribological processes impact all aspects of our daily life. Tribological processes may occur after the implantation of an artificial device in the human body with a wide variety of sliding and frictional interfaces. Blood is a natural bio-lubricant experiencing laminar flow at the lower screw velocities associated with drilling implants into bone, being a viscoelastic fluid with viscous and fluid characteristics. The viscosity comes from the blood plasma, while the elastic properties are from the deformation of red blood cells. In this study, drilling parameters according to material properties obtained by Finite Element Analysis are given. The influence of blood on the resulting friction between the surfaces is demonstrated and correlated with mechanical and biological consequences, identifying an innovative approach to obtaining a new lubricant parameter for bone drilling analysis. The lubrication parameter (HN) found within the limitations of conditions used in this study is 10.7×10^{-7} for both cortical bone (D1) and spongy bone (D4). A thermal-structural analysis of the densities of the soft bone (D4) and hard bone (D1) shows differences in only the equivalent stress values due to the differences in respective Young moduli. The natural occurrences of blood as a lubricant in bone-screw perforations are poorly investigated in the literature and its effects are fundamental in osseointegration. This work aims to elucidate the relevance of the study of blood as a lubricant in drilling and screwing implants into bone at lower speeds.

Keywords: bio-lubricant; lubrication parameter; bone drilling; blood; bioactive kinetic screw

1. Introduction

Blood is a special type of fluid connective tissue derived from mesoderm and composed of plasma (55%) and cellular elements (45%), erythrocytes (red blood cells), leukocytes (white blood cells), and thrombocytes (platelets). Its color changes according to the gas it carries within its structure, being bright red when carrying oxygen, or dark purple when carrying carbon dioxide. It represents 8% of body mass, is slightly alkaline (pH = 7.35–7.45), has a temperature of 37 °C, a viscosity 3 to 4 times greater than that of water, and its average volume in the human body is five liters [1]. Blood transports hormones to organs and causes them to change their physiology, regulates the pH, restricts fluid loss during an injury, acts as a defense against pathogens and toxins, and regulates the body temperature [2]. Plasma is the pale-yellow-colored liquid component of blood that holds its cellular elements in suspension and is constituted of water (91.5%), proteins (7%), namely albumins, globulins, and fibrinogen, and other solutes (1.5%) electrolytic ions, gases, nutrients, and waste products [3]. The function of plasma is to absorb, transport, and release heat through water, maintain osmotic balance through albumins and provide body defense through globulins, blood clotting through fibrinogen, and pH buffering through its electrolytic ions. Red blood cells are circular biconcave non-nucleated cells, measuring 7 to 8 μm in diameter and 2.5 μm in thickness with a life span of 120 days, presenting red color (hemoglobin pigment) [4]. Red blood cells transport oxygen (oxyhemoglobin) from lungs to tissues and carbon dioxide (deoxyhemoglobin) from tissues to lungs via the hemoglobin molecules (Hb) that represent 13 to 15 g per 100 mL of blood. Each molecule of Hb carries four molecules of oxygen [5].

When drilling into bone tissue cuts a blood vessel, the body starts the process to keep homeostasis through hemostasis, which begins with the vascular phase, in which the diameter of the blood vessels decreases, and endothelial cells (the inner layer of blood vessels) releasing chemical factors; next, in the platelet phase, a platelet plug forms and other chemicals are released (ADP, clotting factors); then coagulation or blood clotting occurs, where in addition to platelets, fibrinogen is converted to fibrin to form a net-like structure to form a clot; finally, fibrinolysis occurs, and, after the blood vessel is completely healed and new connective tissue has formed, the now unnecessary blood clot is removed [6].

Blood behaves as a non-Newtonian fluid and its viscosity varies with shear rate, decreasing at high shear rates (shear-thinning fluid) and vice versa. Blood viscosity also increases with increases in red cell aggregability, in coagulating blood, falls with the thrombus formation, while in non-coagulation blood, retains almost the same value, as shown by the activated clotting time and fibrinogen concentration tests. Blood viscosity is determined by plasma viscosity, hematocrit (red blood cell volume), and the mechanical properties of red blood cells, mainly erythrocyte deformability and erythrocyte aggregation [7]. The viscosity, equivalent to friction in fluids, of blood at 37 °C is normally 4×10^{-3} pascal-seconds [8]. The friction arising from bone-implant contact (BIC) during drilling converts kinetic energy into thermal energy. Between bone-implant surfaces, blood flows naturally after the surgical cutting of the bone blood vessels during drilling, and filling this gap with blood is desirable to obtain the initial phase of inflammation and subsequent osseointegration. Hydrophilic features are desired on implant surfaces to attract and adhere blood in the initial process of inflammation in the bone-implant contact healing process [9]. Although surgery damages bone tissue, it also triggers a cascade of wound-healing events that stimulate osseointegration, improving implant stability through bone remodeling [10]. The shear rate (τ_{yx}) for a fluid flowing (blood) [11] between bone and a BKS implant, one moving at a constant speed (BKS) and the other stationary (bone) is determined by the change in pressure (Δp), the distance between fluid flow (L) and the diameter of the bone-implant interface micro gap (y), defined by Equation (1):

$$\tau_{yx} = \frac{\Delta p\, y}{L} \quad (1)$$

The Stribeck curve is a fundamental concept in the field of tribology. It shows that friction in fluid-lubricated contacts is a non-linear function of the contact load, the lubricant viscosity, and the lubricant entrainment speed (sliding speed), differentiating boundary lubrication (bone-implant contact), mixed lubrication (bone-implant contact gap filled by blood) and hydrodynamic lubrication (load supported by hydrodynamic pressure) [12]. For the contact between two fluid-lubricated surfaces, the Stribeck curve shows the relationship between the so-called Hersey Number (HN) [13], a dimensionless lubrication parameter that shows the relationship between viscosity and load, and how friction changes with increasing velocity. The Hersey number is defined as Equation (2):

$$HN = \frac{\eta N}{P} \quad (2)$$

where η is the dynamic viscosity (Pa·s = N·s/m^2) of the fluid, N is the entrainment speed of the fluid, which is equal to the velocity of BKS Implant insertion (m/s), and P is the Insertion Torque applied (Nm).

Boundary lubrication is related to bone-implant contact without the effect of the blood as a lubricant and is commonly analyzed by insertion torque forces [13]. Hydrodynamic lubrication is related to the pressure in the plasma and cells involved in the inflammation process initiated by the surgical cut made by drilling into the bone. Mixed lubrication, the objective of this study, correlates the influence of roughness contact between the bone-implant load, supported by both surfaces and the liquid lubricant (blood) [13]. The mixed lubrication regime can be determined by the (λ) ratio of the film thickness to the root-mean-square (RMS) surface roughness of the two frictional surfaces. When $1 < \lambda < 3$ the lubrication condition is considered mixed lubrication. The RMS surface roughness of Ti6Al4V implants is in the range of 6–14 µm [14–16] depending on the surface treatment applied, and the roughness—the linear dimensions of the bone tissue—range from 5.5 to 6.5 µm, depending on the quality of the bone drilling cut [17]. Both can change either slightly or significantly during drilling wear. To maintain full blood film lubrication, the minimum film thickness must be greater than 15–18 µm, which is generally the case in actual physiological conditions when 150 µm is the distance between the screwed implant and the bone bed site after healing [18]. The analysis of the Stribeck curve shows that the lubricant decreases the coefficient of friction proportionally to the velocity applied, likewise when the lubricant is blood, higher speeds can also aggregate the red blood cells increasing its viscosity and decreasing its lubricant properties. Understanding the ideal speed for insertion torque in bone screw implants can optimize the use of the blood as a lubricant, inherent to the surgical cut of the drilling process, and maintain its biological properties, improving the healing process and predictable results in osseointegration [19].

The mechanical properties of bone tissue are widely studied and discussed in the literature [20]. Several properties can be quantified, including the stiffness (S), the ultimate load that corresponds to the load at failure, the energy or work to failure (U), and ultimate displacement. The elastic region, before yield, represents Young's modulus (material stiffness), and the plastic region, a post-yield nonlinear region that contains the ultimate stress and the failure point. Yield stress is the transition to nonlinear behavior, which means that the stress begins to cause permanent damage to the bone structure. The maximum stress and strain that the bone can sustain are called the ultimate stress (strength) and ultimate strain. These properties are strongly dependent on the loading mode (tensile, compression, bending, or shear) and determine the mechanical response of the bone tissue to drilling operations [21]. Bone density varies between individuals and throughout life. A basic concept accepted in the literature is the structural and functional properties differences between cortical bone and trabecular bone. Trabecular bone has the same structures as compact bone, but they are not arranged in osteons, containing the same components. Instead, it has very distinct trabeculae (small beams of bone) separated by macroscopic spaces filled with red bone marrow or yellow bone marrow. The trabeculae are organized on the long lines of stress and help to reduce the weight of the bone [22]. The less-dense trabecular bone presents larger spaces (lacunae) in its composition, filled with higher blood quantity than cortical bone [23]. Maximum insertion Torque analyses clearly show the influence of different bone densities, and their relationship is robustly described in the literature. However, the lubricating effect of the blood into the bone-implant contact during drilling and screwing, and the lower torque obtained in the insertion of implants into trabecular bone, are not correlated in the literature and may influence these results [21].

The friction coefficient is independent of the applied normal force and displacement rate [24] but depends on the properties of the bone tissue surrounding the implant and on the properties of the implant surface [10]. The test of bone against implant surfaces produced a variety of different force-displacement curves and a wide range of friction coefficients (in the range of 0.19 to 0.78) [25–27].

Maximum insertion torque (MIT) values can range from 15 to 150 Ncm [28] with a mean value of 78.30 Ncm. The mean MIT is typically higher in D1 cortical bone (126.67 Ncm) and lower in D4 spongy bone (40.22 Ncm) [29]. A statistically significant correlation is found between bone volume and MIT values ($r= +0.771$, $p < 0.0001$). No statistically significant correlation is found between implant length and/or diameter and MIT in all bone densities. About 50–80% of bone-implant contact is described in the literature as clinically successful implants. Some results suggest that no matter the initial percentage of BIC, the final Osseointegration is about 58–60% BIC if the bone remodeling equilibrium state is reached [18].

Many studies on BIC are on the secondary stability (biological) of bone implants, and only the values of maximum insertion torque are described in primary or mechanical stability analysis, without the determination of BIC in this initial and fundamental phase to promote healing. Understanding BIC in primary stability, mainly in cases of high (D1) and low (D4) bone density increases our understanding of osseointegration. The interface between the implant and bone tissue presents a dynamic environment expressed by mechanical and biological interactions between the surfaces. The surgical trauma caused by drilling and screwing the screw into the bone promotes hemorrhage, the first and most important step of the healing process in osseointegration [3–7,14–16]. The objective of this work is to use finite element analysis (FEA) of drilling an implant into the bone with specific parameters to introduce innovative theoretical hypotheses of the correlation between blood as a natural biological lubricant, bone densities, maximum insertion torque, and a coefficient of friction that is a result of those interactions. The focus is on mechanical stability or primary stability and its immediate mechanical behaviors after bone plastic and elastic deformation due to the drilling and screwing process. Within the limitations of this study, we found a new lubrication parameter for bone drilling.

2. Materials and Methods

BKS is an innovative mechanical device with inherent biomechanical properties [22] including the bone compacting factor inside the BKS, allowing us to determine the absolute bone density through invasive direct measurement in the region of interest.

Applying simple biomechanical concepts of bone drilling, screwing, biocompatibility, and bone implant, the engineering design of BKS was created to, among other characteristics, optimize the surgical technique and reduce the trauma of bone perforation, with a smaller number of drillings, as seen in Figure 1.

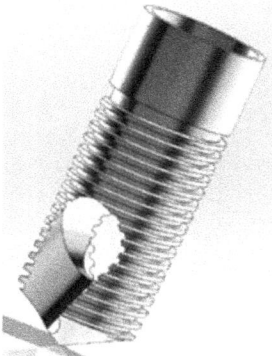

Figure 1. BKS as a dental implant applied in the Finite Element Analysis drilling and screwing into the bone simultaneously.

In this work, three-dimensional finite element modeling and numerical analysis were carried out to facilitate thermal-structural analysis. The 3D models were built in Solidworks ® and ANSYS 2020 R2 ®—Workbench 2020 R2 software programs. The BKS modeling was carried out in Solidworks and imported into ANSYS Workbench, as shown in Figure 1. After importing the Solidworks model into ANSYS, a cortical bone block (workpiece) was constructed, representing the surrounding dental bone.

Based on the geometrical models, finite element meshes were generated. The numerical model was prepared in ANSYS 2020 R2 ®—Workbench 2020 R2. The BKS model and the bone disc were meshed with 3D SOLID elements.

In the presented simulation, the BKS tool was provided with TiAl64V parameters as seen in Table 1, and cortical bone (Table 2) with two distinct parameters to compare bone of density D1 (1.85×10^{-6} kg/mm³) and D4 (0.45×10^{-6} kg/mm³). First, for bone of density D1, an angular velocity of 300 rpm and a feed rate equal to 0.1 mm/s vertically down into the bone were applied. Second, the steps were applied to bone of density D4. In both cases, a thrust load of 80 N was used with a temperature of 39 °C in the absence of irrigation, as it is intended to be used in ongoing research.

Table 1. BKS Implant properties applied in FEA [21,30].

	Ti6Al4V (Grade 5)
Young's Modulus, MPa	2.0×10^5
Poisson's Ratio	0.3
Maximum Yield Stress, MPa	1450
Initial Yield Stress, MPa	850
Density, kg/mm³	4.51×10^{-6}
Coefficient of Thermal Expansion, 1/°C	8.5×10^{-6}

Table 2. Bone properties applied in FEA [21,30].

	Cortical Bone
Poisson's Ratio	0.3
Maximum Yield Stress, MPa	125
Initial Yield Stress, MPa	10
Coefficient of Thermal Expansion, 1/°C	8.9×10^5
Young's Modulus, MPa (D1)	17,000
Young's Modulus, MPa (D4)	175.12
Density, kg/mm³ (D1)	1.85×10^{-6}
Density, kg/mm³ (D4)	0.45×10^{-6}

In the present study, an electric motor EM-12L with a maximum power of 59 W was selected with angular speeds of between 100 and 40,000 rpm [30]. The relation between the torque (M_t in Nm), the maximum electrical power during drilling (P in W), and the speed of rotation (n in rpm) are determined according to Equation (3).

$$M_t = 9.55 \frac{P}{n} \qquad (3)$$

According to this equation, the torque is equal to 187.8 Ncm at a rotational speed of 300 rpm. The FEA results obtained were applied to determine optimal parameters for insertion of the new BKS biomechanical design, as seen in Figure 2, relating them to the mathematical concepts used in tribology to support the proposed hypothesis of the lubricating effect of blood when drilling implants into bone, and the advantages of choosing the drilling parameters based on the geometry and surface of the bone implant.

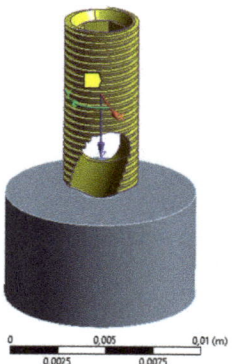

Figure 2. Schematic diagram of BKS Screw in the cortical bone block (workpiece).

3. Results

In previous studies [30] the formation of the plastic strain over different time instants of the bone drilling process was described. As expected, the BKS screw during the drilling process does not present plastic strain. Bone material during perforation presents high plastic strain which increases with the amount of material removed [30–32]. The soft bone (D4) and hard bone (D1) densities used in the thermal-structural analysis show differences in only the equivalent stress values, which, in the case of D1 equals 102.6 MPa, and in the case of D4 equals 1.056 MPa; and normal stress values, which is the case of D1 equals −92.7 MPa, and in the case of D4 equals −0.955 MPa, due to the differences in respective Young moduli. The results for deformation and strain followed the same trend.

3.1. FEA Bone Density D1 (1.85×10^{-6} kg/mm^3, 17,000 MPa)

The results of drilling the implant into bone of density D1 are shown in Figures 3–7:

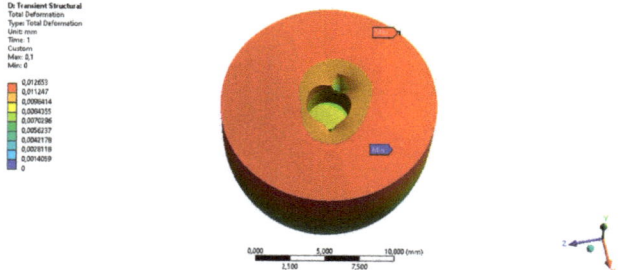

Figure 3. Thermal-Structural Analysis. Bone total deformation 0.013 mm.

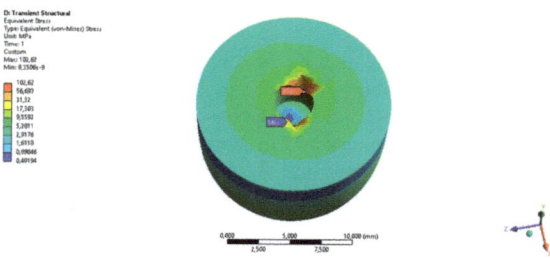

Figure 4. Thermal-Structural Analysis. Equivalent Stress 102.6 MPa.

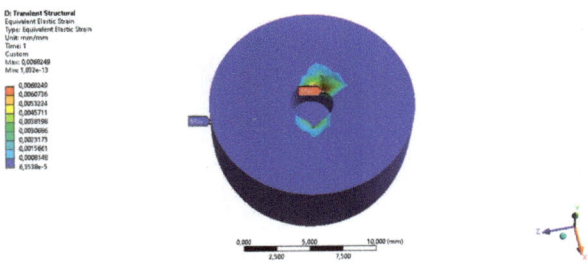

Figure 5. Thermal-Structural Analysis. Equivalent Elastic Strain 0.0068.

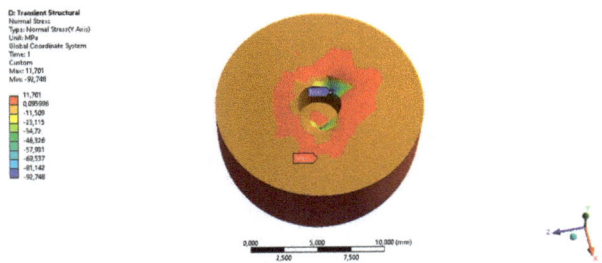

Figure 6. Thermal-Structural Analysis. Y-axis Normal Stress −92.7 MPa.

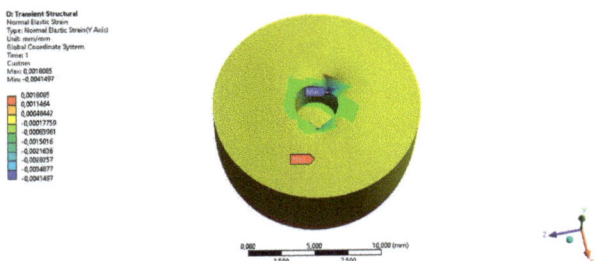

Figure 7. Thermal-Structural Analysis. Y-axis Normal elastic Strain 0.0018.

3.2. FEA Bone Density D4 (0.45×10^{-6} kg/mm^3, 175.12 MPa)

The results of drilling the implant into bone of density D4 only changed in terms of equivalent and normal stress values, since they depend on the Young modulus.

The displacement and deformation are the same because the remaining conditions are equal, as seen in Figures 8 and 9.

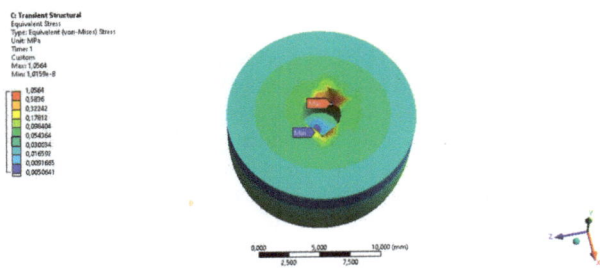

Figure 8. Thermal-Structural Analysis. Equivalent Stress 1.056 MPa.

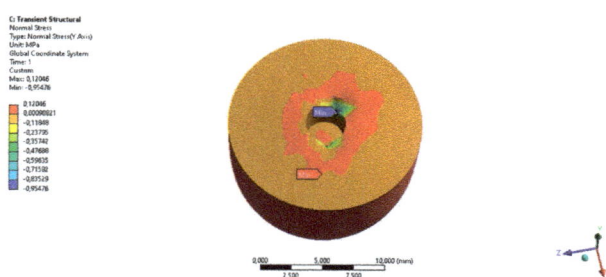

Figure 9. Thermal-Structural Analysis. Y-axis Normal Stress −0.955 MPa.

4. Discussion

Previous studies of BKS implants [22,30–32] obtained by FEA, when analyzed from the biological perspective, describe the plastic deformation promoting bone tissue rupture (osteotomy fracture), blood vessel rupture, the release of salts, enzymes, acids, proteins, macromolecules, and cell death; and the elastic stress/strain of the BKS in the bone, with the blood from cutting and drilling the bone around the screw, and the higher stress/strain obtained in the MIT at the apex of the BKS in contact with the bone at the end of the drilling. As soon as the BKS implant is drilled into the bone, the inflammation process starts through the release of blood adjacent to the cutting, deformation, and stress areas.

Microscopically, the cut bone tissue and blood vessels develop at the interface of the cutting edge of the drilling site, exactly where the bone will be stressed on the threaded walls of the BKS, as analyzed in the results by FEM. Since in the BKS surgical technique, the drilling is not performed by an undersized drill, it is possible to determine and control the plastic and elastic stress/strain, which varies only with the relative bone densities, during the BKS insertion. The coefficient of friction is independent of the applied normal force and the displacement rate [33].

Applying equation (2), where η is the dynamic viscosity of the blood (4×10^{-3} N·s/m²), N is the entrainment speed of the fluid, that is equal to the velocity of BKS Implant insertion (5×10^{-4} m/s), and P is the insertion torque applied (1.87 Nm), we can determine the dimensionless lubrication parameter (HN) where, for a given viscosity and load, the Stribeck curve shows how friction changes with increasing velocity, resulting in:

$$HN = \frac{4 \times 10^{-3} \times 5 \times 10^{-4}}{1.87} \qquad (4)$$

The lubrication parameter (HN) found within the limitations of the conditions employed in this study is 10.7×10^{-7} for both the cortical bone (D1) and spongy bone (D4) properties defined as shown in Table 2, and the BKS Implant properties in Table 1.

The Stribeck Curve helps us to understand the lubrication regimes where the interface between the bone-implant acts [13]. A meta-analysis [24] compared the suitability of various parameters used to characterize wettability in tribological systems and showed the relationship between wettability and the friction factor for multiple lubricant-surface pairings.

The differences in equivalent stress values, 102.6 MPa, and 1.056 MPa for D1 and D4 respectively, and normal stress values, of −92.7 MPa and −0.955 MPa for D1 and D4, respectively, indicate that the bone blood vessels adjacent to the BIC site suffer different stresses under those densities, which has already been proven in the literature to interfere in the healing process, slowing, or preventing, it [34].

The bleeding and clotting time measures the clotting time of the blood and is dependent on the proper functioning of platelets in the blood vessels with normal hemostasis occurring between 2 and 7 min [35]. Most individuals have a bleeding time of less than 4 min, showing that the lubricating capacity of blood, before its clotting, should become active immediately after cutting the bone through the initial drilling.

More time spent with multiple bone drilling not only damages the bone bed [36] but also increases the time between initial bone drilling and final implant screwing, decreasing the benefit of blood as a lubricant and its sliding across the implant surface [34–36]. With the new BKS design, simultaneous drilling and screwing and low applied speed ensure that the blood acts as a lubricant and can maintain its normal functions. The benefits of blood in intimate contact with the bone-implant surface have already been robustly described in the literature, and the optimal surface for this to occur in a controlled manner is still being sought [18,34].

Bone is tensioned and compressed during the drilling and screwing of implants. On the compression side, bone undergoes a cascade of events that result in upregulated osteoclasts absorbing bone, and, on the tension side, bone undergoes a separate cascade of events that result in upregulated osteoblasts, which create bone. These result in resorption on the compression side and apposition on the tension side, remodeling in such a way that enables the implant to develop long-term osseointegration [37]. By understanding and respecting these parameters, we optimize the probability of achieving controlled and successful results.

Within seconds of the drilling and cutting forces being applied, the bone blood vessels are distorted on the compression side, and they will be partially compressed and partially dilated on the tension side. In minutes, with those blood vessels having been distorted, the blood flow is altered, and oxygen and carbon dioxide levels will change. This change in oxygen tension will trigger inflammatory mediators like prostaglandins and RANKL to be released [38].

Limitations in experimental in vivo research and computational modeling due to the not-well-established mixed-lubrication mechanism, the high computational costs required to model the bearing surfaces within a relatively large contact area, and the complexity of geometry analyzing lubrication of biological and non-biological surfaces (drilling bone screws, hip, and knee joints) with biological lubricants, inhibit the development of the field of tribology [27,39].

Highlighting the importance of the inflammatory process and the lubricating effect of the blood during bone drilling, we can promote future studies to determine other blood lubrication parameters at different bone densities, different blood viscosities (pathologies), other bone screw insertion speeds, and different implant geometries, comparing the results and improving the osseointegration prognosis. In addition, biofunctionalization may shorten the healing period of osseointegrated biomaterials [40].

5. Conclusions

A new BKS biomechanism for bone screws and implants was presented as a bone implant screw to show how blood could influence the resulting friction between bone-implant surfaces, correlating with mechanical and biological properties, defining a novel approach to obtain a new lubricant parameter in the analysis of drilling into bone. The natural effect of blood as a lubricant in bone-screw perforations is not investigated in the literature and its effects are paramount in bone healing. This work has elucidated the relevance of blood as a lubricant in drilling and screwing bone at lower speeds with pre-defined parameters.

The lubrication parameter (HN) found within the limitations of the conditions employed in this study is 10.7×10^{-7} for both cortical bone (D1) and spongy bone (D4).

Thermal-structural analysis of soft bone (D4) and hard bone (D1) densities shows differences only in equivalent stress values, due to the differences in respective Young moduli. This is ongoing research and future studies will be able to experimentally determine the advantages and disadvantages of blood as a bio-lubricant.

Author Contributions: Conceptualization, C.A.A.; methodology, C.A.A.; formal analysis, C.A.A.; investigation, C.A.A.; writing—original draft preparation, C.A.A.; writing—review and editing, E.M.M.F.; visualization, E.M.M.F.; supervision, R.N.J. All authors have read and agreed to the published version of the manuscript.

Funding: This research received no external funding.

Data Availability Statement: Not applicable.

Conflicts of Interest: The authors declare no conflict of interest.

References

1. Vahedi, A.; Bigdelou, P.; Farnoud, A.M. Quantitative analysis of red blood cell membrane phospholipids and modulation of cell-macrophage interactions using cyclodextrins. *Sci. Rep.* **2020**, *10*, 15111. [CrossRef] [PubMed]
2. Minton, K. Red blood cells join the ranks as immune sentinels. *Nat. Rev. Immunol.* **2021**, *21*, 760–761. [CrossRef] [PubMed]
3. Mathew, J.; Sankar, P.; Varacallo, M. Physiology, Blood Plasma. In *StatPearls*; StatPearls Publishing: Treasure Island, FL, USA, 2022.
4. Generalov, V.M.; Safatov, A.S.; Kruchinina, M.V. Dielectric Properties of the Human Red Blood Cell. *Meas. Tech.* **2020**, *63*, 580–586. [CrossRef]
5. Ahmed, M.H.; Ghatge, M.S.; Safo, M.K. Hemoglobin: Structure, Function and Allostery. *Subcell. Biochem.* **2020**, *94*, 345–382. [CrossRef]
6. Tutwiler, V.; Singh, J.; Litvinov, R.I.; Bassani, J.L.; Purohit, P.K.; Weisel, J.W. Rupture of blood clots: Mechanics and pathophysiology. *Sci. Adv.* **2020**, *6*, eabc0496. [CrossRef] [PubMed]
7. Li, J.; Sapkota, A.; Kikuchi, D.; Sakota, D.; Maruyama, O.; Takei, M. Red blood cells aggregability measurement of coagulating blood in extracorporeal circulation system with multiple-frequency electrical impedance spectroscopy. *Biosens. Bioelectron.* **2018**, *112*, 79–85. [CrossRef]
8. Stauffer, E.; Loyrion, E.; Hancco, I. Blood viscosity and its determinants in the highest city in the world. *J. Physiol.* **2020**, *598*, 4121–4130. [CrossRef]
9. Makowiecki, A.; Hadzik, J.; Błaszczyszyn, A.; Gedrange, T.; Dominiak, M. An evaluation of superhydrophilic surfaces of dental implants—a systematic review and meta-analysis. *BMC Oral Health* **2019**, *19*, 79. [CrossRef]
10. Florencio-Silva, R.; Sasso, G.R.; Sasso-Cerri, E.; Simões, M.J.; Cerri, P.S. Biology of Bone Tissue: Structure, Function, and Factors That Influence Bone Cells. *Biomed Res. Int.* **2015**, *2015*, 421746. [CrossRef]
11. Raj, A.; Rajak, D.K.; Gautam, S.; Guria, C.; Pathak, A.K. Shear Rate Estimation: A Detailed Review. In Proceedings of the Paper Presented at the Offshore Technology Conference, Houston, TX, USA, 2–5 May 2016. [CrossRef]
12. Gu, C.; Meng, X.; Xie, Y.; Zhang, D. The influence of surface texturing on the transition of the lubrication regimes between a piston ring and a cylinder liner. *Int. J. Eng. Res.* **2017**, *18*, 785–796. [CrossRef]
13. Veltkamp, B.; Velikov, K.P.; Venner, C.H.; Bonn, D. Lubricated Friction and the Hersey Number. *Phys. Rev. Lett.* **2021**, *126*, 044301. [CrossRef] [PubMed]
14. Straumal, B.B.; Gornakova, A.S.; Kiselevskiy, M.V. Optimal surface roughness of Ti6Al4V alloy for the adhesion of cells with osteogenic potential. *J. Mater. Res.* **2022**, *37*, 2661–2674. [CrossRef]
15. Kamynina, O.K.; Kravchuk, K.S.; Lazov, M.A. Effect of Surface Roughness on the Properties of Titanium Materials for Bone Implants. *Russ. J. Inorg. Chem.* **2021**, *66*, 1073–1078. [CrossRef]
16. Boyan, B.D.; Lotz, E.M.; Schwartz, Z. Roughness and Hydrophilicity as Osteogenic Biomimetic Surface Properties. *Tissue Eng. Part A* **2017**, *23*, 1479–1489. [CrossRef] [PubMed]
17. Wang, C.; Zhang, G.; Li, Z.; Zeng, X.; Xu, Y.; Zhao, S.; Hu, H.; Zhang, Y.; Ren, T. Tribological behavior of Ti-6Al-4V against cortical bone in different biolubricants. *J. Mech. Behav. Biomed. Mater.* **2019**, *90*, 460–471. [CrossRef]
18. Lian, Z.; Guan, H.; Ivanovski, S.; Loo, Y.C.; Johnson, N.W.; Zhang, H. Effect of bone to implant contact percentage on bone remodeling surrounding a dental implant. *Int. J. Oral Maxillofac. Surg.* **2010**, *39*, 690–698. [CrossRef] [PubMed]
19. Lee, J.W.Y.; Bance, M.L. Physiology of Osseointegration. *Otolaryngol. Clin. N. Am.* **2019**, *52*, 231–242. [CrossRef]
20. Rahmanpanah, H.; Mouloodi, S.; Burvill, C.; Gohari, S.; Davies, H.M.S. Prediction of load-displacement curve in a complex structure using artificial neural networks: A study on a long bone. *Int. J. Eng. Sci.* **2020**, *154*, 103319. [CrossRef]
21. Maria, G.F.; Elza, M.F.; Renato, M.N. Three-dimensional dynamic finite element and experimental models for drilling processes. *Proc. IMechE. Part L J. Mater. Des. Appl.* **2015**, *232*, 35–43.
22. Andreucci, C.A.; Fonseca, E.M.M.; Jorge, R.N. Increased Material Density within a New Biomechanism. *Math. Comput. Appl.* **2022**, *27*, 90. [CrossRef]
23. Wang, S.-H.; Shen, Y.-W.; Fuh, L.-J.; Peng, S.-L.; Tsai, M.-T.; Huang, H.-L.; Hsu, J.-T. Relationship between Cortical Bone Thickness and Cancellous Bone Density at Dental Implant Sites in the Jawbone. *Diagnostics* **2020**, *10*, 710. [CrossRef] [PubMed]
24. Schertzer, M.J.; Iglesias, P. Meta-Analysis Comparing Wettability Parameters and the Effect of Wettability on Friction Coefficient in Lubrication. *Lubricants* **2018**, *6*, 70. [CrossRef]

25. Shacham, S.; Castel, D.; Gefen, A. Measurements of the static friction coefficient between bone and muscle tissues. *J. Biomech. Eng.* **2010**, *132*, 084502. [CrossRef] [PubMed]
26. Dannaway, J.; Dabirrahmani, D. An investigation into the frictional properties between bone and various orthopedic implant surfaces—implant stability. *J. Musculoskelet.* **2015**, *18*, 1550015. [CrossRef]
27. Haoyu, Z.; Zhang, X.; Jun, S.; Dagang, W. A study of misaligned compliant journal bearings lubricated by non-Newtonian fluid considering surface roughness. *Trib. Int.* **2023**, *179*, 108138. [CrossRef]
28. Halldin, A.; Jinno, Y.; Galli, S.; Ander, M.; Jacobsson, M.; Jimbo, R. Implant stability and bone remodeling up to 84 days of implantation with an initial static strain. An in vivo and theoretical investigation. *Clin. Oral Impl. Res.* **2016**, *27*, 1310–1316. [CrossRef] [PubMed]
29. Makary, C.; Rebaudi, A.; Mokbel, N.; Naaman, N. Peak Insertion Torque Correlated to Histologically and Clinically Evaluated Bone Density. *Impl. Dent.* **2011**, *20*, 182–191. [CrossRef] [PubMed]
30. Andreucci, C.A.; Fonseca, E.M.M.; Natal, R.M.J. Structural analysis of the new Bioactive Kinetic Screw in titanium alloy vs. commercially pure titanium. *J. Comp. Art. Int. Mec. Biomec.* **2022**, *2*, 35–43. [CrossRef]
31. Andreucci, C.A.; Alshaya, A.; Fonseca, E.M.M.; Jorge, R.N. Proposal for a New Bioactive Kinetic Screw in an Implant, Using a Numerical Model. *Appl. Sci.* **2022**, *12*, 779. [CrossRef]
32. Andreucci, C.A.; Fonseca, E.M.M.; Jorge, R.N. 3D Printing as an Efficient Way to Prototype and Develop Dental Implants. *BioMedInformatics* **2022**, *2*, 44. [CrossRef]
33. Trzepiecinski, T. A Study of the Coefficient of Friction in Steel Sheets Forming. *Metals* **2019**, *9*, 988. [CrossRef]
34. Xing, G.; Manon, F.; Guillaume, H. Biomechanical behaviours of the bone–implant interface: A review. *J. R. Soc. Interface* **2019**, *16*, 20190259. [CrossRef]
35. Milillo, L.; Cinone, F.; Lo Presti, F.; Lauritano, D.; Petruzzi, M. The Role of Blood Clot in Guided Bone Regeneration: Biological Considerations and Clinical Applications with Titanium Foil. *Materials* **2021**, *14*, 6642. [CrossRef] [PubMed]
36. Tsiagadigui, J.G.; Ndiwe, B.; Yamben, M.N.; Fotio, N.; Belinga, F.E.; Njeugna, E. The effects of multiple drilling of a bone with the same drill bit: Thermal and force analysis. *Heliyon* **2022**, *8*, e08927. [CrossRef]
37. Pallua, J.D.; Putzer, D.; Jäger, E.; Degenhart, G.; Arora, R.; Schmölz, W. Characterizing the Mechanical Behavior of Bone and Bone Surrogates in Compression Using pQCT. *Materials* **2022**, *15*, 5065. [CrossRef] [PubMed]
38. Anesi, A.; Cavani, F. Editorial for the Special Issue on "Multidisciplinary Insights on Bone Healing". *Biology* **2022**, *11*, 1776. [CrossRef]
39. Anitua, E. Biological drilling: Implant site preparation in a conservative manner and obtaining autogenous bone grafts. *Balk. J. Dent. Med.* **2018**, *22*, 98–101. [CrossRef]
40. Cirera, A.; Manzanares, M.C.; Sevilla, P.; Ortiz-Hernandez, M.; Galindo-Moreno, P.; Gil, J. Biofunctionalization with a TGFβ-1 Inhibitor Peptide in the Osseointegration of Synthetic Bone Grafts: An In Vivo Study in Beagle Dogs. *Materials* **2019**, *12*, 3168. [CrossRef]

Disclaimer/Publisher's Note: The statements, opinions and data contained in all publications are solely those of the individual author(s) and contributor(s) and not of MDPI and/or the editor(s). MDPI and/or the editor(s) disclaim responsibility for any injury to people or property resulting from any ideas, methods, instructions or products referred to in the content.

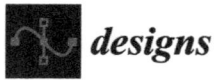

Article

About the Mechanical Strength of Calcium Phosphate Cement Scaffolds

Elisa Bertrand [1,2], Sergej Zankovic [1], Johannes Vinke [2], Hagen Schmal [1] and Michael Seidenstuecker [1,*]

[1] G.E.R.N. Center of Tissue Replacement, Regeneration & Neogenesis, Department of Orthopedics and Trauma Surgery, Medical Center-Albert-Ludwigs-University of Freiburg, Faculty of Medicine, Albert-Ludwigs-University of Freiburg, Hugstetter Straße 55, 79106 Freiburg, Germany; elisa.bertrand@uniklinik-freiburg.de (E.B.)

[2] Institute for Applied Biomechanics, Offenburg University, Badstraße 24, 77652 Offenburg, Germany

* Correspondence: michael.seidenstuecker@uniklinik-freiburg.de; Tel.: +49-761-270-26104

Abstract: For the treatment of bone defects, biodegradable, compressive biomaterials are needed as replacements that degrade as the bone regenerates. The problem with existing materials has either been their insufficient mechanical strength or the excessive differences in their elastic modulus, leading to stress shielding and eventual failure. In this study, the compressive strength of CPC ceramics (with a layer thickness of more than 12 layers) was compared with sintered β-TCP ceramics. It was assumed that as the number of layers increased, the mechanical strength of 3D-printed scaffolds would increase toward the value of sintered ceramics. In addition, the influence of the needle inner diameter on the mechanical strength was investigated. Circular scaffolds with 20, 25, 30, and 45 layers were 3D printed using a 3D bioplotter, solidified in a water-saturated atmosphere for 3 days, and then tested for compressive strength together with a β-TCP sintered ceramic using a Zwick universal testing machine. The 3D-printed scaffolds had a compressive strength of 41.56 ± 7.12 MPa, which was significantly higher than that of the sintered ceramic (24.16 ± 4.44 MPa). The 3D-printed scaffolds with round geometry reached or exceeded the upper limit of the compressive strength of cancellous bone toward substantia compacta. In addition, CPC scaffolds exhibited more bone-like compressibility than the comparable β-TCP sintered ceramic, demonstrating that the mechanical properties of CPC scaffolds are more similar to bone than sintered β-TCP ceramics.

Keywords: calciumphosphate cement; CPC; β-TCP; 3D printing; mechanical properties; sinter ceramics

Citation: Bertrand, E.; Zankovic, S.; Vinke, J.; Schmal, H.; Seidenstuecker, M. About the Mechanical Strength of Calcium Phosphate Cement Scaffolds. *Designs* 2023, 7, 87. https://doi.org/10.3390/designs7040087

Academic Editors: Mahdi Bodaghi and Richard Drevet

Received: 8 May 2023
Revised: 15 June 2023
Accepted: 28 June 2023
Published: 3 July 2023

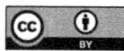

Copyright: © 2023 by the authors. Licensee MDPI, Basel, Switzerland. This article is an open access article distributed under the terms and conditions of the Creative Commons Attribution (CC BY) license (https://creativecommons.org/licenses/by/4.0/).

1. Introduction

Europe and the USA are in the midst of demographic change. The consequences of this are becoming more and more apparent every year [1,2]. In the EU, the average age continues to rise. One in five Europeans are already older than 65 [3]. In Germany, one in two are older than 45 and one in five are older than 66 [4]. In the US, the average age is 38.1 and, according to a study by the U.N. [5], the average age forecast is 43.1 years in 2050. As a result, age-related diseases such as those affecting the musculoskeletal system are continuing to increase in prevalence. For example, the implantation of a hip endoprosthesis is already the sixth most common surgical intervention in Germany [6]. With the increase in the prevalence of such surgeries, the demand for clinically approved bone replacement materials will also continue to grow. However, until now, many problems, e.g., with metallic implants, have been caused by the imbalance in the elasticity moduli between bone and the metals used. This thus results in so-called stress shielding (undesirable or too weak bone growth) [7]. Biodegradable biomaterials are a potential alternative whose support function decreases as the healing process progresses due to their eventual complete degradation, which allows the support function of the bone to eventually take over [8]. In the past, biodegradable calcium phosphate ceramics in particular have stood out due to these characteristics [9–11], especially because they have a similar composition to bone and can be degraded by the bone cells. However, in order for this degradation to function correctly, it is necessary to have sufficient porosity [12]. Both hydroxyapatite (HA) and beta tricalcium phosphate (β-TCP) are suitable for these applications—HA because it is the same material as in bone, and β-TCP because it is also a calcium phosphate like HA but has better solubility [8]. However, there is still a large difference between CaP ceramics and bone, particularly in the fracture elongation of bones, which can be up to 1–2%, compared to ceramics, which break at best at 0.1% [13]. Moreover, the compressive strength and Young's modulus are in some cases (for ceramics) up to a factor of 10-foldgreater [14], which again raises the problem of stress shielding. Bone does not consist exclusively of HA, but rather of nano-crystalline HA platelets packed in collagen strands. Additionally, bone adapts to mechanical loads according to Wolff's law and becomes stronger in stressed areas [15], and no biomaterial has so far been able adapt to the changing forces that bone experiences.

In addition to these issues, ceramics partially shrink during the sintering process, sometimes by even up to 30% [16], which must be taken into account for a precisely fitting shape, e.g., for filling defects in the bone. It is easier to create implants from a larger ceramic block directly on site in the operating room based on the bone defect. It also makes sense to use artificial substitute materials in view of an increasingly aging population, due to the limited availability of natural grafts. Additive manufacturing processes in particular have enormous potential, especially for individual patient care. For example, if bone material is missing after a fracture or after the removal due to infection, this individual lesion can be converted into a digital 3D construct (CAD) using clinical imaging techniques (CT, MRI) [17]. This 3D model of the damaged bone can then be used to produce a bone substitute [18], e.g., by milling it from a sinter ceramic block (HA or β-TCP) or by 3D printing. This bone substitute can then be perfectly adapted to the individual case and can ensure mechanical stability, and can thus take over the function of the damaged bone during the healing period. Additive manufacturing also offers a great opportunity for patient-specific replacement. These replacements can be custom-made from calcium phosphate cement (CPC) using 3D printing [19]. This also has the advantage of being a biodegradable ceramic [19,20], which can be broken down by the body. Ideally, once it has done its job and the bone has healed, it is completely degraded. This eliminates the need for a second surgery to remove the structure, with all of the associated risks. To enable even faster healing and new bone formation, additives such as growth factors and/or antibiotics [21–23] can also be incorporated into the cement. Commercially available CPC especially for injection at defect sites in the bone or for 3D printing do not set until they come into contact with water. For this purpose, an oil phase is usually dispersed, which escapes during the imaging reaction and can be absorbed by the body [20]. As with other cements, the setting reaction with water takes time [24]. During this period, the CPC scaffolds cannot be mechanically loaded. Importantly, printed CPC scaffolds could serve as a support and guidance structure during the bone healing process. In addition, the surface of the printed CPC scaffold plays an important role in regeneration [25]. In this work, both systems, namely sintered ceramics and 3D-printed CPC scaffolds, were to be compared with regard to their mechanical properties [22,26] to determine if 3D-printed scaffolds exhibited similar mechanical properties to bone. To achieve this, we first focused on 3D printing more than 12 layers [27–29] so that we could produce comparably sized specimens. The working hypotheses were that (1) as the number of layers increased, the mechanical strength of the 3D-printed CPC scaffolds would increase and (2) the internal needle diameter would influence the mechanical strength, which would better mimic the mechanical strength of the bone than what is possible with sintered ceramics.

2. Materials and Methods
2.1. Materials

Conical printer needles with 0.2 (article No.: 561751MA) and 0.25 (article No.: 561751MA) mm inner diameters were purchased from VIEWEG GmbH (Kranzberg, Germany). The CPC paste for printing (20 mL, article No.: 087-020-PL) was purchased from Innotere (Radebeul,

Germany). Phosphate buffered saline (PBS) (Thermo Fisher Scientific, Waltham, MA, USA) was purchased from ThermoFisher (article No.: 14190-094).

2.2. β-TCP Ceramics

The β-TCP ceramics used in this work were produced according to our specifications by the Robert Mathys Foundation (RMS) [11,22,23,30]. In this process, 20 g of tricalcium phosphate (Art. No. 102143, Merck, Switzerland) and 80 g of α-tricalcium phosphate (α-TCP; $Ca_3(PO_4)_2$) were mixed with a 60.0 ± 0.2 g solution of 0.2 M Na_2HPO_4 and 1% polyacrylic acid (Art. No. 81132, Fluka, Switzerland; Mw = 5.1 kDa). The paste was stirred intensively for 2.5 min and then transferred to a plastic syringe. The plastic syringe was 70 mm long and had a diameter of 23 mm. After 45 min, the paste was covered with 10 mL of PBS (part no. P5368, Sigma, USA), at pH 7.4, and incubated at a temperature of 60 °C for 3 days. The green bodies were then dried at the same temperature. Sintering was performed at 1250 °C for 4 h with a heating and cooling rate of 1 °C/min. The ceramic cylindrically shaped bodies were then cut to a diameter of 7 mm and a length of 25 mm. In a final step, the ceramic scaffolds were washed in an ethanol bath and calcined at 900 °C to burn away all abrasive particles and organic residues [31].

2.3. Three-Dimensional Printing

We used a 3D bioplotter (EnvisionTec, Gladbeck, Germany) with a low-temperature print head and conical needles made from polypropylene with inner diameters of 0.2 and 0.25 mm to print the round geometry that we developed. The CPC paste used was made by Innotere GmbH (Innotere, Radebeul, Germany). It consisted of synthetic calcium and phosphate salts finely dispersed in a biocompatible oil phase of short-chain triglycerides (caprycil/capric triglycerides) together with two further emulsifiers (polyoxyl-35-castor oil/cetyl phosphate). The triglycerides and the polyoxyl-35-castor oil (castor oil) were both based on pure raw vegetable materials [32].

2.3.1. Optimizing Printing Parameters

The parameters were referred to as optimized if the printed strand width was similar in width to the inner needle diameter of the needle used. In the present case, for an inner needle diameter of 0.20 mm, the desired strand width was 0.20 mm. The same then applied for an inner needle diameter of 0.25 mm. This was important so that the structure did not collapse. The geometry therefore needed to remain the same from layer to layer. To achieve this, the printing parameters were varied. The printing parameters were:

- The pressure (bar);
- The printing speed (mm/s);
- The needle offset (mm);
- The post-flow (s);
- The pre-flow (s).

The 3D printing parameters determined the way the material was printed. They had a special influence on the width of the printed strands. Thus, the first task was to determine the optimal printing parameters. In a previous work, these printing parameters were determined using the "Parameter Tuning" of the "Visual Machines" software [28]. For this purpose, several lines were printed where pressure and speed were varied. However, it was found that the measured widths depended on the printed shape (e.g., circle) and did not correspond in comparison to the printed line using the "Parameter Tuning" function. That is, the printed shapes also played a role in the actual printed strand width. So, to find the optimal printing parameters for the CAD model (see Figure 1), single-layer samples of the CAD model were printed, varying the printing parameters. The pre-flow was kept at 0.15 s. The scaffolds were printed with conical needles (Vieweg GmbH, Kranzberg, Germany) with a diameter of 0.20 (Art. No.: 501611) and 0.25 mm (Art. No.: 501610).

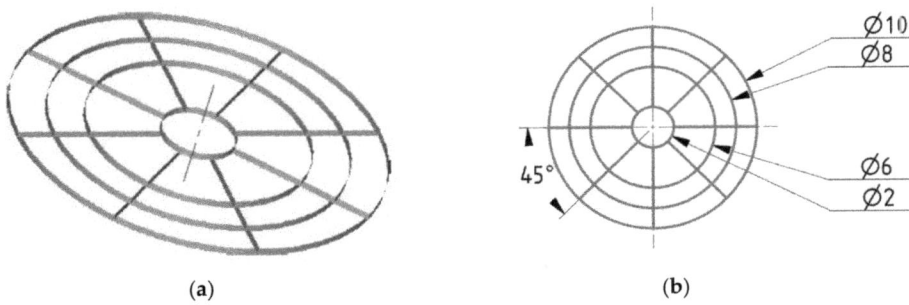

Figure 1. CAD model used for 3D printing; all values in mm; (**a**) 3D model; (**b**) model with dimensions.

2.3.2. Printing the Round Geometries with More Than 12 Layers

In previous works [33,34], cube-shaped geometries were printed using patterns from the Visual Machines software (EnvisionTec, Gladbeck, Germany). In one of our previous works [28], round structures with a layer rotation of 1° showed good results regarding mechanical strength, but were limited to 12 layers. In addition, there were printing errors such as delamination of the layers. The CPC paste itself probably caused this problem. This is because the CPC paste is not solid after printing, which means that the printed strands are not stable and are deformed by their own weight. To counteract this, water was sprayed onto the green body after a defined number of printed layers to add strength to the structure. A preliminary test was conducted to determine when the water needed to be sprayed onto the green bodies and how much time was needed after that for the structure to be sufficiently strong for additional layers. Water was sprayed onto the green bodies every 7 layers for the samples printed with a needle with a 0.20 mm inner diameter and every 5 layers for those printed with a needle with an inner diameter of 0.25 mm (see Table 1). The scaffolds were set for 3 days at 37 °C according to Akkineni et al. [35] in an incubator in a water-saturated atmosphere. After this time, half of the printed scaffolds were additionally incubated in phosphate buffered saline (PBS) for 1 week with daily changes of the PBS.

Table 1. Three-dimensional printing parameters used.

Sample	Pressure (bar)	Printing Speed (mm/s)	Needle Offset (mm)	Post Flow (s)	Water Applied after Layer
020_20layers	1.0	4.5	0.16	0.0	7
020_25layers	1.0	4.5	0.16	0.0	7
020_30layers	1.0	4.0	0.16	0.0	7
020_45layers	1.0	4.0	0.16	0.0	7
025_20layers	0.9	5.2	0.22	−0.05	5
025_25layers	0.8	4.5	0.22	−0.05	5
025_30layers	0.9	4.3	0.22	−0.05	5
025_45layers	0.9	5.3	0.22	−0.05	5

020 = 0.20 mm; 025 = 0.25 mm inner diameter of the needle used.

2.4. Characterization of the Scaffolds: 3D-Printed and Sintered

The dimensions of all scaffolds (3D-printed and sintered) were measured with a digital caliper (Burg-Wächter, Wetter-Volmarstein, Germany). The surface roughness (center roughness) was characterized by means of 3D laser scanning microscopy (Keyence VK-X 200; Keyence, Osaka, Japan) at 200× and 400× magnification. For phase composition analysis, XRD (Bruker D8 Advance, Bruker Corp., Billerica, MA, USA) and ESEM (FEI Quanta 250 FEG, FEI, Hilsboro, OR, USA) with an EDX unit (Oxford Instruments, Abingdon, UK) were used. The measuring conditions of ESEM were 20 kV acceleration voltage, 115 Pa pressure and, for EDX, 10 kV, 5 min counting time (lifetime) and area scan. The measuring conditions of Bruker D8 Advance were as follows: Bragg–Brentano geometry, equipped with a Cu anode and secondary graphite monochromator, scintillation counter, 40 kV/40 mA,

1°2 theta/min, step size 0.02°2 theta. The following Rietveld refinement analysis of the XRD data was performed by using profex 4.3 (freeware, www.profex-xrd.org). The porosity of the β-TCP scaffolds was measured via mercury porosimetry Porotec 140/440 (Porotec GmbH, Hofheim, Germany). The overall porosity of the 3D-printed scaffolds was determined using image analysis with Gimp 2.10.34 (open-source image editor, gimp.org). The mechanical strength, compression modulus and maximum failure load of the different scaffolds were determined using a Zwick Z005 universal testing machine (Zwick/Roell, Ulm, Germany). For this purpose, a compression test was performed with a preload of 1 N applied to the scaffolds, and the maximum failure load was determined at a traverse speed of 1 mm/s in a displacement-controlled manner.

2.5. Statistics

All results are expressed as means ± standard deviations. Measured values were analyzed using one-way analysis of variance (ANOVA) with a significance level of $p < 0.05$. Origin 2022 Professional SR1 (OriginLab, Northampton, MA, USA) was used for all statistical analyses.

3. Results

3.1. Characterization of the Scaffolds

3.1.1. Dimensions

The results of the dimensions of the printed or sintered scaffolds, which were measured with the aid of a caliper gauge, are shown in Table 2. The scaffolds printed with 0.20 and 0.25 mm needles had a diameter of 10.5 ± 0.10 mm. The height varies (depending on the number of layers) from 3.4 to 9.5 ± 0.10 mm. No differences in height were observed between samples incubated for one week in PBS and the samples that were not incubated (please see Table 2 and Figure 2).

Table 2. Comparison of dimensions of the scaffolds (3D-printed and sintered).

Scaffold	Height (mm)	Diameter (mm)
020_20layer	3.4	10.5
020_20layer + PBS	3.4	10.5
020_25layer	4.3	10.5
020_25layer + PBS	4.3	10.5
020_30layer	5.0	10.5
020_30layer + PBS	5.0	10.5
020_45layer	7.5	10.5
020_45layer + PBS	7.5	10.5
025_20layer	4.4	10.5
025_20layer + PBS	4.4	10.5
025_25layer	5.3	10.5
025_25layer + PBS	5.3	10.5
025_30layer	6.4	10.5
025_30layer + PBS	6.4	10.5
025_45layer	9.5	10.5
025_45layer + PBS	9.5	10.5
Sinter ceramics	7	7

020 = 0.20 and 025 = 0.25 mm; +PBS = incubation in PBS for 1 week after 3 days in a water-saturated atmosphere.

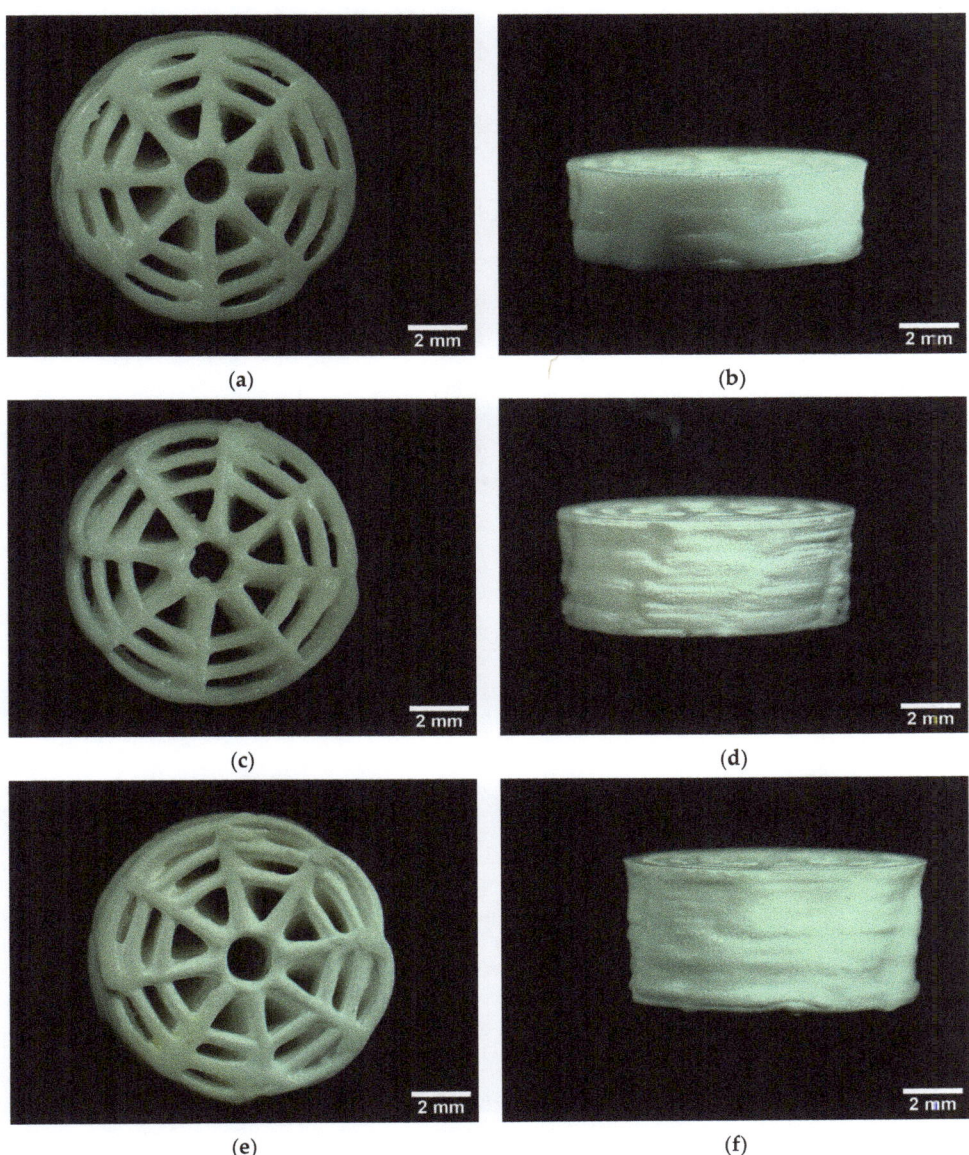

(a)

(b)

(c)

(d)

(e)

(f)

Figure 2. *Cont.*

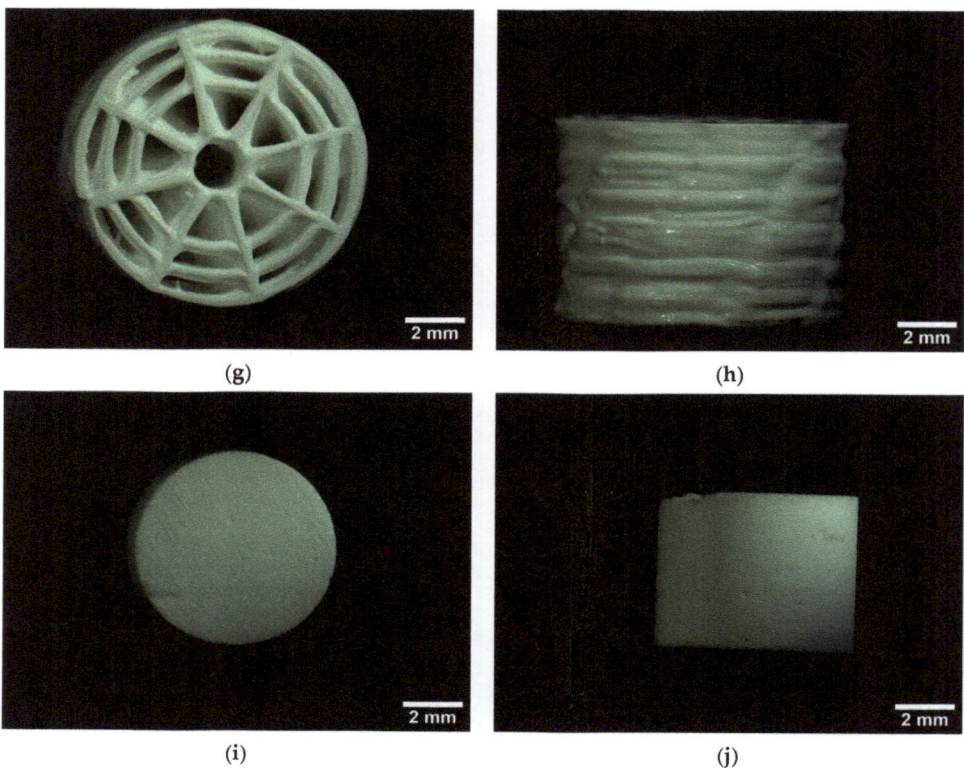

Figure 2. Top (left column) and side view (right column) of the scaffolds used; (**a,b**) 20 layers; (**c,d**) 25 layers; (**e,f**) 30 layers; (**g,h**) 45 layers; (**i,j**) sinter ceramics.

3.1.2. Strand Width and Surface Roughness (S_a)

The strand widths were measured by comparing scaffolds with and without post-consolidation in PBS. For the scaffolds printed with a 0.20 mm needle, the minimum strand width was 267.26 ± 31.83 μm (20 layers) and the maximum was 369.83 ± 32.16 μm (30 layers). There was no significant difference in strand width between the samples with and without PBS post-consolidation. For the scaffolds printed with 0.25 mm needles, the maximum was 475.50 ± 52.98 μm (20 layers) and the minimum was 331.95 ± 26.12 μm (45 layers). Just as for the scaffolds printed with 0.2 mm needles, no significant differences were found between the scaffolds printed with 0.25 mm needles with and without post-consolidation in PBS. In general, however, all strand widths are larger than the inner needle diameters of 0.2 mm and 0.25 mm, respectively (please see Figure 3).

The values of the measured surface roughness S_a for the scaffolds printed with 0.20 mm needles ranged from 4.42 ± 1.79 μm to 7.16 ± 1.76 μm. The samples with incubation in PBS showed a rougher surface. The surface roughness S_a measurements for the scaffolds printed with 0.25 mm needles showed mean values ranging from 4.15 ± 0.97 μm to 6.17 ± 1.55 μm. A comparison is shown in Figure 3.

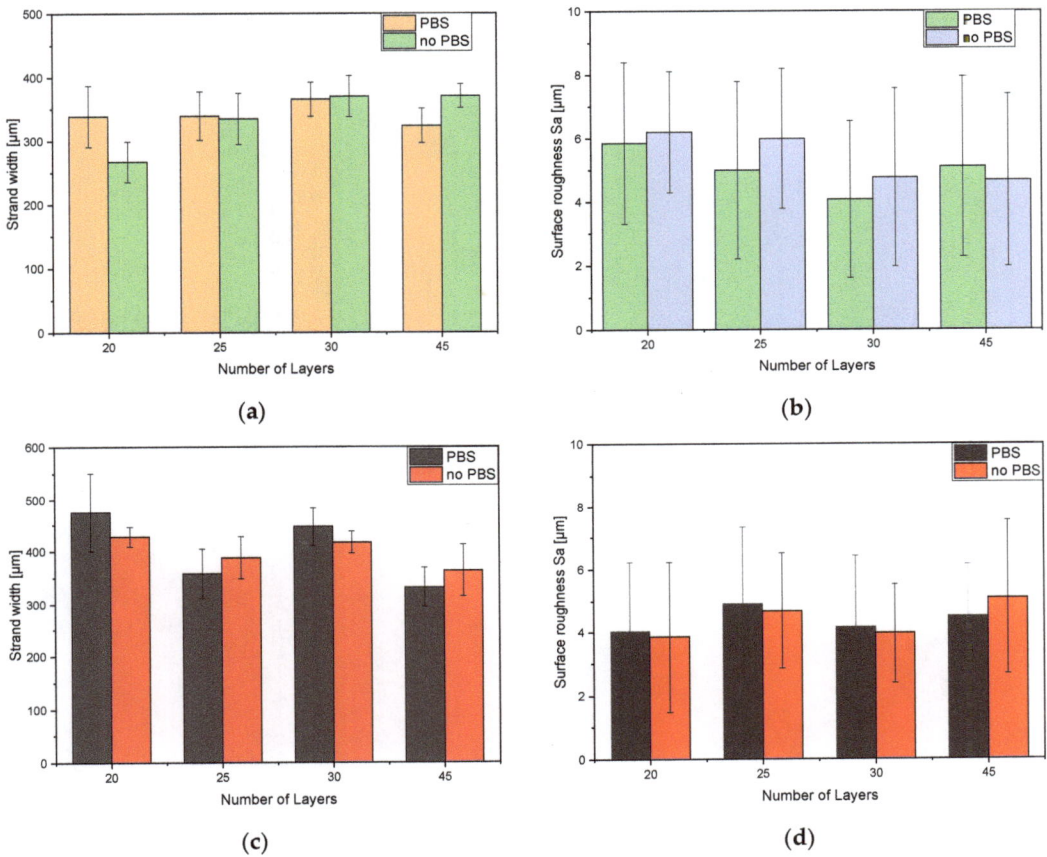

Figure 3. Overview of resulting strand width and surface roughness S_a by using a needle with a (**a**,**b**) 0.20 mm and (**c**,**d**) 0.25 mm inner diameter.

3.1.3. Phase Composition (EDX and XRD)

In the EDX investigation, a calcium phosphate ratio of 1.53 was determined for the sintered ceramic. This means that it is most likely β-TCP [8]. The additional XRD examination (compared to the β-TCP standard, and following Rietveld refinement analysis) confirmed this hypothesis (99.5% β-TCP and traces of CPP). Additional ESEM images of the 3D-printed scaffolds and sinter ceramics are shown in Figure A1. Phase composition analysis of the 3D-printed scaffolds using XRD with subsequent Rietveld refinement analysis revealed a composition of 9% calcium-deficient hydroxyapatite (CDHA), 46% hydroxyapatite (HA), 27% α-TCP and 18% dicalcium phosphate (DCPA). The XRD patterns of the scaffolds used are summarized in Figure 4. The Rietveld refinement analyses can be found in Figure A2 in the Appendix A.

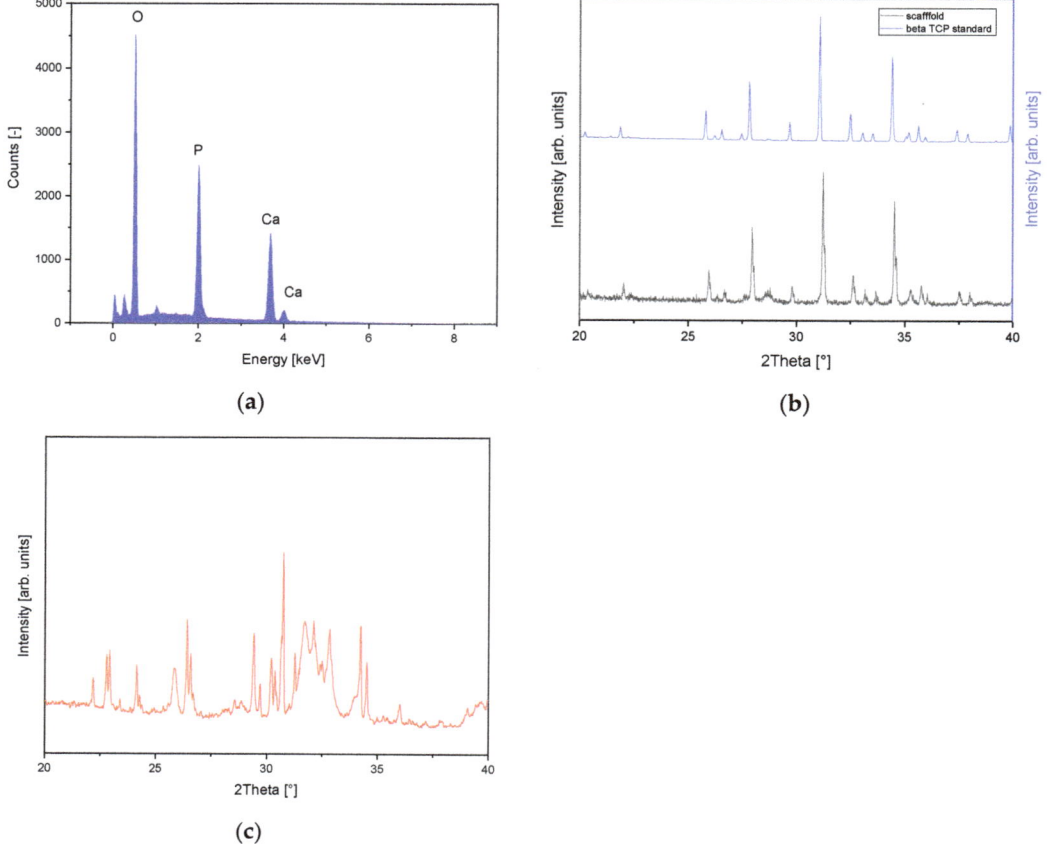

Figure 4. Elemental analysis and phase composition of the β-TCP sinter ceramics; (**a**) EDX spectrum; (**b**) XRD pattern in comparison to the β-TCP standard and (**c**) XRD pattern of the CPC after setting in a water-saturated atmosphere for 3 d. The EDX spectrum was obtained with an Oxford EDX unit for 5 min using the area scan mode, lifetime. The XRD patterns were obtained using Bruker D8 Advance—measurement conditions: 40 kV/40 mA, 1°2 theta/min, step size 0.02°2 theta.

3.1.4. Porosity

Our β-TCP ceramics had pore sizes in the range of 1–5 µm (orange bars in Figure 5a) and were very porous (see also the ESEM images in the Appendix A). The (weighted) pore size distribution was determined with the mercury porosimeters Pascal 140 and 440, as summarized in the following diagram in Figure 5 (purple curve—Pascal 140; red curve—Pascal 440). The average pore diameter was 4.2 ± 0.6 µm. The total porosity was determined with a value of 41.7 ± 2.1%. The total porosity of the 3D-printed scaffolds determined via image analysis was 38.8 ± 2.7%. No significant differences could be observed (see Figure 5b).

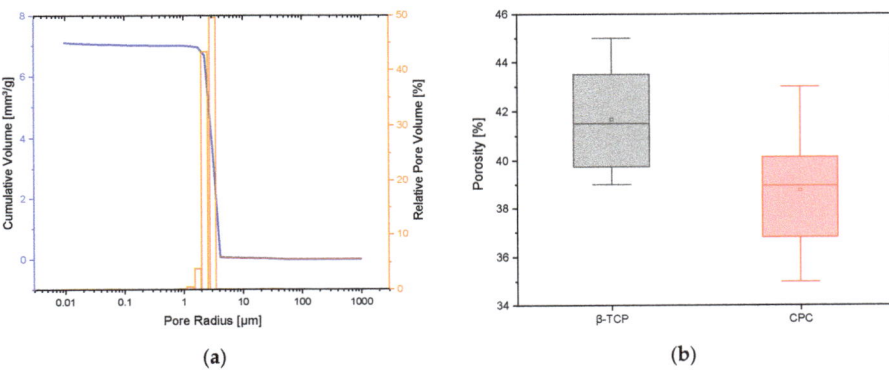

Figure 5. (**a**) Pore size distribution of the β-TCP ceramics determined using Pascal 140 (purple) and 440 (blue curve) mercury porosimeters; (**b**) boxplot of porosity of β-TCP vs. CPC, with no significant differences.

3.1.5. Mechanical Properties

The compressive strength values of the 3D-printed scaffolds ranged from 14.97 ± 1.08 MPa as a minimum to 41.6 ± 7.12 MPa as a maximum. With a few exceptions, there was no difference in the compressive strength of samples with post-incubation or no post-incubation in PBS. There was no significant difference in the compressive strength values of the sintered β-TCP ceramics between native samples or those incubated in PBS. The compressive strength of the sintered β-TCP ceramics was 24.16 ± 4.44 MPa, which was within the compressive strength range of the 3D-printed scaffolds and comparable to the values of the 3D-printed scaffolds with 20 and 25 layers (0.20 mm needle i.d.) with incubation in PBS and the scaffolds with 20, 25 and 30 layers (0.25 mm needle i.d.). Looking at the areas underlying the compressive strength of the 3D-printed scaffolds as well as the β-TCP ceramic, both had similar overall porosities, except for the fact that the pores were more contiguous in the 3D-printed scaffold than in the β-TCP ceramic. Figure 6 shows an overview of the different compressive strengths for the sintered ceramic and 3D-printed scaffolds. Table 3 shows the summary of the compressive moduli for the 3D-printed and sintered scaffolds. There were no significant differences between the samples post-cured in PBS and the samples that were not post-cured. However, a trend can be seen in the samples incubated in PBS where the compression modulus increases as the number of layers increases, while the compression modulus for the sintered ceramics is significantly higher than for the 3D-printed scaffolds.

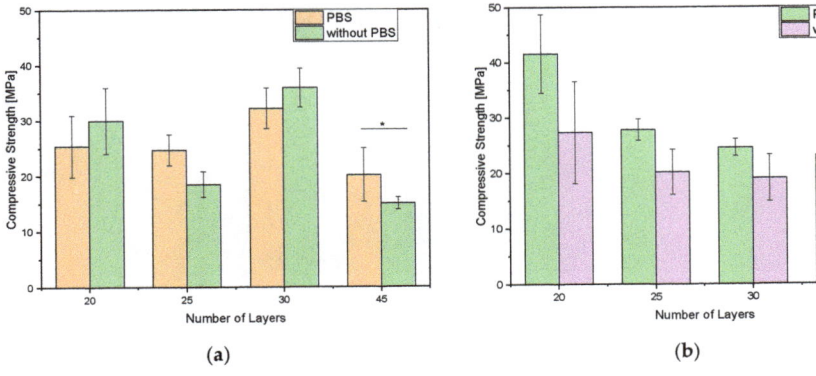

Figure 6. *Cont.*

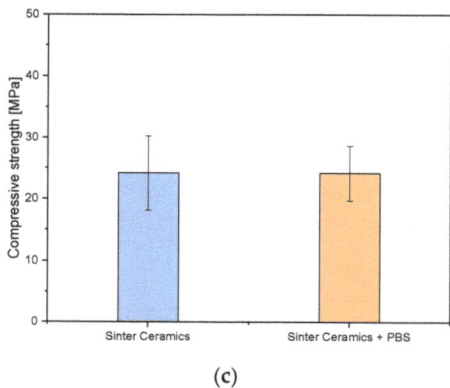

(c)

Figure 6. Comparison of compressive strength for 3D-printed scaffolds regarding needle inner diameter: (**a**) 0.20 mm; (**b**) 0.25 mm; (**c**) sinter ceramics. * $p < 0.05$.

Table 3. Overview of compression moduli for 3D-printed and sintered scaffolds.

Number of Layers	Compression Modulus [MPa]			
	0.20 mm Needle Inner Diameter		0.25 mm Needle Inner Diameter	
	PBS	No PBS	PBS	No PBS
20	5.65 ± 1.19	6.62 ± 0.89	7.87 ± 1.32	6.57 ± 1.93
25	7.46 ± 1.15	5.82 ± 1.25	9.47 ± 2.60	6.06 ± 1.81
30	9.72 ± 0.64	10.75 ± 0.81	8.47 ± 0.99	4.94 ± 1.94
45	10.13 ± 2.54	7.67 ± 0.79	13.42 ± 1.74	9.42 ± 2.84
β-TCP Ceramics	PBS		No PBS	
	50.9 ± 3.81		51.92 ± 4.13	

at $p < 0.05$, there were no significant differences between the PBS/no PBS groups.

Figure 7 shows an example of a CPC scaffold after mechanical testing. It can be seen that the upper outer rings up to the base ring have been blown off, whereas the central rings are still standing. This damage pattern is representative for all tested CPC scaffolds.

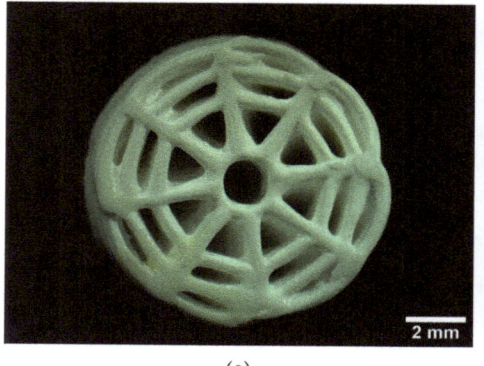
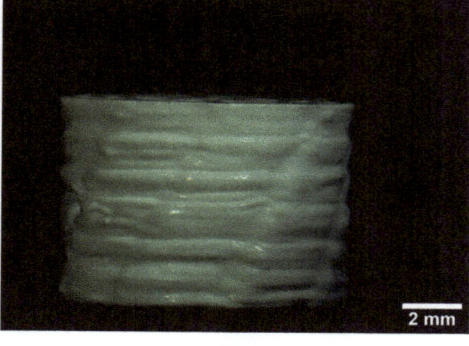

(**a**) (**b**)

Figure 7. *Cont.*

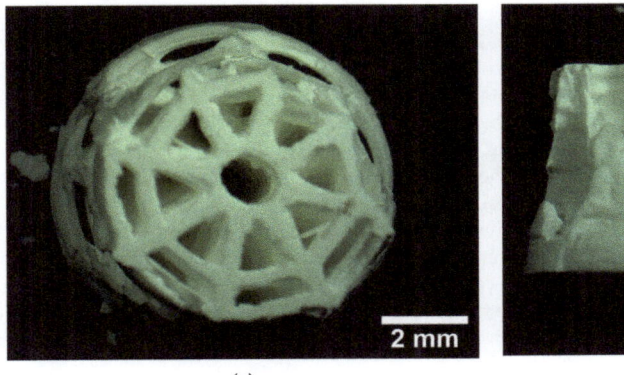
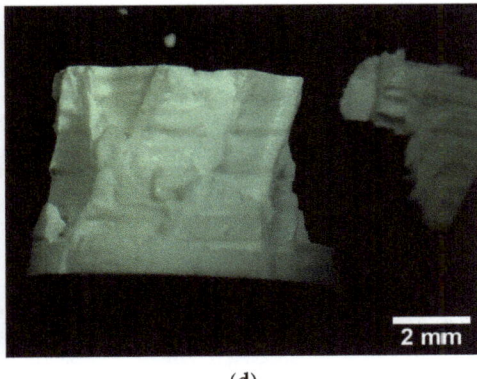

Figure 7. Fracture behavior of 3D-printed CPC scaffolds (**a**,**b**) before and (**c**,**d**) after mechanical tests.

4. Discussion

4.1. Strand Width and Surface Roughness S_a

The characterization of the samples with respect to the strand widths did not show any significant differences whether post-consolidation in PBS was performed after printing or not. This is due to the fact that water was sprayed every five to seven layers during 3D printing for intermediate consolidation of the green bodies in order to prevent the samples from slumping. In the work of Blankenburg et al. [28], only 12 layers of maximum height could be achieved before printing defects such as delamination occurred. By spraying with water, more than 12 layers could be printed. For time reasons, we limited ourselves to 45 layers, because after spraying with water, we waited 30 s before resuming the printing process. The fact that the strand widths were larger than the inner diameter of the needles is not surprising. This was due to the 3D plotting process, in which an overlay of the strands of 10–20% needs to be achieved to obtain the maximum strength of the construct. Raymond et al. [36] described a similar 3D plotting with 10% overlapping strands. As in Blankenburg et al. [28], there were no significant differences in the surface roughness of the scaffolds regardless of whether the samples were incubated in PBS or not. There were also no significant differences in surface roughness between the two needles with a 200 and 250 µm inner diameter.

4.2. Elemental Analysis EDX and XRD and Microstructure by ESEM

Elemental analysis using EDX (Ca/P ratio 1.53) and XRD (Rietveld refinement with profex 4.3) yielded 99% β-TCP, as observed in similar studies by our group followed by Rietveld refinement analysis. We have already performed similar verifications for the sinter ceramics in the past [22,37,38]. The Rietveld refinement analysis of the 3D-printed scaffolds resulted in a main phase of HA of about 46%, followed by 27% α-TCP, 18% DCPA and 9% CDHA. Fathi et al. [39] also describe the formation of a CDHA phase after their CPC was soaked for a week in water. Our ESEM images showed similar fractured surfaces as described by Fathi et al. [39]. The microstructure of the β-TCP is comparable with that previous published by Mayr et al. [40] or Bohner et al. [11].

4.3. Mechanical Properties

The compressive strength of the 3D-printed scaffolds increased with the number of layers for the scaffolds printed with an inner needle diameter of 0.20 mm to a maximum value of 35.86 ± 3.56 MPa at 30 layers. For the scaffolds printed with an inner needle diameter of 0.25 mm, the compressive strength decreased from 41.56 ± 7.12 MPa to 23.12 ± 1.71 MPa as the number of layers increased. From the preliminary tests and previous work [28], it was found that 3D printing with a larger inner needle diameter also increased the compressive strength. Looking at the results in Figure 6 for the 20-layer scaffold only, this assumption is correct. The compressive strength of the 20-layer scaffolds printed with a needle with an inner diameter of 0.25 mm was 39.1 ± 2.3% higher than that of the scaffolds printed with a needle with an inner diameter of 0.20 mm. Our working hypothesis was that, in addition, with an increasing number of layers, an increase in compressive strength would also be expected. Incubation in PBS led to a doubling of the compressive strength in the previous work [28], so we also incubated in PBS in this work. The increase in compressive strength was only noticeable in the scaffolds printed with a 0.25 mm needle inner diameter, at 27.9 ± 7.9%. Only two of four scaffolds showed an increase in compressive strength when printed with a 0.20 mm inner diameter needle. The reason for the deviation in compressive strength in terms of the number of layers is the formation of micro-cracks due to wetting with water during 3D printing. In addition, the bond between the wetted layers and the subsequent printed layer was not as strong as the bond between the non-wetted layers.

Nevertheless, the 3D-printed scaffolds were more compressive than the microporous β-TCP sintered ceramics, with a compressive strength of 24.16 ± 4.44 MPa. Similar values have already been determined in previous studies [22,30,40]. Miyamoto et al. [41] achieved a compressive strength of 4–10 MPa with their CPC scaffolds. Li et al. [42] also used round geometries, but unfortunately they did not perform mechanical tests. Additionally, Raymond et al. [36] only achieved values of 1–6 MPa with their 3D-printed CPC scaffolds depending on geometry. Similarly, Wu et al. [43] reached a compressive strength of 3.57 ± 0.12 MPa with their 3D-printed calcium silicate scaffolds. However, one must considering that the bone tissues for which the scaffolds are intended as a substitute during healing, namely cancellous and compact bone, have compressive strength values (in the upper range) of 6–45 MPa and 80–150 MPa, respectively [44]. Based on the work of other authors such as Olszta et al. [45], our 3D-printed scaffolds achieved values slightly above those for cancellous bone (2–20 MPa) and in the range between cancellous and compact bone [46].

Looking at compressibility (since we were limited to compression testing due to the scaffold geometry) rather than fracture elongation, the 3D-printed scaffolds were able to compress by 4–5% before total failure occurred (without first breaking out parts erupted from the scaffolds), whereas the β-TCP scaffolds broke after compression by only 0.05–0.1%. This is also reflected in the much lower compressive modulus values in Table 3. Thus, at least in terms of fracture elongation and compressibility, the 3D-printed scaffolds are in the range of bone [13].

4.4. Novelty Character and Limitations of the Present Study

Previous 3D printing experiments were limited to 12 layers [27,28] because otherwise the green body would deform under its own weight, which led to printing errors such as stringing, oozing or layer separation when printing more than 12 layers. Wu et al. [47] only studied CPC scaffolds at a 2 mm height. By spraying during printing after five to seven layers, it was possible to prevent the CPC from collapsing. This shows that future CPC scaffolds can be 3D printed as a bone substitute material of any height using the described technique. The limitation of this technique lies in the time factor. Three-dimensionally printing six scaffolds at the same time takes 1 min per layer and, with the breaks for spraying, this results in a pure printing time of 49 min for spraying after five layers and 48 min for spraying after seven layers. Of course, this problem could be circumvented by using a different CPC. However, slow-setting CPCs have not yet been described for 3D printing in the literature. This would also cause another problem: the printing parameters would vary over time as the setting process begins, and the results would no longer be reproducible.

5. Conclusions

In this work, we wanted to compensate for the disadvantages of sintered β-TCP ceramics, namely the fracture elongation, through 3D printing of comparable (external) geometries. We showed that CPCs' 3D printing could be improved so that more layers (above 12) can be printed. Thus, by spraying with water, we were able to print significantly more layers than in previous works [28]. This prevented the green body from collapsing under its own weight during 3D printing. The surface roughness was in a similar range and did not differ significantly from the conical printer wires used. While post-curing in PBS did not lead to a significant increase in the compressive strength as in previous works [28], importantly, thanks to the 3D printing geometry, we were able to double the compressive strength compared to sintered ceramics to achieve values similar to compact bone. Since we were limited to a compression test with our scaffolds, we could not measure fracture elongation, but rather the compressibility of the scaffolds. The 3D-printed scaffolds could be compressed by 4–6% to failure, whereas the β-TCP scaffolds failed after being compressed by 0.05–0.1%. Thus, the mechanical properties of 3D-printed CPC scaffolds are more similar to bone than the sintered β-TCP ceramics. This could be useful for the regeneration of bones in the musculoskeletal system where a load-bearing function is required during bone healing.

Author Contributions: Conceptualization, M.S. and J.V.; methodology, M.S.; software, S.Z.; validation, E.B., S.Z. and M.S.; formal analysis, E.B.; investigation, E.B.; resources, H.S.; data curation, S.Z. and M.S.; writing—original draft preparation, E.B. and M.S.; writing—review and editing, M.S.; visualization, S.Z.; supervision, M.S. and J.V.; project administration, M.S. and H.S.; funding acquisition, M.S.: All authors have read and agreed to the published version of the manuscript.

Funding: The article processing charge was funded by the Baden-Württemberg Ministry of Science, Research and Art and the University of Freiburg in the funding program Open Access Publishing.

Data Availability Statement: The data presented in this article are available on request from the corresponding author.

Acknowledgments: The authors would like to thank Melanie Lynn Hart for the spell check and grammar corrections.

Conflicts of Interest: The authors declare no conflict of interest.

Appendix A

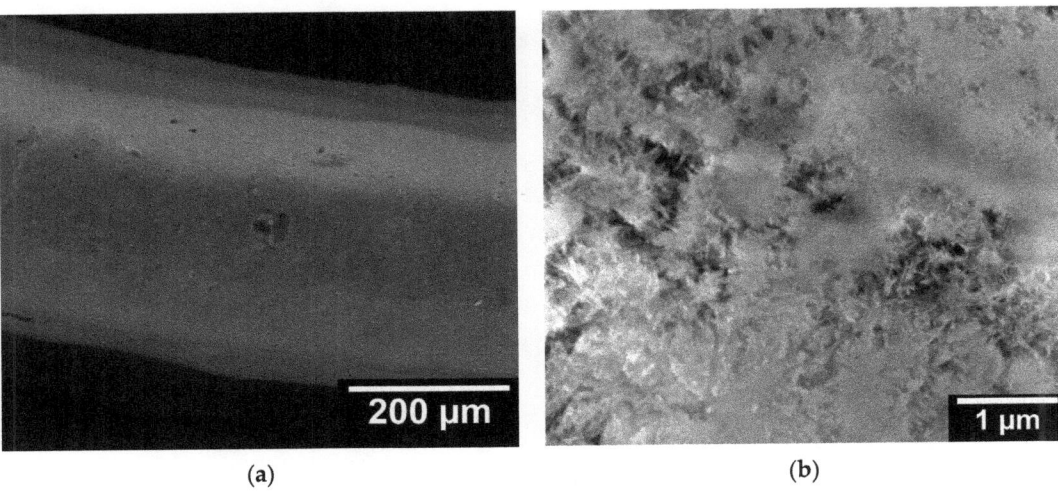

(a)   (b)

Figure A1. *Cont.*

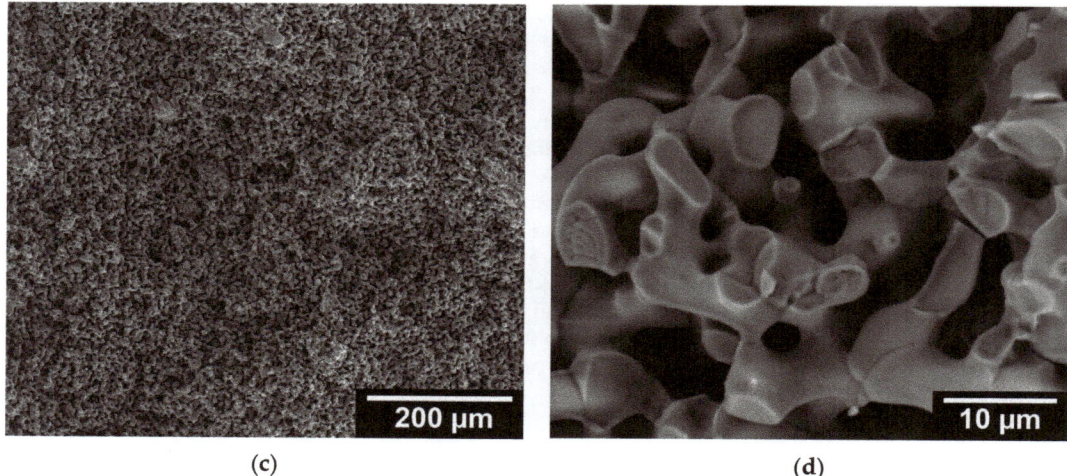

(c)   (d)

Figure A1. ESEM images of the (**a**,**b**) 3D-printed scaffolds and (**c**,**d**) sinter ceramics.

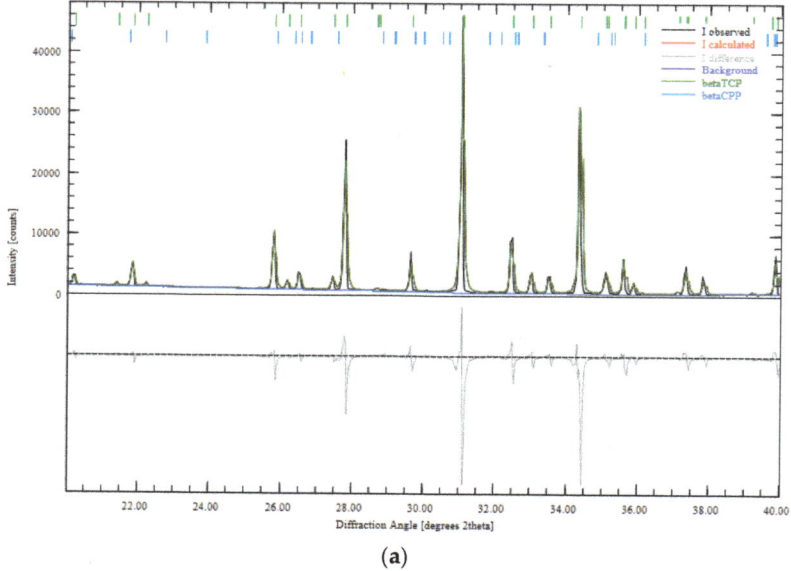

(a)

Figure A2. *Cont.*

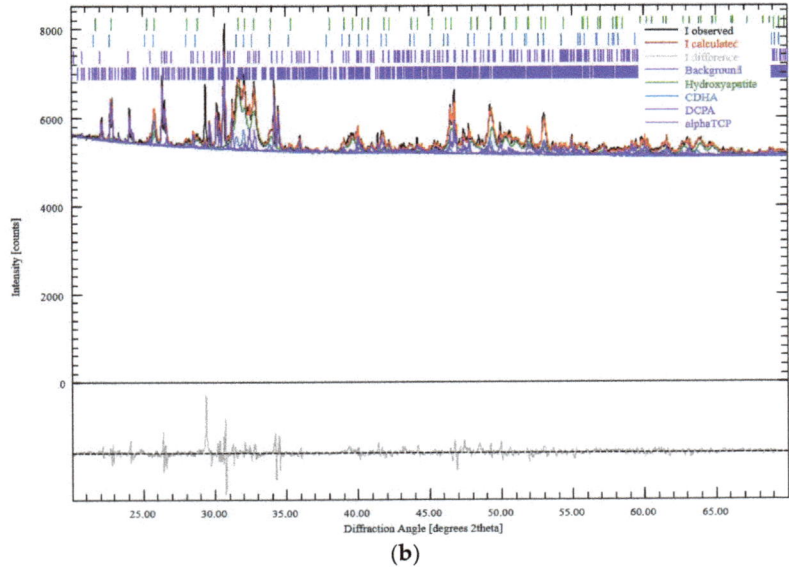

(b)

Figure A2. Rietveld refinement analysis of the XRD pattern of (**a**) β-TCP ceramics; (**b**) CPC (after 3d in water saturated atmosphere); pattern recorded using Bruker D8 Advance with a Cu Kα X-ray source.

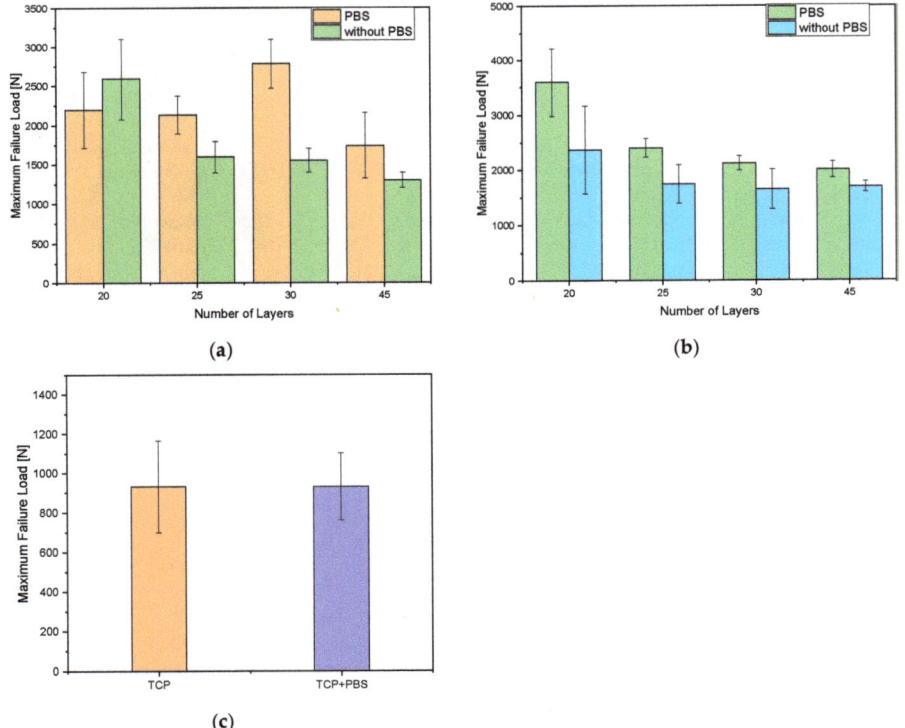

Figure A3. Maximum failure load for scaffolds 3D printed with a (**a**) 0.20 mm needle inner diameter, a (**b**) 0.25 mm needle inner diameter and (**c**) β-TCP sinter ceramics scaffolds.

References

1. Behrendt, H.; Runggaldier, K. [A problem outline on demographic change in the federal republic of germany]. *Notfall + Rettungsmedizin* **2009**, *12*, 45–50. [CrossRef]
2. Peters, E.; Pritzkuleit, R.; Beske, F.; Katalinic, A. Demografischer wandel und krankheitshäufigkeiten. *Bundesgesundheitsblatt Gesundheitsforschung Gesundheitsschutz* **2010**, *53*, 417–426. [CrossRef] [PubMed]
3. Eurostat. European Union: Age Structure in the Member States in 2019. Available online: https://de.statista.com/statistik/daten/studie/248981/umfrage/altersstruktur-in-den-eu-laendern/ (accessed on 25 March 2023).
4. Destatis. Mitten im Demografischen Wandel. Available online: https://www.destatis.de/DE/Themen/Querschnitt/Demografischer-Wandel/demografie-mitten-im-wandel.html (accessed on 2 September 2020).
5. U.N. World Population Prospects 2022. Available online: population.un.org (accessed on 20 February 2023).
6. Destatis. *Gesundheit—Fallpauschalenbezogene krankenhausstatistik (drg-statistik) operationen und prozeduren der vollstationären patientinnen und patienten in krankenhäusern (4-steller)*; Statistisches Bundesamt (Destatis): Wiesbaden, Germany, 2020.
7. Engh, C.A., Jr.; Young, A.M.; Engh, C.A., Sr.; Hopper, R.H., Jr. Clinical consequences of stress shielding after porous-coated total hip arthroplasty. *Clin. Orthop. Relat. Res.* **2003**, *417*, 157–163. [CrossRef] [PubMed]
8. Epple, M. *Biomaterialien und Biomineralisation, eine Einführung für Naturwissenschaftler, Mediziner und Ingenieure*; Teubner: Sonnewalde, Germany, 2003. [CrossRef]
9. Jarcho, M. Calcium phosphate ceramics as hard tissue prosthetics. *Clin. Orthop. Relat. Res.* **1981**, *157*, 259–278. [CrossRef]
10. Ducheyne, P.; Qiu, Q. Bioactive ceramics: The effect of surface reactivity on bone formation and bone cell function. *Biomaterials* **1999**, *20*, 2287–2303. [CrossRef]
11. Bohner, M.; van Lenthe, G.H.; Grünenfelder, S.; Hirsiger, W.; Evison, R.; Müller, R. Synthesis and characterization of porous-tricalcium phosphate blocks. *Biomaterials* **2005**, *26*, 6099–6105. [CrossRef]
12. Karageorgiou, V.; Kaplan, D. Porosity of 3d biomaterial scaffolds and osteogenesis. *Biomaterials* **2005**, *26*, 5474–5491. [CrossRef]
13. Jacob, H.A.C. Materialverhalten (knochen und implantatwerkstoffe) bei mechanischer beanspruchung. In *Orthopädie und Unfallchirurgie: Für Praxis, Klinik und Facharztprüfung*; Grifka, J., Kuster, M., Eds.; Springer: Berlin/Heidelberg, Germany, 2011; pp. 29–47. [CrossRef]
14. Akao, M.; Aoki, H.; Kato, K. Mechanical properties of sintered hydroxyapatite for prosthetic applications. *J. Mater. Sci.* **1981**, *16*, 809–812. [CrossRef]
15. Pearson, O.M.; Lieberman, D.E. The aging of wolff's "law": Ontogeny and responses to mechanical loading in cortical bone. *Yearb. Phys. Anthropol.* **2004**, *125*, 63–99. [CrossRef]
16. Tian, J.; Tian, J. Preparation of porous hydroxyapatite. *J. Mater. Sci.* **2001**, *36*, 3061–3066. [CrossRef]
17. Figliuzzi, M.; Mangano, F.; Mangano, C. A novel root analogue dental implant using ct scan and cad/cam: Selective laser melting technology. *Int. J. Oral Maxillofac. Surg.* **2012**, *41*, 858–862. [CrossRef]
18. Igawa, K.; Mochizuki, M.; Sugimori, O.; Shimizu, K.; Yamazawa, K.; Kawaguchi, H.; Nakamura, K.; Takato, T.; Nishimura, R.; Suzuki, S.; et al. Tailor-made tricalcium phosphate bone implant directly fabricated by a three-dimensional ink-jet printer. *J. Artif. Organs* **2006**, *9*, 234–240. [CrossRef]
19. Xu, H.H.K.; Wang, P.; Wang, L.; Bao, C.; Chen, Q.; Weir, M.D.; Chow, L.C.; Zhao, L.; Zhou, X.; Reynolds, M.A. Calcium phosphate cements for bone engineering and their biological properties. *Bone Res.* **2017**, *5*, 17056. [CrossRef]
20. Vorndran, E.; Geffers, M.; Ewald, A.; Lemm, M.; Nies, B.; Gbureck, U. Ready-to-use injectable calcium phosphate bone cement paste as drug carrier. *Acta Biomater.* **2013**, *9*, 9558–9567. [CrossRef]
21. Ghosh, S.; Wu, V.; Pernal, S.; Uskoković, V. Self-setting calcium phosphate cements with tunable antibiotic release rates for advanced antimicrobial applications. *ACS Appl. Mater. Interfaces* **2016**, *8*, 7691–7708. [CrossRef]
22. Seidenstuecker, M.; Ruehe, J.; Suedkamp, N.P.; Serr, A.; Wittmer, A.; Bohner, M.; Bernstein, A.; Mayr, H.O. Composite material consisting of microporous β-tcp ceramic and alginate for delayed release of antibiotics. *Acta Biomater.* **2017**, 433–446. [CrossRef]
23. Kuehling, T.; Schilling, P.; Bernstein, A.; Mayr, H.O.; Serr, A.; Wittmer, A.; Bohner, M.; Seidenstuecker, M. A human bone infection organ model for biomaterial research. *Acta Biomater.* **2022**, *144*, 230–241. [CrossRef]
24. Takagi, S.; Chow, L.C.; Hirayama, S.; Sugawara, A. Premixed calcium–phosphate cement pastes. *J. Biomed. Mater. Res. Part B Appl. Biomater.* **2003**, *67B*, 689–696. [CrossRef] [PubMed]
25. Lu, J.; Descamps, M.; Dejou, J.; Koubi, G.; Hardouin, P.; Lemaitre, J.; Proust, J.-P. The biodegradation mechanism of calcium phosphate biomaterials in bone. *J. Biomed. Mater. Res.* **2002**, *63*, 408–412. [CrossRef]
26. Seidenstuecker, M.; Mrestani, Y.; Neubert, R.H.H.; Bernstein, A.; Mayr, H.O. Release kinetics and antibacterial efficacy of microporous β-tcp coatings. *J. Nanomater.* **2013**, *2013*, 8. [CrossRef]
27. Huber, F.; Vollmer, D.; Vinke, J.; Riedel, B.; Zankovic, S.; Schmal, H.; Seidenstuecker, M. Influence of 3d printing parameters on the mechanical stability of pcl scaffolds and the proliferation behavior of bone cells. *Materials* **2022**, *15*, 2091. [CrossRef] [PubMed]
28. Blankenburg, J.; Vinke, J.; Riedel, B.; Zankovic, S.; Schmal, H.; Seidenstuecker, M. Alternative geometries for 3d bioprinting of calcium phosphate cement as bone substitute. *Biomedicines* **2022**, *10*, 3242. [CrossRef] [PubMed]
29. Egorov, A.; Riedel, B.; Vinke, J.; Schmal, H.; Thomann, R.; Thomann, Y.; Seidenstuecker, M. The mineralization of various 3d-printed pcl composites. *J. Funct. Biomater.* **2022**, *13*, 238. [CrossRef]

30. Seidenstuecker, M.; Schmeichel, T.; Ritschl, L.; Vinke, J.; Schilling, P.; Schmal, H.; Bernstein, A. Mechanical properties of the composite material consisting of β-tcp and alginate-di-aldehyde-gelatin hydrogel and its degradation behavior. *Materials* **2021**, *14*, 1303. [CrossRef]
31. Stahli, C.; Bohner, M.; Bashoor-Zadeh, M.; Doebelin, N.; Baroud, G. Aqueous impregnation of porous beta-tricalcium phosphate scaffolds. *Acta Biomater.* **2010**, *6*, 2760–2772. [CrossRef]
32. Khairoun, I.; Boltong, M.G.; Driessens, F.C.; Planell, J.A. Effect of calcium carbonate on clinical compliance of apatitic calcium phosphate bone cement. *J. Biomed. Mater. Res.* **1997**, *38*, 356–360. [CrossRef]
33. Seidenstuecker, M.; Schilling, P.; Ritschl, L.; Lange, S.; Schmal, H.; Bernstein, A.; Esslinger, S. Inverse 3d printing with variations of the strand width of the resulting scaffolds for bone replacement. *Materials* **2021**, *14*, 1964. [CrossRef]
34. Muallah, D.; Sembdner, P.; Holtzhausen, S.; Meissner, H.; Hutsky, A.; Ellmann, D.; Assmann, A.; Schulz, M.C.; Lauer, G.; Kroschwald, L.M. Adapting the pore size of individual, 3D-printed cpc scaffolds in maxillofacial surgery. *J. Clin. Med.* **2021**, *10*, 2654. [CrossRef]
35. Akkineni, A.R.; Luo, Y.; Schumacher, M.; Nies, B.; Lode, A.; Gelinsky, M. 3d plotting of growth factor loaded calcium phosphate cement scaffolds. *Acta Biomater.* **2015**, *27*, 264–274. [CrossRef]
36. Raymond, S.; Maazouz, Y.; Montufar, E.B.; Perez, R.A.; González, B.; Konka, J.; Kaiser, J.; Ginebra, M.-P. Accelerated hardening of nanotextured 3D-plotted self-setting calcium phosphate inks. *Acta Biomater.* **2018**, *75*, 451–462. [CrossRef]
37. Seidenstuecker, M.; Kissling, S.; Ruehe, J.; Suedkamp, N.; Mayr, H.; Bernstein, A. Novel method for loading microporous ceramics bone grafts by using a directional flow. *J. Funct. Biomater.* **2015**, *6*, 1085. [CrossRef] [PubMed]
38. Bernstein, A.; Niemeyer, P.; Salzmann, G.; Südkamp, N.P.; Hube, R.; Klehm, J.; Menzel, M.; von Eisenhart-Rothe, R.; Bohner, M.; Görz, L.; et al. Microporous calcium phosphate ceramics as tissue engineering scaffolds for the repair of osteochondral defects: Histological results. *Acta Biomater.* **2013**, *9*, 7490–7505. [CrossRef] [PubMed]
39. Fathi, M.; Kholtei, A.; El Youbi, S.; Chafik El Idrissi, B. Setting properties of calcium phosphate bone cement. *Mater. Today Proc.* **2019**, *13*, 876–881. [CrossRef]
40. Mayr, H.O.; Klehm, J.; Schwan, S.; Hube, R.; Sudkamp, N.P.; Niemeyer, P.; Salzmann, G.; von Eisenhardt-Rothe, R.; Heilmann, A.; Bohner, M.; et al. Microporous calcium phosphate ceramics as tissue engineering scaffolds for the repair of osteochondral defects: Biomechanical results. *Acta Biomater.* **2013**, *9*, 4845–4855. [CrossRef]
41. Miyamoto, Y.; Ishikawa, K.; Fukao, H.; Sawada, M.; Nagayama, M.; Kon, M.; Asaoka, K. In vivo setting behaviour of fast-setting calcium phosphate cement. *Biomaterials* **1995**, *16*, 855–860. [CrossRef]
42. Li, C.; Jiang, C.; Deng, Y.; Li, T.; Li, N.; Peng, M.; Wang, J. RhBMP-2 loaded 3D-printed mesoporous silica/calcium phosphate cement porous scaffolds with enhanced vascularization and osteogenesis properties. *Sci. Rep.* **2017**, *7*, 41331. [CrossRef]
43. Wu, C.; Fan, W.; Zhou, Y.; Luo, Y.; Gelinsky, M.; Chang, J.; Xiao, Y. 3D-printing of highly uniform CaSiO$_3$ ceramic scaffolds: Preparation, characterization and in vivo osteogenesis. *J. Mater. Chem.* **2012**, *22*, 12288–12295. [CrossRef]
44. Richard, H.A.; Kullmer, G. Biomechanik—Definitionen, aufgaben und fragestellungen. In *Biomechanik: Anwendungen Mechanischer Prinzipien auf den Menschlichen Bewegungsapparat*; Richard, H.A., Kullmer, G., Eds.; Springer Fachmedien Wiesbaden: Wiesbaden, Germany, 2020; pp. 1–14. [CrossRef]
45. Olszta, M.J.; Cheng, X.; Jee, S.S.; Kumar, R.; Kim, Y.-Y.; Kaufman, M.J.; Douglas, E.P.; Gower, L.B. Bone structure and formation: A new perspective. *Mater. Sci. Eng. R Rep.* **2007**, *58*, 77–116. [CrossRef]
46. Kaur, G.; Kumar, V.; Baino, F.; Mauro, J.C.; Pickrell, G.; Evans, I.; Bretcanu, O. Mechanical properties of bioactive glasses, ceramics, glass-ceramics and composites: State-of-the-art review and future challenges. *Mater. Sci. Eng. C* **2019**, *104*, 109895. [CrossRef]
47. Wu, Y.; Woodbine, L.; Carr, A.M.; Pillai, A.R.; Nokhodchi, A.; Maniruzzaman, M. 3D printed calcium phosphate cement (cpc) scaffolds for anti-cancer drug delivery. *Pharmaceutics* **2020**, *12*, 1077. [CrossRef]

Disclaimer/Publisher's Note: The statements, opinions and data contained in all publications are solely those of the individual author(s) and contributor(s) and not of MDPI and/or the editor(s). MDPI and/or the editor(s) disclaim responsibility for any injury to people or property resulting from any ideas, methods, instructions or products referred to in the content.

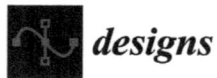

Article

3D Printed Voronoi Structures Inspired by *Paracentrotus lividus* Shells

Alexandros Efstathiadis [1], Ioanna Symeonidou [1], Konstantinos Tsongas [2], Emmanouil K. Tzimtzimis [3] and Dimitrios Tzetzis [3,*]

[1] Department of Architecture, University of Thessaly, 38334 Volos, Greece; alexef@uth.gr (A.E.); symeonidou@uth.gr (I.S.)
[2] Department of Industrial Engineering and Management, School of Engineering, International Hellenic University, 57001 Thessaloniki, Greece; k.tsongas@ihu.edu.gr
[3] Digital Manufacturing and Materials Characterization Laboratory, School of Science and Technology, International Hellenic University, 57001 Thermi, Greece
* Correspondence: d.tzetzis@ihu.edu.gr

Abstract: The present paper investigates the mechanical behavior of a biomimetic Voronoi structure, inspired by the microstructure of the shell of the sea urchin *Paracentrotus lividus*, with its characteristic topological attributes constituting the technical evaluation stage of a novel biomimetic design strategy. A parametric design algorithm was used as a basis to generate design permutations with gradually increasing rod thickness, node count, and model smoothness, geometric parameters that define a Voronoi structure and increase its relative density as they are enhanced. Physical PLA specimens were manufactured with a fused filament fabrication (FFF) printer and subjected to quasi-static loading. Finite element analysis (FEA) was conducted in order to verify the experimental results. A minor discrepancy between the relative density of the designed and printed models was calculated. The tests revealed that the compressive behavior of the structure consists of an elastic region followed by a smooth plateau region and, finally, by the densification zone. The yield strength, compressive modulus, and plateau stress of the structure are improved as the specific geometric parameters are enhanced. The same trend is observed in the energy absorption capabilities of the structure while a reverse one characterizes the densification strain of the specimens. A second-degree polynomial relation is also identified between the modulus, plateau stress, and energy capacity when plotted against the relative density of the specimens. Distinct Voronoi morphologies can be acquired with similar mechanical characteristics, depending on the design requirements and application. Potential applications include lightweight structural materials and protective gear and accessories.

Keywords: biomimicry; strategy; Voronoi; 3D printing; mechanical behavior; compression; finite element analysis; FEM

1. Introduction

Cellular structures can be commonly found in nature and have been observed in bones, seashells, and the plant kingdom [1–3]. Such structures are a product of billions of years of natural evolution and manage to achieve exceptional mechanical properties while maintaining low weight and minimal usage of material and energy [4], traits that are vital for the survival of organisms in nature. More specifically, the shell of the sea urchin *Paracentrotus lividus* has been shown, under scanning electron microscope (SEM) analysis, to be comprised of a porous structure known as the stereom which resembles a foam, as illustrated in Figure 1 [5]. The porous calcite shell provides the urchin with the necessary toughness and impact resistance to protect itself from environmental threats and predators [6–8].

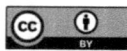

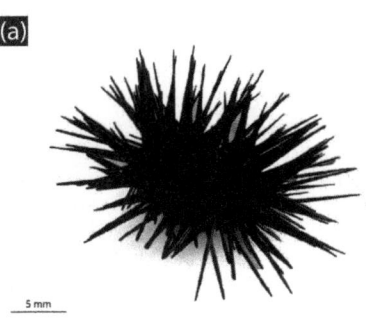
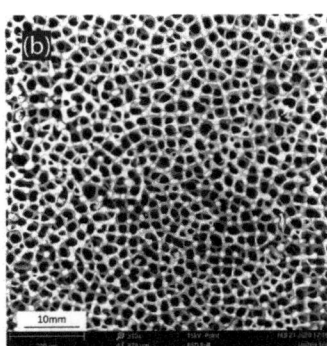

Figure 1. (**a**) A fresh sample of the sea urchin *Paracentrotus lividus*; (**b**) the porous structure of its shell.

Cellular structures have a variety of cells shapes and can generally be categorized as honeycombs [9], closed- or open-cell foams [10], and lattice formations with regularly arranged cells like gyroid [11], truncated cuboctahedron [12], and octet-truss [13] lattices. The natural formation of the urchin's stereom closely resembles the geometric formation of a 3D Voronoi diagram [14]. As a result, Voronoi diagrams have been employed for the design and fabrication of biomimetic porous structures and materials [1,15]. Traditional fabrication techniques include gas injection in melts [16], the co-expansion method of powders, and blowing agents mixtures [17], or foaming by gases produced through a reduction reaction [18], and are mainly used to produce polymer and metal foams [19–21]. Such structures have found application as energy absorption parts in the aeronautic and automotive industries [22], insulators [23], automotive catalysts [24], and in medical applications like orthopedic implants [19,25]. Nevertheless, the above construction techniques have held back the accuracy, the complexity, and the reproducibility of such structures [10,26]. Advancements in 3D printing technologies make it possible to overcome these obstacles and fabricate intricate porous materials efficiently, with high precision and control over their geometry, in a large variety of advanced materials [27–31].

Another constraint for the design and fabrication of cellular structures and materials has been the available Computer Aided Design (CAD) software. Until recently, researchers have generally been limited to simplistic Voronoi design techniques with limited control over the model's geometric parameters and have relied on the overall relative density of the structure as a characterization basis [32–34]. Although relative density has been proven to play an important role in the mechanical performance of such topologies [35,36], several geometric characteristics can alter a sample's relative density [15,17,37]. Progress in algorithmic, parametric design enables designers, nowadays, to create fully customizable algorithms containing several interactive parameters that can control a wide range of the geometric attributes of the cellular structure while requiring little computational power [38–40]. As a result, new approaches to the study and mechanical characterization of such morphologies can be explored based on their topological design.

The present paper aims to examine the technical evaluation of a biomimetic Voronoi structure inspired by the porous microstructure of the stereom of the sea urchin *Paracentrotus lividus* as part of the development of a novel strategy for biomimetic design. More specifically, the goal of the study is to investigate the mechanical performance of the structure in relation to its characteristic geometric properties. A parametric algorithm was implemented for the emulation of the biological structure. The biomimetic digital model was taken as the basis for the generation of a series of models with variable design parameters. The node count, the rod radius, and the smoothness of the geometry were modified, and physical specimens were printed in a fused filament fabrication (FFF) 3D printer. The mechanical properties and fracture behavior of the structure were examined experimentally under quasi-static compression loading and finite element analysis (FEA) was carried out to validate the results.

2. Materials and Methods

2.1. Biomimetic Design Strategy

A novel biomimetic design strategy that was developed as part of the present research serves as a guideline for the technical evaluation of the Voronoi structure inspired by *Paracentrotus lividus* shell microstructure. The strategy consists of three separate stages: "Research and Analysis", followed by "Abstraction and Emulation", and concluded with the "Technical Evaluation" phase. The workflow of the strategy is not linear, but instead consists of bi-directional feedback loops that inform and counter-inform the three stages as seen in Figure 2. More specifically the "Technical Evaluation" phase incorporates the prototyping of the structure with the aid of additive manufacturing technologies and the mechanical characterization through testing of the physical samples combined with finite element analysis (FEA). The printing process was informed by the topological intricacies of the structure while fabrication constraints counter-informed the design. Furthermore, the functional role of the biological structure informed the testing process and FEA.

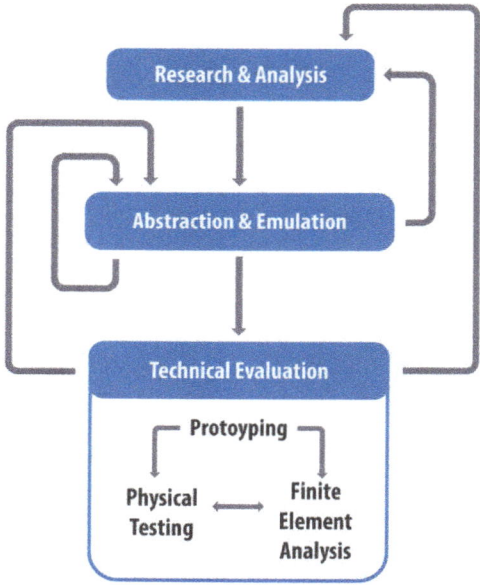

Figure 2. The stages "Research and Analysis", "Abstraction and Emulation", and "Technical Evaluation" of the novel biomimetic strategy are interconnected via bi-directional feedback loops. The Technical Evaluation stage consists of prototyping and mechanical characterization of the biomimetic model.

2.2. Design Parameters and 3D Printing

A parametric design algorithm, emulating the morphogenetic process of a 3D Voronoi diagram [5], was developed with the aid of the computer-aided design (CAD) software Rhinoceros 3D and Grasshopper 3D (v. Rhino 7, 7.1.20343.09491, Robert McNeel & Associates, Seattle, WA, USA) in a previous stage of this research. A custom set of points is created within a bounding geometry. Spheres are drawn around each point and are expanded at the same rate until they come into contact so that planar faces are created that form convex polyhedrons. Their edges are extracted, forming the rods of the Voronoi structure. A custom thickness can be applied to them with the aid of the plug-in Dendro (ECR Labs, Los Angeles, CA, USA). The same tool is used to smooth out the volume. The algorithm was further developed by applying a volume Boolean union between the original Voronoi volume and the volume that is derived after the smoothing process. This was deemed necessary to ensure constant rod thickness beyond the boundaries of the smoothing operation around the volume's nodes, which are the junction points of 2 or more rods. The updated definition is illustrated in Figure 3 as scripted in the Grasshopper environment.

A baseline model (Model 1) was established [5], with XYZ dimensions of 40 mm × 40 mm × 40 mm, node count of 60, rod radius 1.8 mm, and smoothness scale 1. Variations of this model were generated with successive changes in geometric parameters that define a 3D Voronoi structure and have significant impact on its relative density [14]. Initially, the node count was changed to 80 and then to 100. Afterwards, the rod radius was altered to 2 mm and 2.2 mm. Lastly, the smoothness was set to 4 and 7. All the geometric parameters of the models are shown in Table 1. The 3D printing of the specimens was conducted with a Creality Ender 3 Pro printer (Shenzhen Creality 3D Technology Co., Shenzhen, China) using a commercial PLA filament (NEEMA3D, Petroupolis, Greece). The slicing process was carried out on the Ultimaker Cura slicer (v.4.9.1, Ultimaker, Utrecht, The Netherlands). An outer wall speed of 15 mm/s was selected. The speed for inner walls and infill was set at 30 mm/s. The layer thickness was adjusted at 0.2 mm, as a compromise between quality and printing time which ranged from 6 to 7 h. A lines infill pattern was chosen along with 100% infill density. A 0.4 mm diameter nozzle was used which was heated to 205 °C, while the temperature of the build platform was set at 55 °C. No additional support structures were utilized. The complete printing parameters can be found in Table 2. The digital and the 3D printed models are illustrated in Figure 4.

Table 1. Geometric parameters of the printed and tested models.

Model	Node Count	Rod Radius (mm)	Smoothness Scale
1	60	1.8	1
2	60	2	1
3	60	2.2	1
4	80	1.8	1
5	100	1.8	1
6	60	1.8	4
7	60	1.8	7

Table 2. Printer parameters.

Printer Parameter	Value
Nozzle size	0.4 mm
Materials	PLA
Layer Thickness	0.2 mm
Wall Thickness	0.8 mm
Infill Pattern	Lines
Infill Density	100%
Outer Wall Speed	15 mm/s
Inner Wall Speed	30 mm/s
Infill Speed	30 mm/s
Printing Temp.	205 °C
Build Plate Temp.	55 °C
Support	No
Print Time	6–7 h

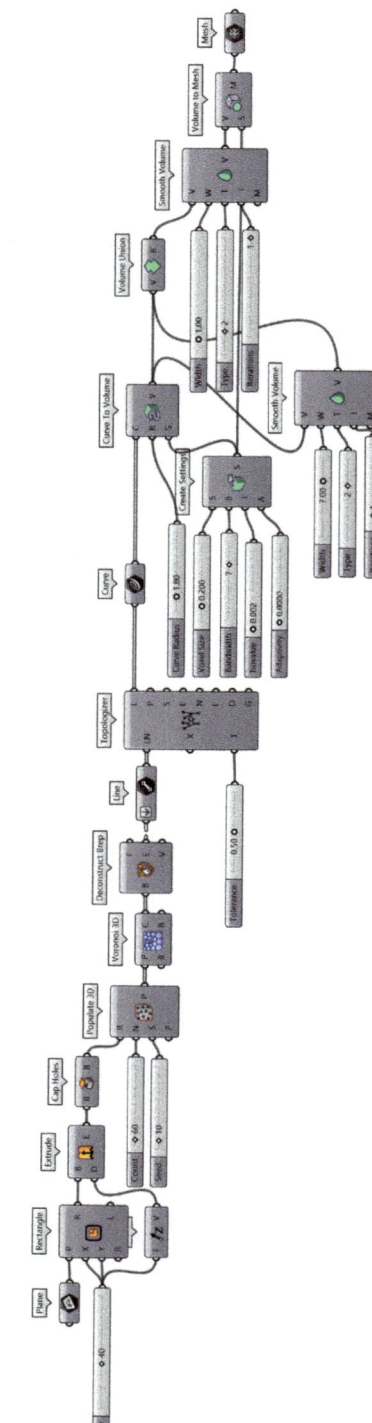

Figure 3. The updated definition in the Grasshopper environment. A volume Boolean union is added to ensure constant rod thickness.

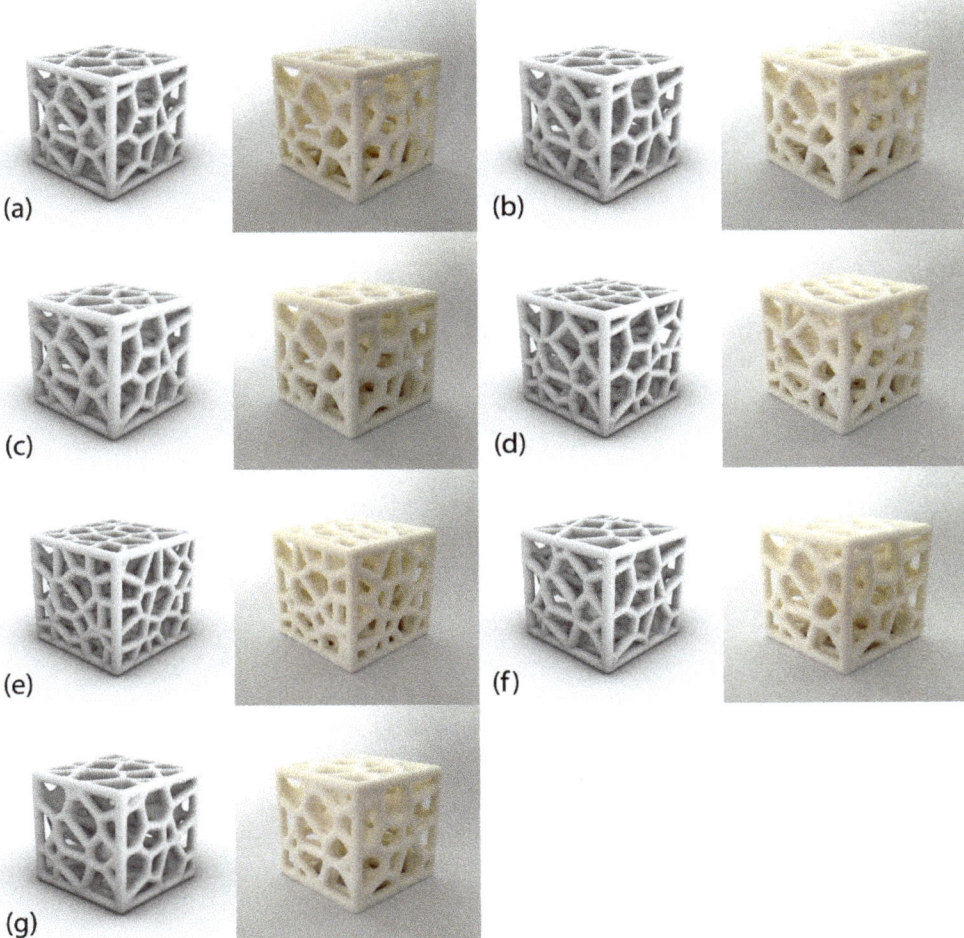

Figure 4. Designed and fabricated samples: (**a**) Model 1; (**b**) Model 2; (**c**) Model 3; (**d**) Model 4; (**e**) Model 5; (**f**) Model 6; and (**g**) Model 7.

2.3. Compression Testing Supported by FEA

Three specimens of each model were printed (for a total of 21) in order to derive a statistical model of the mechanical properties of the Voronoi structure. The compressive behavior of the printed samples was examined on a Testometric M500-50AT system (Testometric company, Rochdale, United Kingdom) and compression tests were conducted with a constant deformation rate of 5mm/min. The ANSYS™ software (Ansys® Academic Research Mechanical, Release 23.1, ANSYS, Inc., Canonsburg, PA, USA) was used to study the mechanical behavior of all the Voronoi lattice structures. An explicit dynamic analysis was conducted to accurately simulate the mechanical response of the lattices which was necessary to capture their large deformations and bi-linear material behavior.

A convergence study was performed to ensure a mesh-independent response, which showed that stress convergence was achieved with nearly 130,000 elements for each verification model. Specific density or relative density is defined as the ratio of the density of a porous material to that of the solid material from which it is made [41]. The porosity P (%) of each sample was determined according to the following equation [18]:

$$P = \left(1 - \frac{\rho}{\rho_s}\right) \times 100 \tag{1}$$

where ρ is the density of the Voronoi structure in g/cm^3 and ρ_s is the density of PLA (1.24 g/cm^3) [42]. Stress σ (MPa) was calculated as the ratio between force F (N) and the apparent cross-sectional area A (mm^2) of the specimens [43]:

$$\sigma = \frac{F}{A}, \tag{2}$$

Strain ε (%) was estimated as the percentage of the ratio between deflection L (mm) and initial height h (mm) of the samples [44]:

$$\varepsilon = \frac{L}{h} 100, \tag{3}$$

In order to calculate the energy absorption capacity of the biomimetic Voronoi structure, the densification strain ε_D must first be determined. Densification strain is the effective strain when the cells of the Voronoi structure have entirely collapsed, and further strain would compress the bulk PLA material. The densification strain ε_D of porous materials is derived based on its energy absorption efficiency [45], which is calculated with the following equation:

$$\eta(\varepsilon) = \frac{1}{\sigma(\varepsilon)} \int_0^\varepsilon \sigma(\varepsilon) d\varepsilon, \tag{4}$$

The densification strain ε_D is the strain that corresponds to the maximum value of the $\eta(\varepsilon)$ curve [32,45]. After this point, the stress increases rapidly, as the bulk material is compressed, resulting in a substantial drop in the efficiency of the structure [32]. A typical energy efficiency curve is illustrated in Figure 5 for Model 1 of the designed and fabricated specimens. The energy absorption efficiency η of the model is plotted against the strain ε. The value of strain corresponding to the maximum value of the efficiency curve is the densification strain ε_D of Model 1 [45].

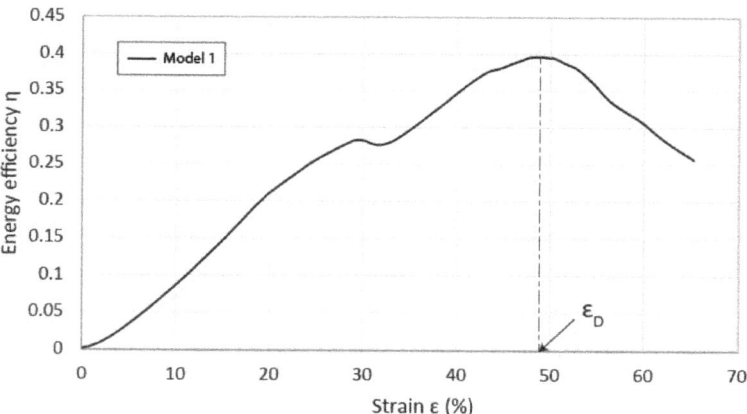

Figure 5. A typical energy efficiency curve $\eta(\varepsilon)$ for Model 1 of the biomimetic Voronoi structure and the respective densification strain.

The plateau stress σ_{pl} is a significant parameter used to assess the compressive performances of porous materials as it describes the plateau region of the stress–strain curve of cellular solids and is calculated by the following equation [46]:

$$\sigma_{pl} = \frac{1}{\varepsilon_D - \varepsilon_y} \int_{\varepsilon_D}^{\varepsilon_y} \sigma(\varepsilon) d\varepsilon, \tag{5}$$

where ε_y is the yield strain, which corresponds to the onset of plastic deformation.

Porous structures absorb energy at an almost constant load until the densification strain, when the load rapidly increases. Thus, the energy absorption capacity W_v (MJ/m^3) of the foams is estimated by the energy absorbed per unit of volume up to the densification strain ε_D. [45]:

$$W_v = \int_0^{\varepsilon_D} \sigma(\varepsilon), \tag{6}$$

And the specific energy absorption W_m (KJ/kg) as the energy absorbed per unit of mass [47]:

$$W_m = \frac{W_v}{\rho} \tag{7}$$

3. Results and Discussion

3.1. Characterization of the Biomimetic Voronoi Structure

In order to examine the mechanical response of the biomimetic Voronoi structures, it is necessary to first evaluate the impact of the changes in the geometric parameters of the structure on the overall relative density of the designed unit cells. It is also important to determine and compare the relative density of the 3D printed samples in relation to the designed ones and identify potential discrepancies. In Table 3, the designed relative density of the digital models is compared to the calculated values of the 3D printed physical models. First of all, it becomes obvious that the relative density of the structure can be increased either by increasing the thickness of the rods, or by raising the number of total nodes or by smoothing the geometry, as more material is added to it. More specifically, the relative density of the baseline Model 1 is 0.44 for the digital model and 0.4 ± 0.004 for the printed one, a discrepancy of 9.09%. In Models 2 and 3, the designed relative density is raised to 0.52 and 0.61, respectively, as the thickness of the rods is also raised to 2 mm and 2.2 mm. The calculated relative density of Model 2 is 0.48 ± 0.005, a difference of 7.69% and relative density of Model 3 is 0.56 ± 0.005, a difference of 8.2%. In Models 4 and 5, as the nodes are increased to 80 and 100, so increases the designed relative density to 0.53 and 0.60. Once again, a discrepancy of 7.55% and 8.33% can be observed in the calculated values which were determined to be 0.49 ± 0.03 and 0.55 ± 0.03, respectively. The designed relative density of Model 6 (smoothness 4) is 0.46 and the relative density of Model 7 (smoothness 7) is 0.5. The value for the printed Model 6 is 0.42 ± 0.08, a deviation of 8.7% and for the printed Model 7 is 0.46 ± 0.02, a discrepancy of 8%. It becomes evident that the difference in relative density between the digital and physical models is consistent among all specimens, a trend that can be attributed to limitations of the fused filament fabrication technology [48].

3.2. Compression Results of the Biomimetic Voronoi Structures

3.2.1. Compressive Behavior, Strength, and Modulus

The compression tests of the biomimetic Voronoi structure reveal a repeated behavior across all specimens which can be distinguished into three separate zones. The first is the elastic zone where the stress increases linearly. It is followed by a long plateau region where the rods of the structure progressively buckle and collapse while absorbing energy up until the densification strain. At this point, all the cells of the Voronoi have completely collapsed and the densification portion begins which is characterized by a sharp increase in stress as the bulk material is compressed. Figure 6 shows frames of the samples during compression. The second and third column of frames document the gradual failure of the rods in the plateau region. The failure mechanism of the rods can be traced to buckling and layer delamination, as shown in Figure 7, a behavior that is characteristic to 3D printed structures [17,32]. The fourth frames column highlights the fully compacted cells at the onset of the densification zone. It becomes evident that a recurring trend emerges across all models despite their geometric discrepancies that is in agreement with the typical mechanical behavior of porous structures as documented in relevant literature [17,32,34].

Table 3. Designed relative density of the models compared to the calculated values of the 3D printed specimens.

Model	Designed Relative Density	Calculated Relative Density	Discrepancy (%)
1	0.44	0.40 ± 0.004	9.09
2	0.52	0.48 ± 0.005	7.69
3	0.61	0.56 ± 0.005	8.2
4	0.53	0.49 ± 0.03	7.55
5	0.6	0.55 ± 0.03	8.33
6	0.46	0.42 ± 0.08	8.7
7	0.5	0.46 ± 0.02	8

The above behavior can also be observed in the stress–strain curves of the models in Figure 8. The curves can be generally considered smooth, with minimal oscillations since the rods compact without fracturing catastrophically. Table 4 shows the mechanical properties of the biomimetic Voronoi models as calculated based on the data derived from the stress–strain curves. Several trends can be identified. As the thickness of the rods increase in Models 2 and 3, so does the strength of the structure. More specifically, the yield strength, σ_y, of Model 1 (baseline) is 6.26 ± 0.12 MPa, 8.80 ± 0.12 MPa for Model 2, and 10.84 ± 0.10 MPa for Model 3. The compressive modulus E of the porous structure is also improved as the rods become thicker. Model 1 has a compressive modulus of 310.29 ± 15.38 MPa, Model 2 has 443.64 ± 1.10 MPa, and Model 3 has 603.66 ± 13.93 MPa. It should be noted that the strength and modulus of the structures are significantly lower than those of PLA because of their porous geometry and anisotropic layer bonding in the rods [49].

Table 4. Mechanical properties of the biomimetic Voronoi structures.

Model	Porosity (%)	Yield Strength (MPa)	Compressive Modulus (MPa)	Densification Strain (%)	Plateau Stress (MPa)	Energy Capacity (MJ/m^3)	Specific Energy Capacity (KJ/kg)
1	60.43 ± 0.43	6.26 ± 0.12	310.29 ± 15.30	49.39 ± 1.28	6.15 ± 0.09	2.94 ± 0.11	6.01 ± 0.30
2	52.03 ± 0.47	8.80 ± 0.12	443.64 ± 1.10	47.61 ± 1.14	9.38 ± 0.14	4.32 ± 0.14	7.26 ± 0.31
3	44.25 ± 0.50	10.84 ± 0.10	603.66 ± 13.93	47.43 ± 0.47	12.64 ± 0.22	5.78 ± 0.09	8.38 ± 0.20
4	50.99 ± 0.28	9.47 ± 0.13	498.31 ± 8.83	48.68 ± 1.30	10.31 ± 0.02	4.85 ± 0.14	7.98 ± 0.19
5	44.69 ± 0.32	11.55 ± 0.40	658.07 ± 80.29	46.57 ± 0.42	13.55 ± 0.55	6.07 ± 0.19	8.85 ± 0.27
6	58.04 ± 0.85	7.40 ± 0.06	381.33 ± 11.40	48.88 ± 1.59	7.42 ± 0.08	3.51 ± 0.14	6.75 ± 0.37
7	54.23 ± 0.21	8.57 ± 0.45	443.01 ± 14.37	45.07 ± 0.83	8.94 ± 0.40	3.89 ± 0.19	6.85 ± 0.31

The yield strength of Model 4 is 9.47 ± 0.13 MPa and the yield strength of Model 5 is 11.55 ± 0.40 MPa. Their compressive modulus is 498.31 ± 8.83 MPa and 658.07 ± 80.29 MPa, respectively. It can be concluded that as the number of nodes of a Voronoi structure is raised, so increases the structure's strength and stiffness. Furthermore, Model 6 has a yield strength of 7.40 ± 0.06 MPa and compressive modulus of 381.33 ± 11.40 MPa, and Model 7 has 8.57 ± 0.45 MPa and 443.01 ± 14.37 MPa, respectively. It becomes obvious that when smoothing out the overall geometry, and essentially filleting its sharp edges, its strength and stiffness are improved, a principle that generally applies to design and engineering [50,51].

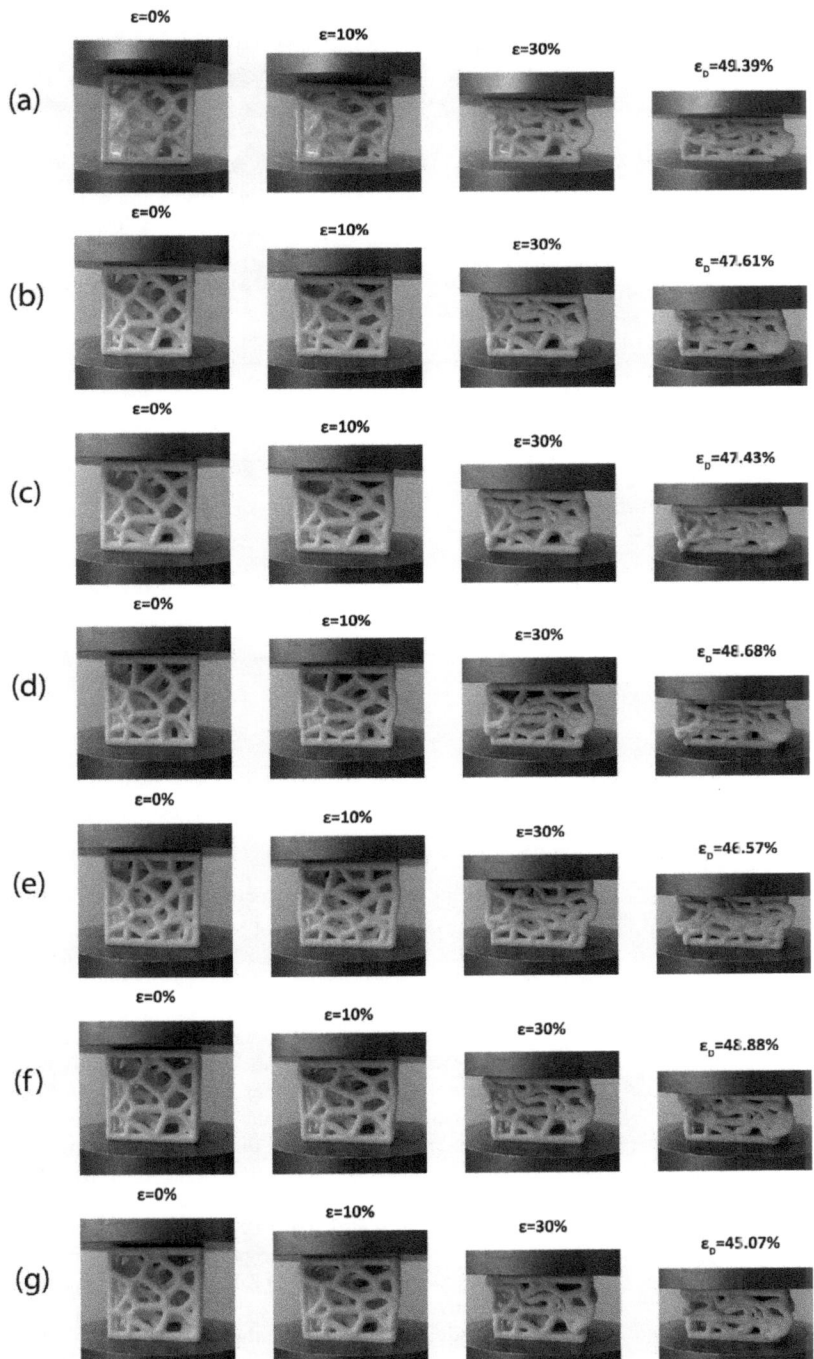

Figure 6. Compressive behavior up until the densification point of: (**a**) Model 1; (**b**) Model 2; (**c**) Model 3; (**d**) Model 4; (**e**) Model 5; (**f**) Model 6; and (**g**) Model 7.

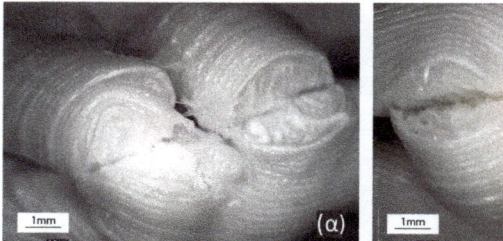 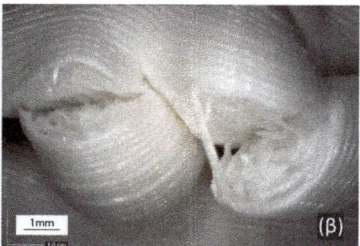

Figure 7. Microscopic images in (α,β) show typical failure points of the rods as they buckle under compressive load and the bonded 3D printed layers are separated.

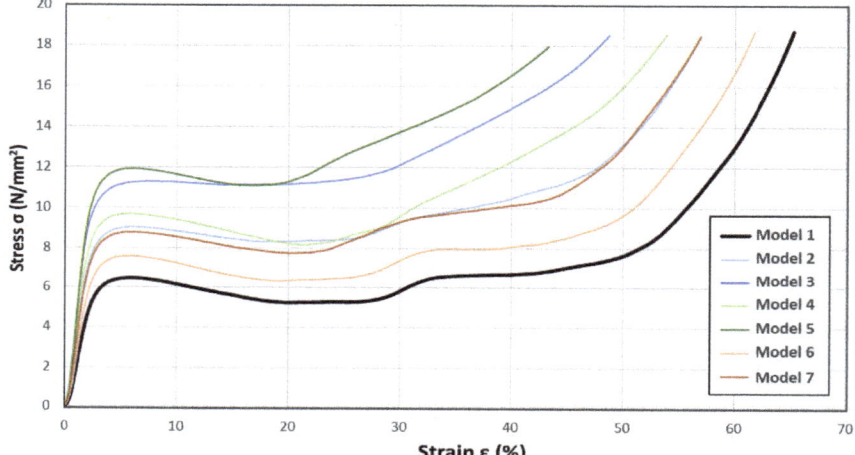

Figure 8. Stress–strain curves of the biomimetic Voronoi models.

3.2.2. Densification Strain, Plateau Stress, and Energy Absorption

The densification strain, ε_D, of Model 1 is 49.39 ± 1.28%. Model 2 has a densification strain of 47.61 ± 1.14%, and Model 3, 47.43 ± 0.47%. The densification strain of Model 4 is 48.68 ± 1.30% and Model 5, 46.57 ± 0.42%. Models 6 and 7 have a densification strain of 48.88 ± 1.59% and 45.07 ± 0.83%, respectively. A reverse trend can be identified in these results. As the thickness of the rods, the number of nodes, and the smoothness of the structure are raised, the densification strain gradually decreases. This can be attributed to the additional PLA material that increases its overall compressible volume, allowing for smaller densification strain values and the observed decline. The plateau stress, σ_{pl}, of Model 1 is 6.15 ± 0.09 MPa, while the plateau stress for Models 2 and 3 were calculated at 9.38 ± 0.14 MPa and 12.64 ± 0.22 MPa, indicating a rising trend as the struts become thicker. A similar trend is noticed as the node count is raised according to the values of Models' 4 and 5 plateau stress which are 10.31 ± 0.02 MPa and 13.55 ± 0.55 MPa, respectively. The same can be said for enhancing the smoothness of the structure, since Models 6 and 7 demonstrate plateau stresses of 7.42 ± 0.08 MPa and 8.94 ± 0.41 MPa, respectively. A correlation between the strength of the structure and plateau stress can be traced. Thicker rods, more nodes, and smoother edges increase not only the compressive strength of the Voronoi structure but also the sustained stress at which the structure progressively collapses up until the densification point is reached.

The baseline Model 1 has an energy capacity W_v of 2.94 ± 0.11 MJ/m^3 and specific energy capacity W_m of 6.01 ± 0.30 KJ/kg. The calculated energy capacity and specific energy capacity for Model 2 are 4.32 ± 0.14 MJ/m^3 and 7.26 ± 0.31 KJ/kg and Model 3 are

5.78 ± 0.09 MJ/m^3 and 8.38 ± 0.20 KJ/kg, respectively. Similarly, to yield strength and plateau stress, the energy absorption capability of the structure increases as the radius of the rods is raised. Model 4 is characterized by an energy capacity of 4.85 ± 0.14 MJ/m^3 and a specific capacity of 7.98 ± 0.19 KJ/kg while Model 5 shows 6.07 ± 0.19 MJ/m^3 and 8.85 ± 0.27 KJ/kg, respectively. Thus, it becomes obvious that the Voronoi structure can absorb more energy when the count of its nodes is increased. Lastly, the capacities of Models 6 and 7 are 3.51 ± 0.14 MJ/m^3 and 3.89 ± 0.19 MJ/m^3 and their specific capacities are 6.75 ± 0.37 KJ/kg and 6.85 ± 0.31 KJ/kg; therefore, smoother Voronoi geometries have superior energy absorption. Overall, enhanced geometric parameters result in higher energy dissipation through rod buckling and collapse at higher constant stress rates.

3.2.3. Correlation of Mechanical Properties to Relative Density

When the modulus of the different samples is plotted against their relative density, a second-degree polynomial correlation is revealed ($R^2 = 0.9596$), as illustrated in Figure 9a. The same relation can be observed when the energy absorption capacity ($R^2 = 0.9783$) of the samples is plotted against their respective relative densities, as shown in Figure 9b. A second-degree polynomial expression ($R^2 = 0.9804$) also describes the relation between plateau stress and relative density in Figure 9c. This trend can be translated as an accelerated increase in the mechanical properties of the structure as more material is added to it and its relative density is raised. It becomes obvious that such an improvement can be achieved either by increasing the thickness of the rods, or by raising the number of the nodes, or by smoothing the geometry, depending on the design requirements or technical and fabrication constraints.

3.3. FEA Validation of Experimental Results

The verified material model from the FEA-supported nanoindentation method [5] has been introduced into the FE model to assess the compression performance of the Voronoi structures. Furthermore, a computational model was utilized to assess the stress response of the 3D printed specimens when subjected to compression. A thorough explicit dynamic analysis was carried out to precisely replicate the mechanical behavior of the lattice structures. This was crucial to accurately represent their substantial deformations and material behavior characterized by a bi-linear pattern. A study has been conducted to confirm that the results were consistent regardless of the mesh density, finding that stress convergence was obtained with approximately 130,000 elements in each model used for verification. The Voronoi structures were subjected to a stepwise vertical velocity applied to the top plate, while the reaction force was measured at the bottom with a fixed boundary condition. The experimental results were used to obtain actual values of the vertical displacement. The force values were determined from the deformation and compared to the experimental results.

The meshing was produced with hexahedral elements for the top compression plate and tetrahedral elements for more complex geometries. Figure 10a displays the force-displacement behavior obtained through finite element analysis (FEA), which demonstrates good agreement between the force-displacement data generated by the FEA simulations and the experimental compression tests for the 3D printed specimens. However, at larger displacements, the experimental curves deviate more from the FEA simulation because of the greater influence of 3D printing defects on the bending response. The material model parameters were analyzed to minimize the differences between the simulated and experimental force-displacement data. Thus, the deformation and equivalent von Mises stress distribution results for the 3D printed Voronoi lattice structures under compressive load, presented in Figure 10b,c, may accurately identify the regions of high stress in the structures. In contrast to previous research [52–62], lattice structures similar to those in our current study exhibited improved physical and mechanical characteristics, particularly in terms of a more significant enhancement in compressive strength and energy absorption. Based on the mechanical test results, it can be concluded that using computationally generated (FEA) compression test data, combined with actual measurements, could be an effective method for characterizing the mechanical deformation behavior of 3D printed Voronoi configurations.

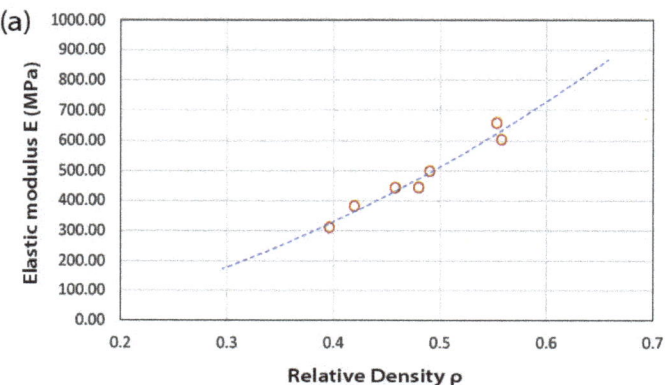

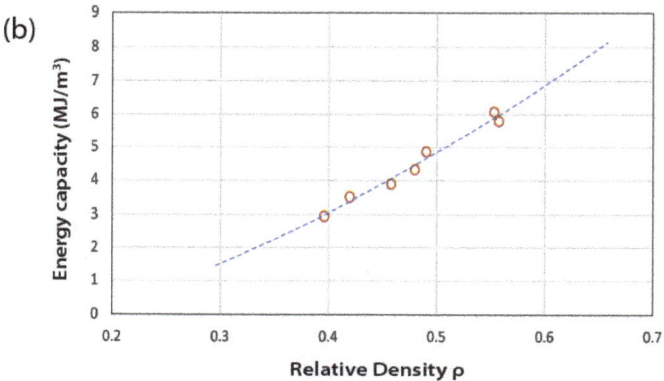

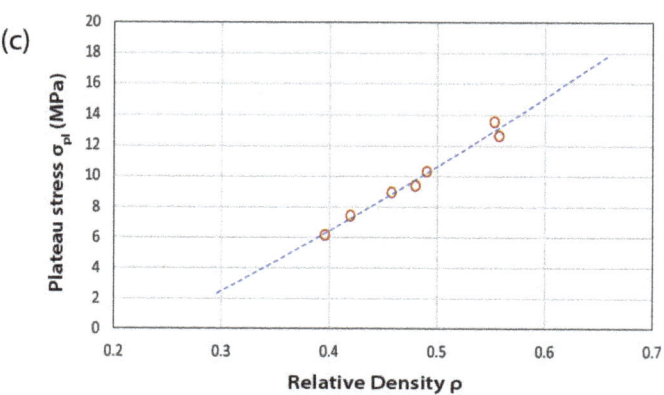

Figure 9. A second-degree polynomial correlation is discernible when the following factors are plotted against their relative densities: (**a**) Elastic modulus; (**b**) energy capacity; and (**c**) plateau stress of the Voronoi structures.

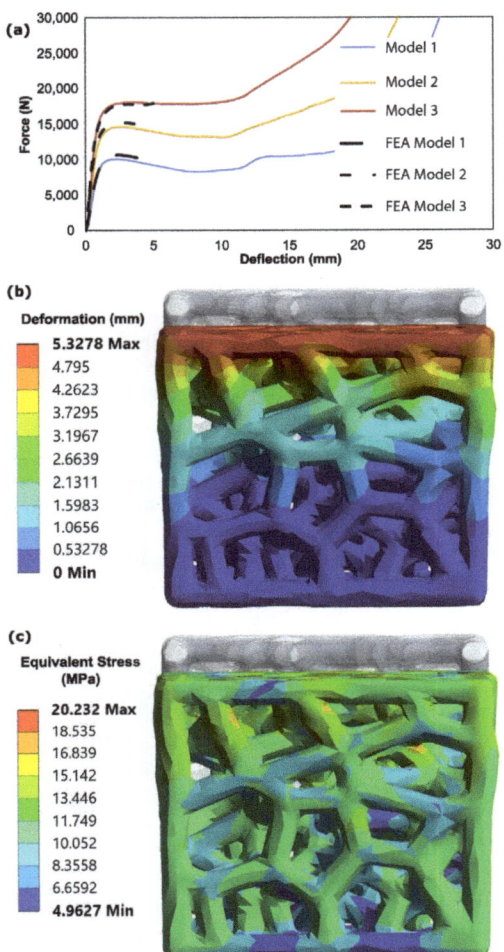

Figure 10. (**a**) Experimental load–displacement response for the Voronoi lattice structures curve-fitted by FEA generated data; (**b**) vertical deformation and (**c**) stress distribution of the Voronoi structure under compression load, utilizing the PLA material properties in the FE model.

4. Conclusions

The technical evaluation stage of a Voronoi structure, inspired by the shell of the sea urchin *Paracentrotus lividus*, has been the focus of the present paper. The stage entails 3D printing the structure followed by mechanical characterization through testing of the physical samples combined with finite element analysis. It is part of a novel biomimetic design strategy that consists of three separate stages: "Research and Analysis", "Abstraction and Emulation", and "Technical Evaluation" that are interconnected via bi-directional loops of feedback.

A parametric algorithm was utilized for the generation of seven different structures with progressive changes in the geometric parameters of rod thickness, node count, and edge smoothness. All the physical specimens were printed with the aid of FFF technology and commercial PLA filament. A consistent divergence was observed between the designed and fabricated relative density of the models which can be attributed to limitations of the 3D printing technology. Compression testing of the physical specimens reveals a common behavior, characterized by an initial linear elastic zone, followed by a long plateau region of progressive collapse of the structure until the densification point is reached in which the cellular structure has completely collapsed, and the bulk material starts to compress. The yield strength and Elastic modulus of the structure increases as the rod thickness, node count, and smoothness are increased. The plateau stress is also raised as the geometric parameters of the structure are enhanced. However, a reverse trend is detected in the densification strain which can be explained by the additional PLA material that increases the overall compressible volume of the material.

The energy capacity and specific energy capacity of the biomimetic structure is also improved as the rod thickness, node count, and smoothness are increased. A second-degree polynomial relation between the Elastic modulus, plateau stress, and energy capacity of the structure and its relative density is detected which is due to accelerated enhancement of its mechanical properties as more material is added. The present research has shown that the relative density and, subsequently, the material properties of a biomimetic Voronoi structure can be enhanced, with great accuracy and reproducibility, through diverse design strategies, either by increasing the thickness of the rods, raising the node count, or by smoothing out sharp edges, depending on the application or design requirements. The conducted finite element analysis validates the above results through good agreement between the force–displacement data generated by the simulations and the experimental compression tests.

Potential applications of the biomimetic Voronoi structure include lightweight structural materials in architectural applications, protective gear and accessories like helmets, or automotive parts. Further research includes the implementation and validation of the biomimetic strategy of analysis, emulation, and technical evaluation in other cases of biological shells to development a series of biomimetic solutions that could serve as the basis of a comprehensive database of biomimetic design concepts.

Author Contributions: Conceptualization, A.E. and I.S.; methodology, A.E., I.S., K.T. and D.T.; software, A.E., I.S. and K.T.; investigation, A.E. and E.K.T.; visualization, A.E.; writing—original draft preparation, A.E. and K.T.; supervision, I.S. and D.T.; funding acquisition, A.E.; validation, E.K.T. formal analysis, A.E. and E.K.T.; data curation, A.E., E.K.T. and K.T. writing—review and editing, I.S., A.E., K.T. and D.T. project administration, I.S. All authors have read and agreed to the published version of the manuscript.

Funding: The research is conducted in the operating framework of the Center of Research Innovation and Excellence of University of Thessaly (Invitation to submit applications for the grant of scholarships to doctoral candidates of University of Thessaly) and was funded by the Special Account of Research Grants of University of Thessaly.

Data Availability Statement: Not applicable.

Conflicts of Interest: The authors declare no conflict of interest.

References

1. Fantini, M.; Curto, M.; De Crescenzio, F. A Method to Design Biomimetic Scaffolds for Bone Tissue Engineering Based on Voronoi Lattices. *Virtual Phys. Prototyp.* **2016**, *11*, 77–90. [CrossRef]
2. Grun, T.B.; Nebelsick, J.H. Structural Design of the Echinoid's Trabecular System. *PLoS ONE* **2018**, *13*, e0204432. [CrossRef] [PubMed]
3. Department of Mathematics, Physics and Descriptive Geometry, Faculty of Civil Engineering, University of Belgrade; Čučaković, A.; Jović, B.; Komnenov, M.; Department of Landscape Architecture and Horticulture, Faculty of Forestry. Biomimetic Geometry Approach to Generative Design. *Period. Polytech. Archit.* **2016**, *47*, 70–74. [CrossRef]
4. Silva, E.C.N.; Walters, M.C.; Paulino, G.H. Modeling Bamboo as a Functionally Graded Material: Lessons for the Analysis of Affordable Materials. *J. Mater. Sci.* **2006**, *41*, 6991–7004. [CrossRef]
5. Efstathiadis, A.; Symeonidou, I.; Tsongas, K.; Tzimtzimis, E.K.; Tzetzis, D. Parametric Design and Mechanical Characterization of 3D-Printed PLA Composite Biomimetic Voronoi Lattices Inspired by the Stereom of Sea Urchins. *J. Compos. Sci.* **2022**, *7*, 3. [CrossRef]
6. Vermeij, G.J. *A Natural History of Shells*; Princeton University Press: Princeton, NJ, USA, 1993; ISBN 978-0-691-08596-8.

7. Grunenfelder, L.K.; Suksangpanya, N.; Salinas, C.; Milliron, G.; Yaraghi, N.; Herrera, S.; Evans-Lutterodt, K.; Nutt, S.R.; Zavattieri, P.; Kisailus, D. Bio-Inspired Impact-Resistant Composites. *Acta Biomater.* **2014**, *10*, 3997–4008. [CrossRef]
8. Smith, A.B. Stereom Microstructure of the Echinoid Test. *Spec. Pap. Palaeontol.* **1980**, *25*, 1–81.
9. Compton, B.G.; Lewis, J.A. 3D-Printing of Lightweight Cellular Composites. *Adv. Mater.* **2014**, *26*, 5930–5935. [CrossRef]
10. Wang, S.; Zheng, Z.; Zhu, C.; Ding, Y.; Yu, J. Crushing and Densification of Rapid Prototyping Polylactide Foam: Meso-Structural Effect and a Statistical Constitutive Model. *Mech. Mater.* **2018**, *127*, 65–76. [CrossRef]
11. Pelanconi, M.; Ortona, A. Nature-Inspired, Ultra-Lightweight Structures with Gyroid Cores Produced by Additive Manufacturing and Reinforced by Unidirectional Carbon Fiber Ribs. *Materials* **2019**, *12*, 4134. [CrossRef]
12. Amin Yavari, S.; Ahmadi, S.M.; Wauthle, R.; Pouran, B.; Schrooten, J.; Weinans, H.; Zadpoor, A.A. Relationship between Unit Cell Type and Porosity and the Fatigue Behavior of Selective Laser Melted Meta-Biomaterials. *J. Mech. Behav. Biomed. Mater.* **2015**, *43*, 91–100. [CrossRef] [PubMed]
13. Ling, C.; Cernicchi, A.; Gilchrist, M.D.; Cardiff, P. Mechanical Behaviour of Additively-Manufactured Polymeric Octet-Truss Lattice Structures under Quasi-Static and Dynamic Compressive Loading. *Mater. Des.* **2019**, *162*, 106–118. [CrossRef]
14. Li, K.; Gao, X.-L.; Subhash, G. Effects of Cell Shape and Strut Cross-Sectional Area Variations on the Elastic Properties of Three-Dimensional Open-Cell Foams. *J. Mech. Phys. Solids* **2006**, *54*, 783–806. [CrossRef]
15. Fantini, M.; Curto, M. Interactive Design and Manufacturing of a Voronoi-Based Biomimetic Bone Scaffold for Morphological Characterization. *Int. J. Interact. Des. Manuf. IJIDeM* **2018**, *12*, 585–596. [CrossRef]
16. Banhart, J. Aluminium Foams for Lighter Vehicles. *Int. J. Veh. Des.* **2005**, *37*, 114. [CrossRef]
17. Ben Ali, N.; Khlif, M.; Hammami, D.; Bradai, C. Mechanical and Morphological Characterization of Spherical Cell Porous Structures Manufactured Using FDM Process. *Eng. Fract. Mech.* **2019**, *216*, 106527. [CrossRef]
18. Murakami, T.; Ohara, K.; Narushima, T.; Ouchi, C. Development of a New Method for Manufacturing Iron Foam Using Gases Generated by Reduction of Iron Oxide. *Mater. Trans.* **2007**, *48*, 2937–2944. [CrossRef]
19. Wang, Y.; Shen, Y.; Wang, Z.; Yang, J.; Liu, N.; Huang, W. Development of Highly Porous Titanium Scaffolds by Selective Laser Melting. *Mater. Lett.* **2010**, *64*, 674–676. [CrossRef]
20. Malewska, E.; Prociak, A. Porous Polyurethane-Polystyrene Composites Produced in a Co-Expansion Process. *Arab. J. Chem.* **2020**, *13*, 37–44. [CrossRef]
21. Utsunomiya, T.; Yamaguchi, R.; Hangai, Y.; Kuwazuru, O.; Yoshikawa, N. Estimation of Plateau Stress of Porous Aluminum Based on Mean Stress on Maximum-Porosity Cross Section. *Mater. Trans.* **2013**, *54*, 1182–1186. [CrossRef]
22. Jung, A.; Diebels, S.; Koblischka-Veneva, A.; Schmauch, J.; Barnoush, A.; Koblischka, M.R. Microstructural Analysis of Electrochemical Coated Open-Cell Metal Foams by EBSD and Nanoindentation: Microstructural Analysis of Electrochemical Coated Open-Cell Metal Foams. *Adv. Eng. Mater.* **2014**, *16*, 15–20. [CrossRef]
23. Degischer, H.-P.; Kriszt, B. *Handbook of Cellular Metals: Production, Processing, Applications*, 1st ed.; Wiley: Hoboken, NJ, USA, 2002; ISBN 978-3-527-30339-7.
24. Agrafiotis, C. Deposition of Nanophase Doped-Ceria Systems on Ceramic Honeycombs for Automotive Catalytic Applications. *Solid State Ion.* **2000**, *136–137*, 1301–1306. [CrossRef]
25. Wang, X.; Xu, S.; Zhou, S.; Xu, W.; Leary, M.; Choong, P.; Qian, M.; Brandt, M.; Xie, Y.M. Topological Design and Additive Manufacturing of Porous Metals for Bone Scaffolds and Orthopaedic Implants: A Review. *Biomaterials* **2016**, *83*, 127–141. [CrossRef] [PubMed]
26. Bates, S.R.G.; Farrow, I.R.; Trask, R.S. 3D Printed Polyurethane Honeycombs for Repeated Tailored Energy Absorption. *Mater. Des.* **2016**, *112*, 172–183. [CrossRef]
27. Yang, Y.; Song, X.; Li, X.; Chen, Z.; Zhou, C.; Zhou, Q.; Chen, Y. Recent Progress in Biomimetic Additive Manufacturing Technology: From Materials to Functional Structures. *Adv. Mater.* **2018**, *30*, 1706539. [CrossRef] [PubMed]
28. Song, X.; Tetik, H.; Jirakittsonthon, T.; Parandoush, P.; Yang, G.; Lee, D.; Ryu, S.; Lei, S.; Weiss, M.L.; Lin, D. Biomimetic 3D Printing of Hierarchical and Interconnected Porous Hydroxyapatite Structures with High Mechanical Strength for Bone Cell Culture. *Adv. Eng. Mater.* **2019**, *21*, 1800678. [CrossRef]
29. Gong, P.; Zhai, S.; Lee, R.; Zhao, C.; Buahom, P.; Li, G.; Park, C.B. Environmentally Friendly Polylactic Acid-Based Thermal Insulation Foams Blown with Supercritical CO_2. *Ind. Eng. Chem. Res.* **2018**, *57*, 5464–5471. [CrossRef]
30. Lehmhus, D.; Vesenjak, M.; Schampheleire, S.; Fiedler, T. From Stochastic Foam to Designed Structure: Balancing Cost and Performance of Cellular Metals. *Materials* **2017**, *10*, 922. [CrossRef]
31. Maiti, A.; Small, W.; Lewicki, J.P.; Weisgraber, T.H.; Duoss, E.B.; Chinn, S.C.; Pearson, M.A.; Spadaccini, C.M.; Maxwell, R.S.; Wilson, T.S. 3D Printed Cellular Solid Outperforms Traditional Stochastic Foam in Long-Term Mechanical Response. *Sci. Rep.* **2016**, *6*, 24871. [CrossRef]
32. Wang, S.; Ding, Y.; Yu, F.; Zheng, Z.; Wang, Y. Crushing Behavior and Deformation Mechanism of Additively Manufactured Voronoi-Based Random Open-Cell Polymer Foams. *Mater. Today Commun.* **2020**, *25*, 101406. [CrossRef]
33. Tang, L.; Shi, X.; Zhang, L.; Liu, Z.; Jiang, Z.; Liu, Y. Effects of Statistics of Cell's Size and Shape Irregularity on Mechanical Properties of 2D and 3D Voronoi Foams. *Acta Mech.* **2014**, *225*, 1361–1372. [CrossRef]
34. Almonti, D.; Baiocco, G.; Tagliaferri, V.; Ucciardello, N. Design and Mechanical Characterization of Voronoi Structures Manufactured by Indirect Additive Manufacturing. *Materials* **2020**, *13*, 1085. [CrossRef] [PubMed]

35. Gibson, L.J.; Ashby, M.F. *Cellular Solids: Structure and Properties*, 2nd ed.; Cambridge University Press: Cambridge, UK, 1997; ISBN 978-0-521-49911-8.
36. Gaitanaros, S.; Kyriakides, S. On the Effect of Relative Density on the Crushing and Energy Absorption of Open-Cell Foams under Impact. *Int. J. Impact Eng.* **2015**, *82*, 3–13. [CrossRef]
37. Siegkas, P. A Computational Geometry Generation Method for Creating 3D Printed Composites and Porous Structures. *Materials* **2021**, *14*, 2507. [CrossRef] [PubMed]
38. Nordin, A.; Hopf, A.; Motte, D. Generative Design Systems for the Industrial Design of Functional Mass Producible Natural-Mathematical Forms. In Proceedings of the 5th International Congress of International Association of Societies of Design Research, IASDR, Tokyo, Japan, 26–30 August 2013; pp. 2931–2941.
39. Aish, R.; Woodbury, R. Multi-Level Interaction in Parametric Design. In *Smart Graphics*; Butz, A., Fisher, B., Krüger, A., Olivier, P., Eds.; Lecture Notes in Computer Science; Springer: Berlin/Heidelberg, Germany, 2005; Volume 3638, pp. 151–162. ISBN 978-3-540-28179-5.
40. Bertacchini, F.; Bilotta, E.; Demarco, F.; Pantano, P.; Scuro, C. Multi-Objective Optimization and Rapid Prototyping for Jewelry Industry: Methodologies and Case Studies. *Int. J. Adv. Manuf. Technol.* **2021**, *112*, 2943–2959. [CrossRef]
41. Bose, S.; Vahabzadeh, S.; Bandyopadhyay, A. Bone Tissue Engineering Using 3D Printing. *Mater. Today* **2013**, *16*, 496–504. [CrossRef]
42. Sharma, P.; Pandey, P.M. Morphological and Mechanical Characterization of Topologically Ordered Open Cell Porous Iron Foam Fabricated Using 3D Printing and Pressureless Microwave Sintering. *Mater. Des.* **2018**, *160*, 442–454. [CrossRef]
43. Zein, I.; Hutmacher, D.W.; Tan, K.C.; Teoh, S.H. Fused Deposition Modeling of Novel Scaffold Architectures for Tissue Engineering Applications. *Biomaterials* **2002**, *23*, 1169–1185. [CrossRef]
44. Anitha, R.; Arunachalam, S.; Radhakrishnan, P. Critical Parameters Influencing the Quality of Prototypes in Fused Deposition Modelling. *J. Mater. Process. Technol.* **2001**, *118*, 385–388. [CrossRef]
45. Tan, P.J.; Reid, S.R.; Harrigan, J.J.; Zou, Z.; Li, S. Dynamic Compressive Strength Properties of Aluminium Foams. Part I—Exp. Data Observations. *J. Mech. Phys. Solids* **2005**, *53*, 2174–2205. [CrossRef]
46. Li, Q.M.; Magkiriadis, I.; Harrigan, J.J. Compressive Strain at the Onset of Densification of Cellular Solids. *J. Cell. Plast.* **2006**, *42*, 371–392. [CrossRef]
47. Ren, H.; Shen, H.; Ning, J. Effect of Internal Microstructure Distribution on Quasi-Static Compression Behavior and Energy Absorption of Hollow Truss Structures. *Materials* **2020**, *13*, 5094. [CrossRef]
48. Vicente, M.F.; Canyada, M.; Conejero, A. Identifying Limitations for Design for Manufacturing with Desktop FFF 3D Printers. *Int. J. Rapid Manuf.* **2015**, *5*, 116. [CrossRef]
49. Pinto, V.C.; Ramos, T.; Alves, S.; Xavier, J.; Tavares, P.; Moreira, P.M.G.P.; Guedes, R.M. Comparative Failure Analysis of PLA, PLA/GNP and PLA/CNT-COOH Biodegradable Nanocomposites Thin Films. *Procedia Eng.* **2015**, *114*, 635–642. [CrossRef]
50. Xing, J.; Qie, L. Fillet Design in Topology Optimization. In Proceedings of the 2020 7th International Conference on Information Science and Control Engineering (ICISCE), Changsha, China, 18–20 December 2020; IEEE: Piscataway, NJ, USA, 2020; pp. 639–643.
51. Singh, A.; Chauhan, P.S.; Pandit, P.P.; Narwariya, M. Effect of Notch Fillet Radius on Tensile Strength of 817M40 Notched Bar. *IOP Conf. Ser. Mater. Sci. Eng.* **2021**, *1136*, 012070. [CrossRef]
52. Kladovasilakis, N.; Tsongas, K.; Kostavelis, I.; Tzovaras, D.; Tzetzis, D. Effective Mechanical Properties of Additive Manufactured Strut-Lattice Structures: Experimental and Finite Element Study. *Adv. Eng. Mater.* **2021**, *24*, 2100879. [CrossRef]
53. Kladovasilakis, N.; Tsongas, K.; Kostavelis, I.; Tzovaras, D.; Tzetzis, D. Effective mechanical properties of additive manufactured triply periodic minimal surfaces: Experimental and finite element study. *Int. J. Adv. Manuf. Technol.* **2022**, *121*, 7169–7189. [CrossRef]
54. Zoumaki, M.; Mansour, M.T.; Tsongas, K.; Tzetzis, D.; Mansour, G. Mechanical Characterization and Finite Element Analysis of Hierarchical Sandwich Structures with PLA 3D-Printed Core and Composite Maize Starch Biodegradable Skins. *J. Compos. Sci.* **2022**, *6*, 118. [CrossRef]
55. Kladovasilakis, N.; Tsongas, K.; Tzetzis, D. Finite Element Analysis of Orthopedic Hip Implant with Functionally Graded Bioinspired Lattice Structures. *Biomimetics* **2020**, *5*, 44. [CrossRef]
56. Giarmas, E.; Tsongas, K.; Tzimtzimis, E.K.; Korlos, A.; Tzetzis, D. Mechanical and FEA-Assisted Characterization of 3D Printed Continuous Glass Fiber Reinforced Nylon Cellular Structures. *J. Compos. Sci.* **2021**, *5*, 313. [CrossRef]
57. Kladovasilakis, N.; Charalampous, P.; Boumpakis, A.; Kontodina, T.; Tsongas, K.; Tzetzis, D.; Kostavelis, I.; Givissis, P.; Tzovaras, D. Development of biodegradable customized tibial scaffold with advanced architected materials utilizing additive manufacturing. *J. Mech. Behav. Biomed. Mater.* **2023**, *141*, 105796. [CrossRef] [PubMed]
58. Mansour, M.T.; Tsongas, K.; Tzetzis, D. Carbon-Fiber- and Nanodiamond-Reinforced PLA Hierarchical 3D-Printed Core Sandwich Structures. *J. Compos. Sci.* **2023**, *7*, 285. [CrossRef]
59. Mansour, M.T.; Tsongas, K.; Tzetzis, D. 3D Printed Hierarchical Honeycombs with Carbon Fiber and Carbon Nanotube Reinforced Acrylonitrile Butadiene Styrene. *J. Compos. Sci.* **2021**, *5*, 62. [CrossRef]
60. Kladovasilakis, N.; Tsongas, K.; Karalekas, D.; Tzetzis, D. Architected Materials for Additive Manufacturing: A Comprehensive Review. *Materials* **2022**, *15*, 5919. [CrossRef] [PubMed]

51. Fu, T.; Hu, X.; Yang, C. Impact Response Analysis of Stiffened Sandwich Functionally Graded Porous Materials Doubly-Curved Shell with Re-Entrant Honeycomb Auxetic Core. *Appl. Math. Model.* **2023**, *124*, 553–575. [CrossRef]
52. Zhao, G.; Fu, T.; Li, J. Study on Concave Direction Impact Performance of Similar Concave Hexagon Honeycomb Structure. *Materials* **2023**, *16*, 3262. [CrossRef]

Disclaimer/Publisher's Note: The statements, opinions and data contained in all publications are solely those of the individual author(s) and contributor(s) and not of MDPI and/or the editor(s). MDPI and/or the editor(s) disclaim responsibility for any injury to people or property resulting from any ideas, methods, instructions or products referred to in the content.

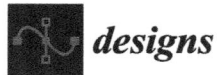

Article

Investigating the Performance of Gammatone Filters and Their Applicability to Design Cochlear Implant Processing System

Rumana Islam * and Mohammed Tarique

Department of Electrical and Computer Engineering, University of Science and Technology of Fujairah, Fujairah P.O. Box 2202, United Arab Emirates; m.tarique@ustf.ac.ae
* Correspondence: r.islam@ustf.ac.ae; Tel.: +971-50-973-6727

Abstract: Commercially available cochlear implants are designed to aid profoundly deaf people in understanding speech and environmental sounds. A typical cochlear implant uses a bank of bandpass filters to decompose an audio signal into a set of dynamic signals. These filters' critical center frequencies f_0 imitate the human cochlea's vibration patterns caused by audio signals. Gammatone filters (GTFs), with two unique characteristics: (a) an appropriate "pseudo resonant" frequency transfer function, mimicking the human cochlea, and (b) realizing efficient hardware implementation, could demonstrate them as unique candidates for cochlear implant design. Although GTFs have recently attracted considerable attention from researchers, a comprehensive exposition of GTFs is still absent in the literature. This paper starts by enumerating the impulse response of GTFs. Then, the magnitude spectrum, $|H(f)|$, and bandwidth, more specifically, the equivalent rectangular bandwidth (ERB) of GTFs, are derived. The simulation results suggested that optimally chosen filter parameters, e.g., critical center frequencies, f_0; temporal decay parameter, b; and order of the filter, n, can minimize the interference of the filter bank frequencies and very likely model the filter bandwidth (ERB), independent of $\frac{f_0}{b}$. Finally, these optimized filters are applied to delineate a filter bank for a cochlear implant design based on the Clarion processor model.

Keywords: basilar membrane; clarion processor; cochlear implant; equivalent rectangular bandwidth (ERB); gammatone filter (GTF) bank; pseudo-resonant frequency

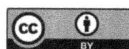

1. Introduction

Speech communication is an integral part of our daily life. During speech production, a speaker encodes information into a continuously time-varying wave propagated through a medium [1]. The wave propagates from a speaker to a listener through the vibration of air particles. Finally, a listener perceives the information contained in the sound wave.

The human peripheral auditory system is one of the most critical components of speech perception. The human peripheral auditory system consists of three major parts [2]: the outer, middle, and inner ears, as shown in Figure 1. Sound enters the outer ear through the pinna, travels down to the auditory canal, and vibrates the eardrum. The middle ear, consisting of three bones, transports the vibration of the eardrum to the inner ear. The main component of the inner ear is the snail-shaped cochlea, a coiled tube filled with fluid [3]. Within the cochlear fluid, there exists a basilar membrane. The sound vibration at the eardrum ultimately generates a compressed sound wave in the cochlear fluid and causes a vertical vibration in the basilar membrane. The basilar membrane is mechanically tuned at different frequencies. It plays a vital role in distributing sound energy in frequencies along the cochlea's length, as shown in Figure 2. The wavelengths of audible sound can cover a wide range of scales. As depicted in this figure, the lower frequencies are located near the 'apex'. In contrast, the higher frequencies are at the far end, called 'base'. The low-frequency waves can have wavelengths of up to 17 m (20 Hz), while the highest frequencies can be as small as 1.7 cm (20,000 Hz).

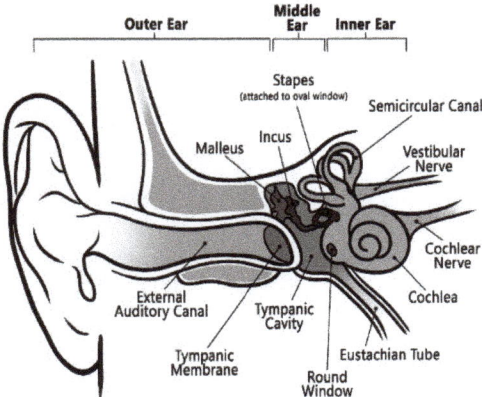

Figure 1. The components of human ear [1]. Sound enters the outer ear through the pinna and travels down to the middle and inner ears. Finally, it reaches the cochlea and vibrates the basilar membrane.

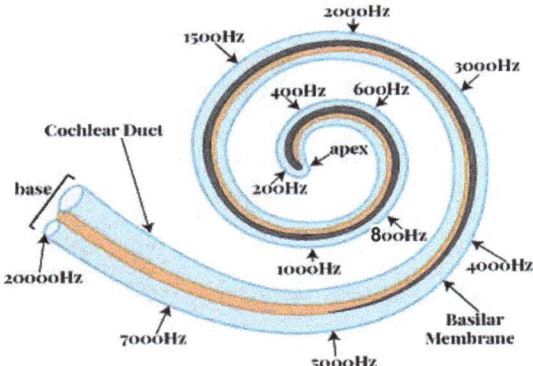

Figure 2. The tuning frequencies of the basilar membrane [4]. The basilar membrane is tuned to different frequencies from the apex to the base. The lower frequencies are near the apex, whereas the higher frequencies are near the base. The tuning frequency spacing also increases towards the base.

In conjunction with the basilar membrane, the hair cells translate mechanical information into neural information. If the hair cells are damaged, the auditory system cannot transform sound into neural impulses. The sound never reaches the brain because of the damaged hair cells. Many causes can damage hair cells, including diseases, congenital disorders, and specific drug treatments. Damaged hair cells can degenerate adjacent auditory neurons, too. Damaged neurons and hair cells can make a person profoundly deaf. However, recent research [5] has shown that the most common cause of deafness is the loss of hair cells rather than the loss of auditory neurons.

Hearing loss is the third most common health problem affecting the elderly population after heart disease and arthritis, according to some statistics [6]. Hair cells can be damaged over time, being open to continuous mechanical stress from environmental issues, including sounds. Various factors, e.g., aging, genetic defects, and ototoxic drugs, also cause additional risks of cell damage [7]. This damage can be mild to severe, causing even the death of hair cells. Unfortunately, human hair cells do not regenerate. The repair of hair cells is crucial for continued auditory function throughout life. Clinicians recommend several drugs to restore the proper functioning of hair cells when the damage is minor. Sudden hearing loss resulting from viral infection is medically treated with corticosteroids. Corticosteroids may also be used to reduce cochlear hair cell swelling and inflammation when exposed to loud noise. However, clinical restoration of damaged hair cells from aging and genetic causes remains a research issue. Recently, gene therapy has been proven effective in restoring the functionality of damaged hair cells due to genetic factors in several animal models [8]. Even the perceptual quality of voice signals is greatly affected by hearing mechanisms [9]. A degraded voice can, in turn, be a biomarker of a human's health status, including both structural and neurological malfunctions in speech and hearing mechanisms [10–13].

A cochlear implant can play an important role here as it can excite the neurons through electrical stimulation to restore the hearing ability of a deaf person. The main idea is bypassing the standard hearing mechanism and electrically stimulating the auditory neurons.

Researchers have proved that frequency analysis performed concerning the cochlea can be modeled as a bandpass filter bank. Various filters have been proposed to implement bandpass filter banks. One of the earliest proposed filters is the rounded exponential function ('roex') [14]. The authors have shown that an exponential function can represent the auditory filter shape successfully. A novel reverse correlation technique has been introduced to better model the auditory filter [15]. Another function called 'revcor' has been introduced to define the impulse response of the peripheral auditory filters. Peculiarly, this function provides the impulse response of a sharp bandpass filter. Consequently, the GTF has been introduced in [16] to provide an analytic mathematical function approximating the 'revcor' function. Other researchers have further developed the GTF to make it suitable for practical design purposes [17,18]. One of the main merits of the GTF is its convenient mathematical form. Hence, its properties can be easily derived analytically compared to similar filters, including 'roex' filters. One of the pioneering works that investigated various properties of the GTF has been presented in [19]. The authors have defined the GTF as an infinite impulse response (IIR) filter in the time domain and described its provenance and some of its elementary properties. They also examined the behavior of the GTF in the frequency domain. They provided a way of calculating the parameters needed for a GTF to have a specified ERB. The authors provided an efficient digital implementation of the GTF on a general-purpose computer. A digital multiple-pass IIR filter technique has also been proposed to implement the GTF [20] for practical designs.

Recently, the GTF has drawn researchers' attention to sound event detection, speech signal processing, voice pathology detection, and speech recognition. In [21], the authors have proposed a GTF-based automatic speech recognition (ASR) technique. They demonstrated that GTFs are promising in terms of improving the robustness of ASR systems against noise compared to the Mel-Frequency Cepstral Coefficient (MFCC) and Perceptual Linear Prediction (PLP). GTF-based parametric filter banks have been proposed in [22] to detect speech. Three filter banks based on Mel, Gammatone, and Gaussian filters have been investigated in that work. The comparative investigation showed that the GTFs provided the highest speech detection accuracy compared to the Gaussian and Mel filters. A GTF-based sound event detection and localization (SEDL) system has been presented in [23]. The authors demonstrated that GTFs could boost the performance of state-of-the-art SEDL algorithms. In [24], the authors have applied the GTF to produce an image representation of sound signals for audio surveillance. They called this image representation a Cochleagram. The authors have shown that the proposed Cochleagram provided more noise robustness than cepstral features, namely Mel-Frequency Cepstral Coefficients and the spectrogram image feature (SIF). A learnable GTF bank is proposed to classify environmental sounds in [25]. The authors demonstrated that the learnable filter parameters of the GTFs could preserve the spectro-temporal domain features of environmental sound and can achieve high classification accuracy. In [26], the authors have shown that the GTF could enhance the performance of hearing aids. They concluded that the GTFs could provide a high hearing aid speech quality index (HASQI). A GTF-based speaker recognition system has been proposed in [27]. The authors have argued that conventional speaker recognition systems perform poorly under noisy conditions. They introduced a novel spectral feature called the Gammatone frequency cepstral coefficient (GFCC). They showed that this feature captured speaker characteristics and performed substantially better than conventional spectral features under noisy conditions. The results showed significant performance improvements over related systems under a wide range of signal-to-noise ratios. In [28], the performances of the cochlear implants (CIs) have been investigated by using three different filters, namely GTF, DAPGF (Differentiated All-Pole GTF), OZGF (One-Zero GTF) and BUTF (Butterworth). Filter parameters, including the filter order (N), the filter quality factor (Q), and the number of channels (C) and their combinations, were tested using objective and subjective metrics in that work. The simulation results concluded that the Q and N parameters are crucial for designing cochlear implants.

Although the GTF has attracted considerable attention from researchers, as mentioned above, a comprehensive exposition on the GTF is still absent in the literature other than the work presented in [29]. That work has provided a tutorial introduction to the GTF without much detail. The main goals of this investigation are as follows:

a. Explore the effects of filter parameters: order n, carrier frequency f_c, carrier phase φ, temporal decay coefficient b, and Gammatone distribution function $r(t)$, on the impulse response $h(t)$ of the GTF.
b. Derive the transfer function of the GTF from the definition of the $h(t)$ by using the Fourier transform and its properties.
c. Investigate the effects of the above filter parameters on the transfer function $H(f)$ of the GTF.
d. Derive the expression for ERB of the GTF.
e. Design a filter bank using the GTF for a given pseudo-resonant f_c.
f. Demonstrate the application of the GTF in cochlear implant design.

The structure of this investigation is organized as follows: Section 2 explains the impulse response and spectrum of GTFs. Section 3 elaborates on the ERBs. Section 4 describes the possible application of GTFs in cochlear implant design. Section 5 addresses some underlying design issues and challenges. Finally, the paper concludes with a synopsis of key findings and explores possible routes for future research.

2. Impulse Response and Spectrum of GTFs

In [30], a Gammatone function has been used to model the basilar membrane displacement in the human ear. It has been further investigated, and it was shown that a GTF can be used to approximate responses recorded from the cochlear nucleus in cats [16]. In a similar work [31], a Gammatone function was used to model the impulse responses based on the auditory nerve fiber recordings in cats. Finally, the term "Gammatone filter" was introduced in [32], and its impulse response was defined as follows:

$$h(t) = ct^{n-1}e^{-2\pi bt}\cos(2\pi f_c t + \varphi)u(t) \quad (1)$$

where c is the proportionality constant, n is the filter order, b the temporal decay constant, f_c is the carrier frequency, φ is the carrier phase, and $u(t)$ is the unit step function. The expression of $h(t)$ can be broken down into two components, namely the carrier component and the Gamma distribution function.

Let us assume that the carrier component is denoted by

$$c(t) = \cos(2\pi f_c t + \varphi) \quad (2)$$

and the Gammatone distribution function is defined by

$$r(t) = t^{n-1}e^{-2\pi bt}u(t) \quad (3)$$

Hence, the impulse response of the GTF can be expressed as

$$h(t) = cs(t)r(t) \quad (4)$$

Figure 3 shows the plot for $h(t)$ of the GTF with its constituent components. In the plot, factor c has been set to $\frac{b^n}{(n-1)!}$ to make the integration under the curve of Gamma distribution equal to one. The other parameters are arbitrarily set to $b = 125$, and $f_c = 1000$ Hz. The filter order n of a GTF is an important design parameter. It controls the relative shape of the filter impulse response, as demonstrated in Figure 4. The relative shape becomes less skewed as the filter order n increases. The carrier phase, φ is also an important property that determines the relative position of the envelope.

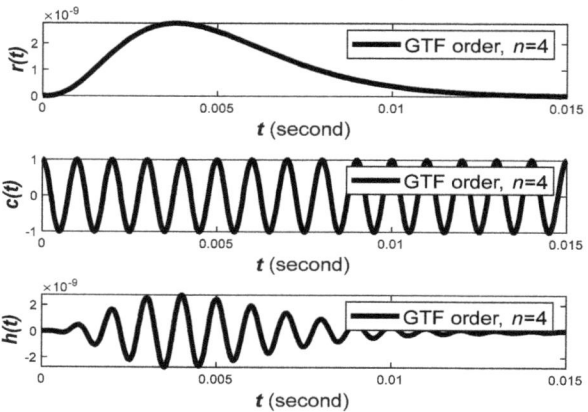

Figure 3. The components of a GTF impulse response: Gammatone distribution $r(t)$ (**top**), the carrier tone $c(t)$ (**middle**), and the impulse response $h(t)$ (**bottom**). The amplitude of the carrier tone is modulated according to the Gammatone distribution function.

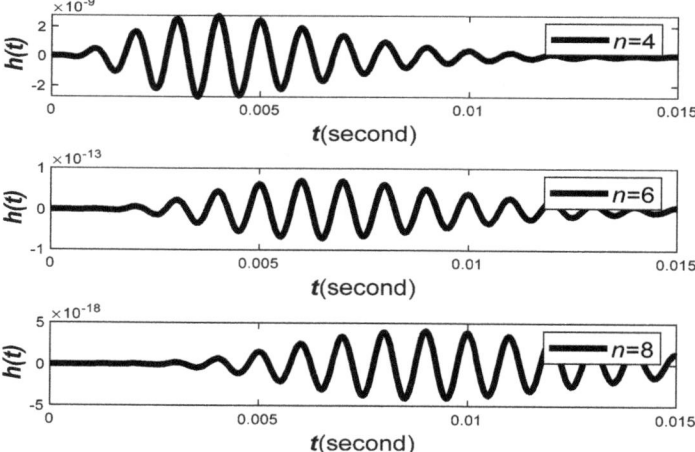

Figure 4. The Gammatone impulse response, $h(t)$ of the GTF with varying order, n. The relative shape becomes less skewed as the filter order n increases.

Observation 1. *When the filter order is higher, the impulse response of the GTF becomes less skewed and vice versa.*

The Fourier transform of the GTF's impulse response $h(t)$ will be derived to investigate its frequency domain behaviors. From the convolution property of the Fourier transform, we know that if $z(t) = x(t)y(t)$, then $Z(f) = X(f) * Y(f)$ (Appendix A). By applying this property to (4), we can express $H(f)$ as

$$H(f) = c[S(f) * R(f)] \tag{5}$$

where $S(f)$ is the Fourier transform of $s(t)$, $R(f)$ is the Fourier transform of $r(t)$, and $H(f)$ is the Fourier transform of $h(t)$. We can find the Fourier transform of $r(t)$ by using the Fourier transform identity, $x(t) = e^{-a(t)}u(t) \leftrightarrow X(f) = \frac{1}{a+j2\pi f}$ (Appendix B). Substituting $a = 2\pi b$, we can find the Fourier transform of $x(t)$ as

$$x(t) = e^{-2\pi bt}u(t) \leftrightarrow X(f) = \frac{1}{2\pi b + j2\pi f} \tag{6}$$

From the property of the Fourier transform (Appendix A), we also know that if

$$x(t) \leftrightarrow X(f), \text{ then } t^m x(t) \leftrightarrow (-j2\pi)^{-m} \frac{d^m}{df^m} X(f).$$

By substituting $m = (n-1)$, we can express the Fourier transform of $r(t)$ as

$$r(t) = t^{n-1} e^{-j2\pi bt} u(t) \leftrightarrow R(f) = (-j2\pi)^{-(n-1)} \frac{d^{n-1}}{df^{n-1}} \left(\frac{1}{2\pi b + j2\pi f} \right) \tag{7}$$

If we substitute $n = 2$ in (7), we can find $te^{-j2\pi bt}u(t) \leftrightarrow \frac{1}{(2\pi b + j2\pi f)^2}$. Similarly, if we substitute $n = 3$, we can find, $t^2 e^{-j2\pi bt}u(t) \leftrightarrow \frac{(2)!}{(2\pi b + j2\pi f)^3}$. Proceeding in the same way, we can find the Fourier transform of $r(t)$ as

$$r(t) = t^{n-1} e^{-j2\pi bt} u(t) \leftrightarrow R(f) = \frac{(n-1)!}{(2\pi b + j2\pi f)^4} \tag{8}$$

The Fourier transform of $r(t)$ can be alternatively expressed as

$$R(f) = (n-1)!(2\pi b)^{-n} \left(1 + j\frac{f}{b} \right)^{-n} \tag{9}$$

Now, let us find the Fourier transform of the carrier signal, $c(t)$. The carrier signal is given by $c(t) = \cos(2\pi f_c t + \varphi)$, which can be alternatively expressed as $c(t) = \frac{1}{2} e^{j2\pi f_c t} e^{j\varphi} + \frac{1}{2} e^{-j2\pi f_c t} e^{-j\varphi}$. By using the Fourier transform identities $e^{j2\pi f_c} \leftrightarrow \delta(f - f_c)$, and $e^{-j2\pi f_0} \leftrightarrow \delta(f + f_0)$, the Fourier transform of $c(t)$ can be expressed as

$$C(f) = \frac{1}{2} e^{j\varphi} \delta(f - f_c) + \frac{1}{2} e^{-j\varphi} \delta(f - f_c) \tag{10}$$

Substituting the Fourier transform of $s(t)$ and $r(t)$ in (5), we can determine the expression of $H(f)$ as

$$H(f) = c(n-1)!(2\pi b)^{-n} \left(1 + j\frac{f}{b} \right)^{-n} * \left[\frac{1}{2} e^{j\varphi} \delta(f - f_c) + \frac{1}{2} e^{-j\varphi} \delta(f + f_c) \right] \tag{11}$$

By using the convolutional property of the delta Dirac function (Appendix C),

$$x(f) * \delta(f - f_c) = x(f - f_c),$$

We can find the final expression of the $H(f)$ as

$$H(f) = c(n-1)!(2\pi b)^{-n}\left[\frac{1}{2}e^{j\varphi}\left(1+j\frac{f-f_c}{b}\right)^{-n}\right] + c(n-1)!(2\pi b)^{-n}\left[e^{-j\varphi}\left(1+j\frac{f+f_c}{b}\right)^{-n}\right] \quad (12)$$

The plots for the $R(f)$ and $H(f)$ are shown in Figure 5. This figure shows that the $H(f)$ produces two copies of the $R(f)$ separated by the two times the carrier frequency, f_c.

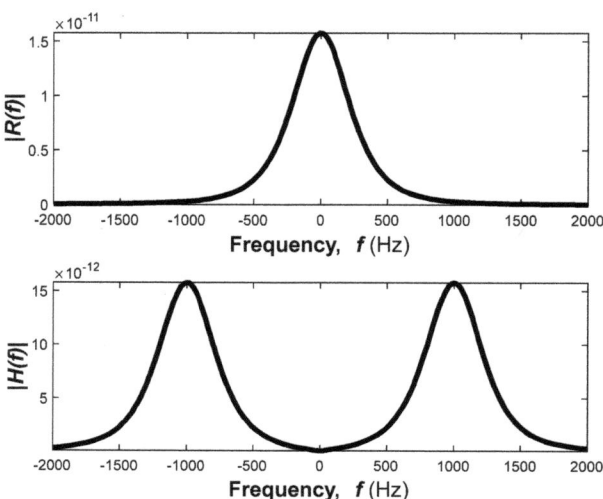

Figure 5. The magnitude spectrum of $r(t)$, i.e., $R(f)$ (**top**) and the magnitude spectrum of $h(t)$, i.e., $H(f)$ (**bottom**). $R(f)$ has a maximum value at, $f = 0$. On the other hand, $H(f)$ has two maxima, and they are located at $\pm f_c$.

Observation 2. *The Fourier transform of the Gamma distribution component of the GTF impulse response has one maximum value at $f_0 = 0$ Hz. However, the Fourier transform of the impulse response has two maxima, and the location of these two maxima depends on the carrier frequency. To avoid interference, these two frequency components shall be sufficiently separated by selecting a high carrier frequency.*

The Fourier transform of $h(t)$ can be expressed in terms of the Fourier transform of $r(t)$. From (5), we can write

$$H(f) = c\left[R(f) * \left\{\frac{1}{2}e^{j\varphi}\delta(f-f_c) + \frac{1}{2}e^{-j\varphi}\delta(f+f_c)\right\}\right] \quad (13)$$

$$H(f) = \frac{1}{2}\left[\left\{e^{j\varphi}R(f-f_c) + e^{-j\varphi}R(f+f_c)\right\}\right] \quad (14)$$

where $R(f)$ is given by (9) and can be alternatively expressed as

$$R(f) = \frac{(n-1)!}{[2\pi b + j2\pi f]^n} \quad (15)$$

The expression of $H(f)$ can be further simplified by assuming

$$k = \frac{c}{2}(n-1)!(2\pi b)^{-n} \quad (16)$$

$$P(f) = e^{j\varphi}[1+j(f-f_c)/b]^{-n} \quad (17)$$

$$P^*(f) = e^{-j\varphi}[1 - j(f - f_c)/b]^{-n} \tag{18}$$

Replacing f with $-f$, we can modify (18) as

$$P^*(-f) = e^{-j\varphi}[1 + j(f + f_c)/b]^{-n} \tag{19}$$

Then, we can express $H(f)$ as

$$H(f) = k[P(f) + P^*(-f)] \tag{20}$$

The impulse response of the GTFs and their transfer functions are plotted in Figure 6 for varying parameters of f_c/b. The figure shows that, f_c/b is another critical parameter that affects the decaying behavior of the filter impulse response and filter transfer function.

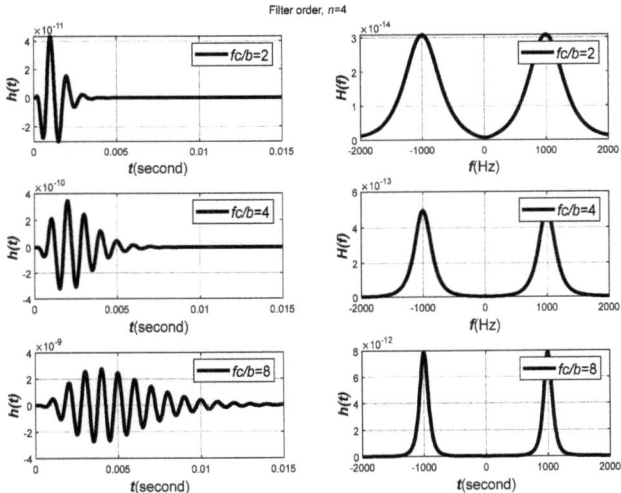

Figure 6. The filter impulse responses, $h(t)$, and their spectrums $H(f)$, with the varying magnitude of f_c/b. The value of $\frac{f_c}{b} \geq 4$ ensures that the two frequency components of GTF do not interfere with each other.

Observation 3. *When b is small (i.e., f_c/b is large), $h(t)$ will decay slowly. On the other hand, $|H(f)|$ will decay more rapidly and vice versa.*

Observation 4. *The larger the ratio f_c/b, the less the components of $KP(f)$ and $KP^*(f)$ overlap, and less interference between $KP(f)$ and $KP^*(f)$ will occur.*

In general, $H(f)$ can be expressed in terms of magnitude and phase spectrum as $H(f) = |H(f)|e^{-j\varnothing}$, where $|H(f)|$ is the magnitude of $H(f)$, and $\varnothing$ = phase spectrum of $H(f)$. The power spectrum of $H(f)$ is expressed by

$$\begin{aligned}|H(f)|^2 &= H(f)H^*(f) \\ &= k^2[P(f) + P^*(-f)][P^*(f) + P(-f)]] \\ &= k^2[P(f)P^*(f) + P^*(f)P^*(-f) + P(f)P(-f) + P^*(-f)P(-f)]\end{aligned} \tag{21}$$

By using the Fourier transform property (Appendix B), we can simplify the following expressions as $P(f)P^*(f) = |P(f)|^2$ and $P^*(-f)P(-f) = |P(-f)|^2$. Hence, $P(f)P(-f) +$

$P^*(f)P^*(-f) = P(f)P(-f) + [P(f)P(-f)]^* = 2Re[P(f)P(-f)]$ and $|H(f)|^2$ can be expressed as

$$|H(f)|^2 = k^2 \left[|P(f)|^2 + |P^*(-f)|^2 + 2Re\{P(f)P(-f)\} \right] \qquad (22)$$

Assume $Q(f) = 1 + j(f - f_c)/b$. The $Q(f)$ can be expressed in terms of magnitude and phase as $Q(f) = |Q(f)|e^{j\theta_1(f)}$, where the magnitude is defined by $|Q(f)| = \sqrt{1 + \frac{(f-f_c)^2}{b^2}}$, and the phase spectrum is defined by $\theta_1(f) = \tan^{-1}\left[\frac{f-f_c}{b}\right]$, now, $P(f)$ can be expressed in terms of $Q(f)$, as

$$P(f) = e^{j\varphi}[Q(f)]^{-n} = e^{j\varphi}\left[|Q(f)|e^{j\theta_1(f)}\right]^{-n} \qquad (23)$$

Substituting f with $-f$, we can find the expression of $Q(-f)$ as $Q(-f) = 1 + j(-f - f_c) = 1 - j(f + f_c)/b$. Now, $Q(-f)$ can be expressed in terms of magnitude and phase as follows $Q(-f) = |Q(-f)|e^{j\theta_2(f)}$, where the magnitude of $Q(f)$ is defined as $|Q(-f)| = \sqrt{1 + \frac{(f-f_c)^2}{b^2}}$, and the phase $\theta_2(f) = \tan^{-1}\left[-\frac{f-f_c}{b}\right]$. Now, $P(-f)$ can be expressed in terms of $Q(-f)$ as

$$\begin{aligned} P(-f) &= e^{j\varphi}[Q(-f)]^{-n} = e^{j\varphi}\left[|Q(-f)|e^{j\theta_2(f)}\right]^{-n} \\ &= e^{j\varphi}|Q(-f)|^{-n}e^{-jn\theta_2(f)} \end{aligned} \qquad (24)$$

We can express the terms presented in (22) as follows

$$\begin{aligned} |P(f)|^2 &= |Q(f)|^{-2n} = \sqrt{1 + (f-f_c)^2/b^2}^{-2n} \\ &= \left[1 + (f-f_c)^2/b^2\right]^{-n} \end{aligned} \qquad (25)$$

Similarly,

$$|P(-f)|^2 = |Q(-f)|^{-2n} = \sqrt{1 + (f+f_c)^2/b^2}^{-2n} = \left[1 + \frac{(f+f_c)^2}{b^2}\right]^{-n} \qquad (26)$$

$$P(f)P(-f) = e^{j\varphi}[Q(f)]^{-n}e^{j\varphi}[Q(-f)]^{-n} = [Q(f)Q(-f)]^{-n}e^{j2\varphi} \qquad (27)$$

Let us find the expression of $Q(f)Q(-f)$ by

$$\begin{aligned} Q(f)Q(-f) &= [1 + j(f - f_c)/b][1 - j(f - f_c)/b] \\ &= 1 - \frac{j(f-f_c)}{b} - j^2\frac{f-f_c}{b}\frac{f+f_c}{b} + j\frac{f-f_c}{b} \\ &= 1 + j\frac{f-f_c-f+f_c}{b} + \frac{f^2-f_c^2}{b^2} \\ &= 1 + \frac{f^2-f_c^2}{b^2} - j2\frac{f}{b} \end{aligned} \qquad (28)$$

The expression of $Q(f)Q(-f)$ can be expressed in terms of magnitude and phase as $Q(f)Q(-f) = |A(f)|e^{j\theta(f)}$, where the magnitude $|A(f)|$ can be expressed as $|A(f)| = \sqrt{\left[1 + \frac{f^2-f_c^2}{b^2}\right]^2 + \left[\frac{2f_c}{b}\right]^2}$ and $\theta(f) = \tan^{-1}\left[\frac{-2f_c/b}{1+\frac{f^2-f_c^2}{b^2}}\right]$. Hence, $P(f)P(-f)$ can be expressed as

$$P(f)P(-f) = \left[\left(1 + \frac{f^2-f_c^2}{b^2}\right)^2 + \left(\frac{2f_c}{b^2}\right)^2\right]^{-n/2} e^{j[2\varphi-n\theta(f)]} \qquad (29)$$

Taking the real part of $P(f)P(-f)$, we can write

$$Re[P(f)P(-f)] = \left[\left(1 + \frac{f^2 - f_c^2}{b^2}\right)^2 + \left(\frac{2f_c}{b^2}\right)^2\right]^{-n/2} \cos[2\varphi - n\theta(f)] \quad (30)$$

Substituting all the derived terms in (22) we write the final expression of the power spectrum as

$$|H(f)|^2 = k^2 \left\{ \left[\frac{1}{1 + \frac{(f-f_c)^2}{b^2}}\right]^n + \left[\frac{1}{1 + \frac{(f+f_c)^2}{b^2}}\right]^n + 2\left[\frac{1}{\sqrt{\left(1 + \frac{f^2 - f_c^2}{b^2}\right)^2 + \left(\frac{2f_c}{b}\right)^2}}\right]^n \cos[2\varphi - n\theta(f)] \right\} \quad (31)$$

$$= k^2 \left\{ \left[\frac{b^2}{b^2 + (f - f_c)^2}\right]^n + \left[\frac{b^2}{b^2 + (f + f_c)^2}\right]^n + 2\left[\frac{b}{\sqrt{(b^2 + f^2 - f_c^2)^2 + (2f_c b)^2}}\right]^n \cos[2\varphi - n\theta(f)] \right\} \quad (32)$$

The power spectrum, $|H(f)|^2$ is plotted in Figure 7 for varying f_c/b. Based on the expression of $|H(f)|^2$ in (32) and the plot in Figure 7, we can make the following observations:

Observation 5. *When b is small, h(t) will decay slowly; however, $|H(f)|^2$ will decay more rapidly.*

Observation 6. *Although $KP(f)$ and $KP^*(f)$ have their maximum at $\pm f_c$, the power spectrum $|H(f)|^2$ does not necessarily have a maximum at $\pm f_c$ Hz.*

Observation 7. *When $KP(f)$ and $KP^*(f)$ overlap significantly for small f_c/b, $|H(f)|^2$ has the character of a low pass filter with the peak at the origin.*

Observation 8. *As f_c/b is increased (for fixed order), the single peak splits and the maxima move outwards and eventually converges to $\pm f_c$.*

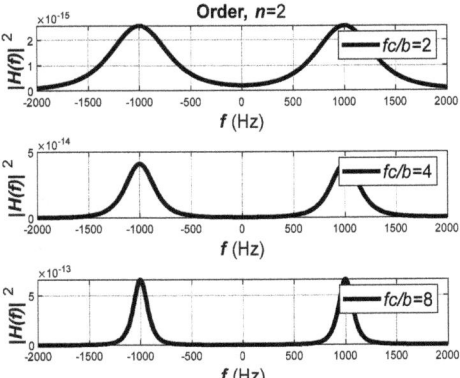

Figure 7. The plot of the power spectrum of the GTF, $|H(f)|^2$ with varying $\frac{f_c}{b}$ for $n = 2$. The plot shows that the power spectrum decays rapidly with a higher value of $\frac{f_c}{b}$. This faster decay reduces the interference between the frequency components of the GTF.

Since the purpose of the GTF in auditory modeling is to model a bandpass filter, the components $KP(f)$ and $KP^*(f)$ must be well separated, and it is required to make f_c/b large enough. In this case, we can simplify the expression of $H(f)$ as

$$H(f) = KP(f) \text{ when } f \geq 0 \quad (33)$$

$$= KP^*(-f) \text{ when } f < 0 \tag{34}$$

In addition, $P(f)P^*(-f) \approx 0$. The power spectrum expressed in (32) will be simplified as

$$|H(f)|^2 \approx k^2\left[|P(f)|^2\right] \text{ when } f \geq 0 \tag{35}$$

$$|H(f)|^2 \approx k^2\left\{\left[\frac{1}{1+\frac{(f-f_c)^2}{b^2}}\right]^n\right\} \text{ when } f \geq 0 \tag{36}$$

Similarly, we can find

$$|H(f)|^2 \approx k^2\left[|P^*(-f)|^2\right] \text{ when } f < 0 \tag{37}$$

$$|H(f)|^2 \approx k^2\left\{\left[\frac{1}{1+\frac{(f+f_c)^2}{b^2}}\right]^n\right\} \text{ when } f < 0 \tag{38}$$

For large f_c/b, the carrier phase φ does not have any effect on the maximum value of the power spectrum. For small f_c/b, the carrier phase φ influences where the maximum power spectrum occurs. Holdsworth shows that the optimum range of f_c/b should be $4 < f_c/b < 8$ for auditory modeling [15].

3. Equivalent Rectangular Bandwidth (ERB)

The ERB is a measure commonly used in psychoacoustics that approximates the bandwidth of the filters in human hearing. The ERB of a filter $H(f)$ is typically defined as the width of a rectangular filter whose height equals the maximum of the power spectrum of $H(f)$ and possesses the same amount of power. Based on this definition, the rectangular bandwidth H_{ERB} can be expressed as

$$H_{ERB} = \frac{\int_{-\infty}^{+\infty}|H(f)|^2 df}{2|H(f_0)|^2} \tag{39}$$

where $|H(f_0)|^2$ is the maximum value of the power spectrum, which occurs at $\pm f_0$. By using Perseval's theorem, the energy of a signal, $h(t)$, can be expressed as

$$E = \int_{-\infty}^{+\infty}|H(f)|^2 df = \int_{-\infty}^{+\infty}|h(t)|^2 dt \tag{40}$$

Hence, the expression of the rectangular bandwidth can be expressed as

$$H_{ERB} = \frac{\int_{-\infty}^{+\infty}|H(f)|^2 df}{2|H(f_0)|^2} = \frac{\int_{-\infty}^{+\infty}|h(t)|^2 dt}{2|H(f_0)|^2} \tag{41}$$

Let us assume $\check{h}(t) = |h(t)|^2$; hence, H_{ERB} can be expressed as

$$H_{ERB} = \frac{\int_{-\infty}^{+\infty}\check{h}(t) dt}{2|H(f_0)|^2} = \frac{\int_{-\infty}^{+\infty}|h(t)|^2 dt}{2|H(f_0)|^2} \tag{42}$$

From the definition of the Fourier transform of $\check{h}(t)$, we can write

$$\check{H}(f) = \int_{-\infty}^{+\infty}\check{h}(t)e^{-j2\pi ft} dt \tag{43}$$

The dc component of $\check{H}(f)$ can be found by substituting $f = 0$ in (43) and can be expressed as

$$\check{H}(0) = \int_{-\infty}^{+\infty} \check{h}(t)dt \qquad (44)$$

By substituting $\int_{-\infty}^{+\infty} \check{h}(t)dt$ by $\check{H}(0)$ in (39), we can find an alternative expression for the equivalent rectangular bandwidth, H_{ERB} as

$$H_{ERB} = \frac{\int_{-\infty}^{+\infty} |H(f)|^2 df}{2|H(f_0)|^2} = \frac{\int_{-\infty}^{+\infty} |h(t)|^2 dt}{2|H(f_0)|^2} = \frac{\check{H}(0)}{2|H(f_0)|^2} \qquad (45)$$

Squaring the (4), we can find the expression of $\check{h}(t)$ as

$$\check{h}(t) = [cr(t)s(t)]^2 \\ = c^2 r^2(t) s^2(t) \qquad (46)$$

This expression can be further simplified as

$$\check{h}(t) = c^2 \check{r}(t)\check{s}(t) \qquad (47)$$

where

$$\check{r}(t) = r^2(t) \\ = \left[t^{n-1} e^{-2\pi bt}\right]^2 \qquad (48) \\ = t^{2n-2} e^{-j4\pi bt} u(t)$$

and

$$\check{s}(t) = s^2(t) = \cos^2(2\pi f_c t + \varphi) \qquad (49)$$

By taking the Fourier transform of both sides of (47) and applying the convolution property of the Fourier transform, we can write

$$\check{H}(f) = c^2 \left[\check{R}(f) * \check{S}(f)\right] \qquad (50)$$

where $\check{R}(f)$ = Fourier transform of $\check{r}(t)$, and $\check{S}(f)$ = Fourier transform of $\check{s}(t)$. Now, we need to find the Fourier transform of $\check{r}(t)$ and $\check{s}(t)$ and substitute in (50). Applying the Fourier transform property $t^m e^{-at} u(t) \leftrightarrow m!(a + j2\pi f))^{-(m+1)}$. Substituting $m = 2n - 2$, and $a = 4\pi b$, we can find the $\check{r}(t) = t^{2n-2} e^{-4\pi bt} u(t) \leftrightarrow \check{R}(f) = (2n-2)!(4\pi b + j2\pi f)^{-(2n-1)}$. This expression can be further simplified as

$$\check{R}(f) = (2n-2)! \left[4\pi b \left(1 + j\frac{2\pi f}{4\pi b}\right)\right]^{-(2n-1)}$$

$$\check{R}(f) = (2n-2)!(4\pi b)^{-(2n-1)} \left[1 + j\frac{f}{2b}\right]^{-(2n-1)} \qquad (51)$$

Now, the expression of $\check{s}(t)$ can be simplified as

$$\check{s}(t) = \cos^2(2\pi f_c t + \varphi) \\ = \tfrac{1}{2}[1 + \cos(4\pi f_c t + 2\varphi)] \\ = \tfrac{1}{2} + \tfrac{1}{2}\left[\frac{e^{j(4\pi f_c t + 2\varphi)} + e^{-j(4\pi f_c t + 2\varphi)}}{2}\right] \\ = \tfrac{1}{2} + \frac{e^{j2\varphi}}{4} e^{j2(2\pi f_c t)} + \frac{e^{-j2\varphi}}{4} e^{-j2(2\pi f_c t)}$$

Taking the Fourier transform, we can express the Fourier transform of $š(t)$ as

$$\check{S}(f) = \frac{1}{2}\delta(f) + \frac{1}{4}e^{j2\varphi}\delta(f - 2f_c) + \frac{1}{4}e^{-j\varphi}\delta(f + 2f_c) \tag{52}$$

Substituting the value of $\check{R}(f)$ and $\check{S}(f)$ in (50), we find the expression of $\check{H}(f)$ as

$$\check{H}(f) = c^2(2n-2)!(4\pi b)^{-(2n-1)}\left[1+j\frac{f}{2b}\right]^{-(2n-1)} * \left[\frac{1}{2}\delta(f) + \frac{1}{4}e^{j2\varphi}\delta(f-2f_c) + \frac{1}{4}e^{-j2\varphi}\delta(f+2f_c)\right]$$

By using the convolution property of the delta dirac function, the above expression can be further simplified as

$$\check{H}(f) = c^2(2n-2)!(4\pi b)^{-(2n-1)}\left\{\left[\frac{1}{2}\left(1+j\frac{f}{2b}\right)\right]^{-(2n-1)} + \frac{1}{4}e^{j2\varphi}\left[1+j\frac{(f-2f_c)}{2b}\right]^{-(2n-1)}\right.$$
$$\left. + \frac{1}{4}e^{-j2\varphi}\left[1+j\frac{(f+2f_c)}{2b}\right]^{-(2n-1)}\right\} \tag{53}$$

By substituting $f = 0$, we can find the expression of $\check{H}(0)$ as

$$\check{H}(0) = c^2(2n-2)!(4\pi b)^{-(2n-1)}\left\{\begin{array}{l}\frac{1}{2} + \frac{1}{4}e^{j\varphi}\left[1-j\frac{f_c}{b}\right]^{-(2n-1)}\\ +\frac{1}{4}e^{-j\varphi}\left[1+j\frac{f_c}{b}\right]^{-(2n-1)}\end{array}\right\} \tag{54}$$

Let us assume $X = \frac{e^{j2\varphi}}{4}\left[1-j\frac{f_c}{b}\right]$ and $X^* = \frac{e^{-j2\varphi}}{4}\left[1+j\frac{f_c}{b}\right]$. We can express X as

$$X = \frac{e^{j2\varphi}}{4}\left[1-j\frac{f_c}{b}\right], \text{ substituting } \theta_1(f) = \tan^{-1}\left[-\frac{f_c}{b}\right]$$
$$= \frac{e^{j2\varphi}}{4}\left[\sqrt{1+\frac{f_c^2}{b^2}}\right]e^{\theta_1(f)} \tag{55}$$

$$= \frac{1}{4}\left[\sqrt{1+\frac{f_c^2}{b^2}}\right]e^{\theta_1(f)+j2\varphi}$$
$$= \frac{1}{4}\left[\sqrt{1+\frac{f_c^2}{b^2}}\right]e^{j[2\varphi+\theta_1(f)]} \tag{56}$$

Similarly, it can be proved that X^* can be expressed as

$$X^* = \frac{1}{4}\left[\sqrt{1+\frac{f_c^2}{b^2}}\right]e^{j[-2\varphi+\theta_2(f)]}$$

where $\theta_2(f) = \tan^{-1}\left[\frac{f_c}{b}\right]$. However, $\theta_2(f) = \pi - \theta_1(f)$. Hence, X^* can be expressed as

$$X^* = \frac{1}{4}\left[\sqrt{1+\frac{f_c^2}{b^2}}\right]e^{-j[2\varphi+\theta_1(f)]}$$

By using the complex variable identity $X^m + (X^*)^m = 2Re[X^m] = 2|X|^m\cos(m\theta)$. We can write the expression of $\check{H}(0)$ as

$$\check{H}(0) = c^2(2n-2)!(4\pi b)^{-(2n-1)}\left\{\begin{array}{l}\frac{2}{4}\left(1+\frac{f_c^2}{b^2}\right)^{-\frac{2n-1}{2}}\\ \cos[2\varphi-(2n-1)\theta_1(f)]+\frac{1}{2}\end{array}\right\} \tag{57}$$

Substituting $f = f_0$ in (32) we can find the expression of $|H(f_0)|^2$ as

$$|\vec{H}(f_0)|^2 = k^2 \left\{ \left[\frac{1}{1+\frac{(f_0-f_c)^2}{b^2}} \right]^n + \left[\frac{1}{1+\frac{(f_0+f_c)^2}{b^2}} \right]^n + 2 \left[\frac{1}{\sqrt{\left(1+\frac{f_0^2-f_c^2}{b^2}\right)^2 + \left(\frac{2f_c}{b}\right)^2}} \right]^n \cos[2\varphi - n\theta(f)] \right\} \quad (58)$$

Substituting $\check{H}(0)$ and $|H(f_{0)}|$ in (45), we can find the final expression of the H_{ERB} as

$$H_{ERB} = \frac{\check{H}(0)}{2|H(f_0)|^2} = \frac{c^2(2n-2)!(4\pi b)^{-(2n-1)} \left\{ \frac{2}{4}\left(1+\frac{f_c^2}{b^2}\right)^{-(2n-1)/2} \cos[2\varphi - (2n-1)\theta_1(f)] + \frac{1}{2} \right\}}{k^2 \left\{ \left[\frac{1}{1+\frac{(f_0-f_c)^2}{b^2}} \right]^n + \left[\frac{1}{1+\frac{(f_0+f_c)^2}{b^2}} \right]^n + 2 \left[\frac{1}{\sqrt{\left(1+\frac{f_0^2-f_c^2}{b^2}\right)^2 + \left(\frac{2f_c}{b}\right)^2}} \right]^n \cos[2\varphi - n\theta(f)] \right\}} \quad (59)$$

According to the definition of the H_{ERB}, we substitute $f_c = f_0$ in (59) and can find the final expression of H_{ERB} as

$$H_{ERB} = \frac{c^2(2n-2)!(4\pi b)^{-(2n-1)} \left\{ \frac{2}{4}\left(1+\frac{f_c^2}{b^2}\right)^{-(2n-1)/2} \cos[2\varphi - (2n-1)\theta_1(f)] + \frac{1}{2} \right\}}{2k^2 \left\{ 1 + \left[\frac{1}{1+\frac{(2f_c)^2}{b^2}} \right]^n + 2 \left[\frac{1}{\sqrt{1+\left(\frac{2f_c}{b}\right)^2}} \right]^n \cos[2\varphi - n\theta(f)] \right\}} \quad (60)$$

Defining two more design parameters η and μ as

$$\eta = \frac{c^2(2n-2)!(4\pi b)^{-(2n-1)}}{2k^2} \quad (61)$$

$$\mu = \frac{\left\{ \frac{2}{4}\left(1+\frac{f_c^2}{b^2}\right)^{-(2n-1)/2} \cos[2\varphi - (2n-1)\theta_1(f)] + \frac{1}{2} \right\}}{\left\{ 1 + \left[\frac{1}{1+\frac{(2f_c)^2}{b^2}} \right]^n + 2 \left[\frac{1}{\sqrt{1+\left(\frac{2f_c}{b}\right)^2}} \right]^n \cos[2\varphi - n\theta(f)] \right\}} \quad (62)$$

Substituting $k = \frac{c}{2}(n-1)!(2\pi b)^{-n}$ (61), we can find the final expression for η as

$$\eta = \frac{c^2(2n-2)!(4\pi b)^{-(2n-1)}}{2\left(\frac{c}{2}(n-1)!(2\pi b)^{-n}\right)^2}$$
$$= \frac{c^2(2n-2)!(4\pi b)^{-(2n-1)}}{2\frac{c^2}{2^2}[(n-1)!(2\pi b)]^2} \quad (63)$$
$$= \frac{(2n-2)!}{[(n-1)!]^2}(\pi b)2^{3-2n}$$

The variation in H_{ERB} with $\frac{f_0}{b}$ is plotted in Figure 8. The maximum value of μ is $1/2$ when $\frac{f_c}{b}$ is sufficiently large. With this value of μ, $H_{ERB} = \eta\mu$ becomes approximately

$$H_{ERB} \approx \eta/2$$

$$H_{ERB} \approx \frac{(2n-2)!(\pi b)2^{2-2n}}{[(n-1)!]^2} \quad (64)$$

Hence, H_{ERB} becomes proportional to b and independent of f_0. As mentioned above, the resonant frequencies along the basilar membrane vary from 20 Hz at the apex to

20,000 Hz at the base. Hence, it is essential to make the bandwidth of the filter independent of the carrier frequency, f_0. This makes the GTF a unique candidate for auditory modeling in cochlear implants.

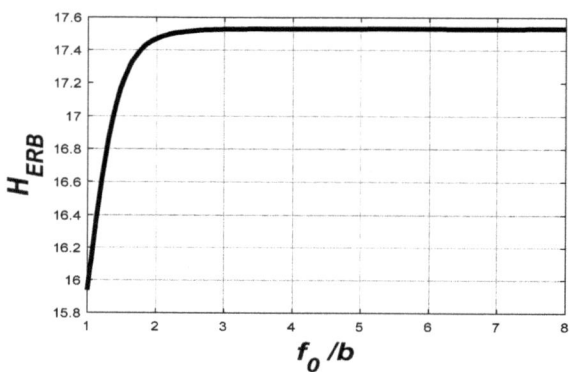

Figure 8. The variation in H_{ERB} with $\frac{f_0}{b}$. This figure shows that H_{ERB} remains independent of $\frac{f_0}{b}$, for $\frac{f_0}{b} > 3$, and $\mu \approx 1/2$.

4. Application of GTFs in Cochlear Implant Design

Almost 40 years ago, researchers initiated the restoration of normal hearing in deaf people via electrical stimulation of the auditory nerve [33]. Since then, they have been investigating different techniques for delivering electrical stimuli to the auditory nerve so that profoundly deaf people understand normal speech. Advances in signal processing largely contribute to the continuous and steady improvement of cochlear implant users. Several review papers on this topic have been published [34–37]. Recently, prosthetic devices [38–41], called cochlear implants [42,43], can be implanted in the inner ear to restore the partial hearing ability of profoundly deaf people. By using cochlear implants, some individuals can now communicate like normal people.

Initially, single-channel implants were tested in human subjects in the early 1970s [44–46]. Single-channel implants provide electrical stimulation at a single site in the cochlea using a single electrode. These implants are of interest because of their simplicity in design, as they do not require much hardware. The first experiments were discouraging as the patients reported unintelligible perception of speech. Later, related research works have been focused on multi-channel implants. Unlike single-channel implants, multi-channel implants provide electrical stimulation at multiple sites in the cochlea using an array of electrodes. An electrode array is used to stimulate different auditory nerve fibers at various places in the cochlea. Different electrodes are stimulated depending on the frequency of the signal. Electrodes near the base of the cochlea are stimulated with high-frequency signals, while electrodes near the apex are stimulated with low-frequency signals, as shown in Figure 2. In multi-channel cochlear implants, signal processing is the most important component [47], and a bank of bandpass filters is used to split the input sound signals into a set of parallel signals [47]. In this work, we are proposing to use GTFs instead.

To investigate the application of GTFs in cochlear implantation, a commercially available cochlear implant processor model called Clarion [33,42], as shown in Figure 9, is used in this work. The Clarion processor uses a microphone, worn at ear level, to capture the incoming sound. The sound is digitized and analyzed by a processor. The processor divides the signal into several channels based on frequency and translates the information in each channel into instructions that are transmitted to and control an implanted receiver that drives the implanted electrode array. The array of electrodes consists of 6–22 intra-cochlear electrodes distributed along the length of the cochlea. Stimuli delivered to an electrode preferentially excite the nerve fibers nearby.

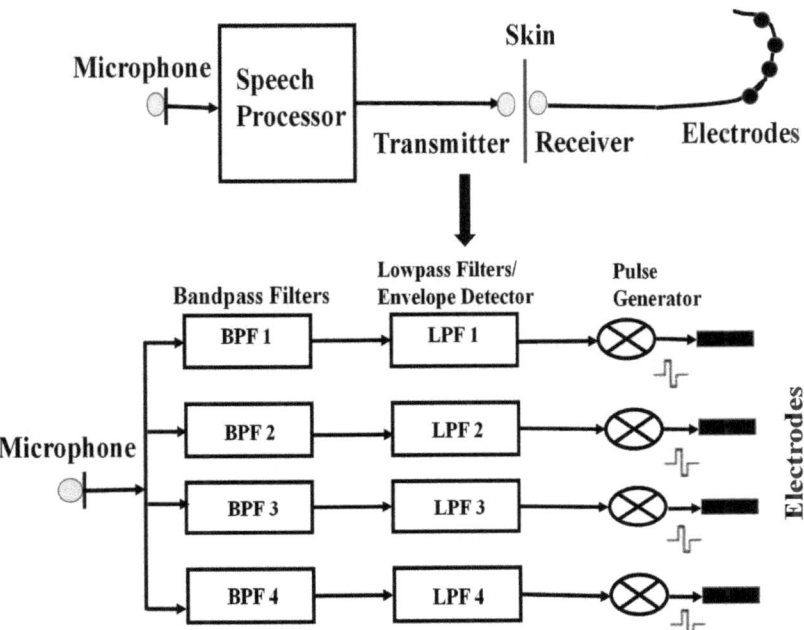

Figure 9. The signal processing steps in the Clarion processor. The main components of a cochlear implant are the microphone, speech processors and the electrodes. The speech processor consists of a bank of bandpass filters that split the incoming sounds into parallel components that are subsequently processed by a bank of lowpass filters. The pulse generator produces non-linearly mapped pulses to excite the electrodes.

The proposed model slightly varies from the Clarion processor. In the proposed model, the audio signal is first pre-emphasized [48] to boost the higher frequency components, as shown in Figure 10. The signal is then divided into channels by a set of GTFs instead of bandpass filters that are used in the Clarion processor. The main reason is that the bandpass filters do not represent the way the human auditory system responds to sounds. In addition, the hardware implementation of the bandpass filters is not as straightforward as the GTF. The next stage in the implant's processing is the extraction of the envelope of the signal from each channel. This is achieved by rectification and lowpass filtering. Full-wave rectification is used in this model. A dc component is introduced during the rectification methods, and the harmonics that typically fall above the Nyquist frequency are aliased to lower frequencies. The rectified signal is lowpass filtered using a 16th-order moving-average filter [49]. In a cochlear implant, the amplitude envelopes of each channel modulate a biphasic pulse train, which has a repetition rate of 800 to 4000 pulses per second (pps). Each modulated pulse train is delivered to a separate electrode, emulating the tonotopic arrangement of the cochlea. The GTFs are designed to cover a range of frequencies representing the basilar membrane [50–54]. In this work, these filters were designed based on the specifications mentioned in [21]. The center frequency and the bandwidth of these eight GTFs are listed in Table 1, and the magnitude spectrum of the GTF bank is shown in Figure 11. Those GTFs perform spectral analysis and convert an acoustic wave into a multichannel representation by mimicking the basilar membrane motion [55]. These GTFs have been designed in a way that $\frac{f_0}{b} = 4$, as mentioned above. The filter order n was set to 4.0. The shape of the magnitude characteristic of the GTFs with order 4 is very similar to that of the *roex* function [56] that is commonly used to represent the magnitude response of the human auditory filter [57].

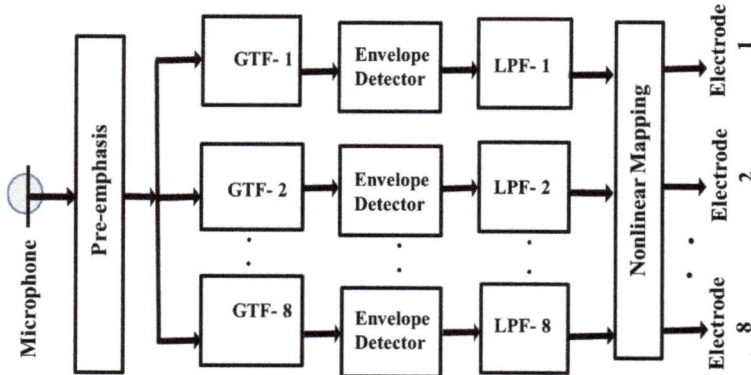

Figure 10. The proposed model uses GTF. The sound signal is pre-emphasized and is split into eight parallel signals by the GTF bank. The envelope detectors extract the signal envelops, which pass through the lowpass filter. Non-linear mapping is performed to reduce the interference among the electrodes.

Table 1. The center frequency and the bandwidth of the GTFs.

Bandwidth (Hz)	Center Frequency (Hz)
158	50
173	186
276	389
478	690
788	1139
1249	1807
1936	2802
2960	4282

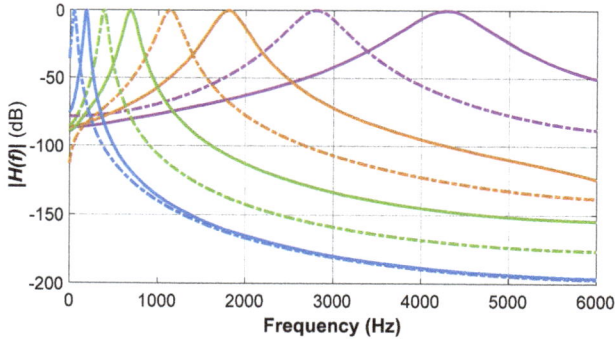

Figure 11. The magnitude spectrum of the GTF. The tuning frequencies and the bandwidth of the filters are determined by the specifications mentioned in Table 1. As depicted in this figure, the filter's bandwidth increases with the tuning frequency. The eight filters are identified with different colors and line styles.

5. Design Issues and Challenges

Despite the impressive ability of cochlear implants to improve sound audibility and speech understanding in profoundly deaf people, several significant challenges remain to address to maximize the benefits of this device. One major challenge is the substantial variability of audio perception among different gender groups, demographics, and ages. Research is still ongoing to correlate neural and cognitive function in cochlear implant users.

There is a need to devise simple assessment measures to evaluate the perceptional outcomes of cochlear implant users. Poorer frequency discrimination abilities and neural deficits resulting from long-term deafness pose extra challenges to audio perception for cochlear implant users [58,59]. Rather than a physiologic point of view, some technological issues also need future investigation. A healthy cochlea transmits temporal-frequency information of audible sounds through around 3000 inner hair cells, but an implanted version could deliver a degraded version of such information resulting from signal processing (e.g., signal compression, bandpass filtering, temporal envelope extraction) and only a small number (up to eight) of electrodes in this design. As mentioned above, the number of spectral channels used for most CI users is likely less than eight due to factors including channel interactions. Signal processing also removes delicate temporal structures that may hinder normal hearing regarding melody contents [60].

While cochlear implants have proven to be beneficial for many individuals with profound hearing loss, there are some potential drawbacks to consider:

Cost: The potential physiological design challenges mentioned above could make cochlear implants expensive, and the cost may not always be fully covered by insurance. This financial aspect can be a barrier for some individuals.

Surgical Risks: Though the implantation process involves a mild surgery, like any surgical procedure, there are inherent risks like infections, bleeding, and issues related to anesthesia.

Learning Curve: Adjusting to hearing with a cochlear implant requires time and effort. Some individuals may find the initial period challenging as they learn to interpret the new auditory signals.

Maintenance and Upkeep: Cochlear implants require ongoing maintenance, including regular checks and adjustments. The external components also need to be cared for to ensure optimal functioning.

It is essential for individuals considering cochlear implants to discuss these aspects with their healthcare providers and audiologists. Despite these considerations, many people with cochlear implants experience significant improvements in their ability to hear and communicate.

6. Conclusions

The design and optimization of GTFs are proposed for cochlear implants. The complex spectrum and equivalent rectangular bandwidth of GTFs have been derived and investigated. One of the key findings is that the frequency domain behavior of the GTF strongly depends on $\frac{f_c}{b}$. Additionally, the optimal choice of a design parameter, i.e., $f_c/b \geq 4$ could minimize the interferences of the filter frequency components. A smaller value of b can cause the power spectrum, $|H(f)|^2$ to decay faster and hence can reduce the interference of the filter output. It is concluded that the ERB of the GTF has a strong influence on b, and becomes independent of f_c for $f_c/b \geq 4$.

This research provides a theoretical and simulation-based analysis of GTFs to explore their applicability for cochlear implants. The details of the hardware implementation are yet to be investigated. The presented filter bank is designed with eight filters. However, the number of filters (and hence the number of electrodes) to optimize the cochlear implants is still an open issue. Reducing the interferences among the electrodes also needs future investigation.

Author Contributions: Conceptualization, analysis, mathematical modeling, simulation, and manuscript writing—R.I.; mathematical modeling, editing, and manuscript writing—M.T. All authors have read and agreed to the published version of the manuscript.

Funding: This research is partially funded by University of Science and Technology of Fujairah (USTF), Fujairah, UAE.

Data Availability Statement: Data are contained within the article.

Conflicts of Interest: The authors declare no conflict of interest.

Appendix A Properties of Fourier Transform

Operation	$x(t)$	$X(f)$
Time Convolution	$x(t) * y(t)$	$X(f)Y(f)$
Multiplication by t	$t^m x(t)$	$(-j2\pi)^{-m} \frac{d^m}{df^m} X(f)$
Modulation	$x(t)\cos 2\pi f_0 t$	$0.5 X(f - f_0) + 0.5 X(f + f_0)$
Frequency Convolution	$x(t)y(t)$	$X(f)Y(f)$
Time Shifting	$x(t - t_0)$	$X(f) e^{-j2\pi f t_0}$
Frequency Shifting	$x(t) e^{j2\pi f_0 t}$	$X(f - f_0)$

Appendix B Short Table of Fourier Transform

$x(t)$	$X(f)$
$e^{-a(t)} u(t)$	$\frac{1}{a + j2\pi f}$
$e^{j2\pi f_0 t}$	$\delta(f - f_0)$
$e^{-j2\pi f_0 t}$	$\delta(f + f_0)$
$\cos 2\pi f_0 t$	$0.5\delta(f - f_0) + 0.5\delta(f + f_0)$
$\cos(2\pi f_0 t + \varphi)$	$0.5 e^{j\varphi} \delta(f - f_0) + 0.5 e^{-j\varphi} \delta(f - f_0)$

Appendix C Some Important Formulae

$$X(f) = \int_{-\infty}^{+\infty} x(t) e^{-j2\pi f t} dt$$

$$x(t) = \int_{-\infty}^{+\infty} X(f) e^{+j2\pi f t} df$$

$$x(t) * \delta(t - t_0) = x(t - t_0)$$

$$E = \int_{-\infty}^{+\infty} |x(t)|^2 dt = \int_{-\infty}^{+\infty} |X(f)|^2 df$$

$$X(f) X(f)^* = |X(f)|^2$$

References

1. Rabiner, L.R.; Schafer, R.W. Auditory, and Speech Perception. In *Theory and Applications of Digital Speech Processing*, 1st ed.; Prentice-Hall: Upper Saddle River, NJ, USA, 2011; pp. 138–145.
2. Chittka, L.; Brockmann, A. Perception Space—The Final Frontier. *PLoS Biol.* **2015**, *3*, 564–568. [CrossRef]
3. Quateri, T.E. Production and Classification of Speech Sounds. In *Discrete-Time Speech Signal Processing: Principles and Practices*; Prentice-Hall: Upper Saddle River, NJ, USA, 2001; pp. 72–76.
4. Islam, R.; Abdel-Raheem, E.; Tarique, M. A Novel Pathological Voice Identification Technique through Simulated Cochlear Implant Processing Systems. *Appl. Sci.* **2022**, *12*, 2398. [CrossRef]
5. Hinojosa, R.; Marion, M. Histopathology of profound sensorineural deafness. *Ann. N. Y. Acad. Sci.* **1983**, *405*, 459–484. [CrossRef]
6. Blackwell, D.L.; Lucas, J.W.; Clarke, T.C. *Summary Health Statistics for US Adults: National Health Interview Survey*; Vital and Health Statistics, Series: 10; Number 260; National Health Survey; National Library of Medicine: Bethesda, MD, USA, 2014; pp. 1–161.
7. Wagner, E.L.; Shin, J.B. Mechanisms of Hair Cell Damage and Repair. *Trends Neurosci.* **2019**, *42*, 414–424. [CrossRef]
8. Taiber, S.; Cohen, R.; Yizhar-Barnea, O.; Sprinzak, D.; Holt, J.R.; Avraham, K.B. Neonatal AAV gene therapy rescues hearing in a mouse model of SYNE4 deafness. *EMBO Mol. Med.* **2021**, *13*, e13259. [CrossRef] [PubMed]
9. Antje, H.; Helen, H.; Melanie, A.F. The relationship of speech intelligibility with hearing sensitivity, cognition, and perceived hearing difficulties varies for different speech perception tests. *Front. Psychol.* **2015**, *6*, 782. [CrossRef]
10. Islam, R.; Tarique, M.; Abdel-Raheem, E. A Survey on Signal Processing Based Pathological Voice Detection Techniques. *IEEE Access* **2020**, *8*, 66749–66776. [CrossRef]
11. Islam, R.; Tarique, M. A novel convolutional neural network based dysphonic voice detection algorithm using chromagram. *Int. J. Electr. Comput. Eng.* **2022**, *12*, 5511–5518. [CrossRef]

12. Islam, R.; Abdel-Raheem, E.; Tarique, M. A study of using cough sounds and deep neural networks for the early detection of COVID-19. *Biomedical. Eng. Adv.* **2022**, *3*, 100025. [CrossRef] [PubMed]
13. Islam, R.; Abdel-Raheem, E.; Tarique, M. Voiced Features and Artificial Neural Networks to Diagnose Parkinson's Disease Patients. In Proceedings of the International Conference on Electrical and Computing Technologies and Applications, Ras Al Khaimah, UAE, 23–25 November 2022; pp. 132–136. [CrossRef]
14. Patterson, R.D.; Moore, B.J.C. Auditory filters and excitation patterns as representations of frequency resolution. In *Frequency Selectivity in Hearing*; Moore, B.C.J., Ed.; Academic Press: Cambridge, MA, USA, 1986; pp. 123–177.
15. Boer, E.D.; Kuyper, P. Triggered Correlation. *IEEE Trans. Biomed. Eng.* **1968**, *BME-15*, 169–179. [CrossRef]
16. Johannesma, P.I.M. The pre-response stimulus ensemble of neurons in the cochlear nucleus. In Proceedings of the Symposium on Hearing Theory, Eindhoven, The Netherlands, 22–23 June 1972; pp. 58–69.
17. Boer, E.D.; Jongh, H.R.D. On cochlear encoding: Potentialities and limitations of the reverse-correlation technique. *J. Acoust. Soc. Am.* **1978**, *63*, 115–135. [CrossRef] [PubMed]
18. Boer, E.D.; Kruidenier, C. On ringing limits of the auditory periphery. *Biol. Cybern.* **1990**, *63*, 433–442. [CrossRef] [PubMed]
19. Holdsworth, J.; Patterson, R.; Nimmo-Smith, I.; Rice, P. Implementing a Gammatone Filter Bank. In *SVOS Final Report Part A: The Auditory Filterbank*; MRC Applied Psychology Unit: Cambridge, UK, 1988.
20. Patterson, R.; Nimmo-Smith, I.; Holdsworth, J.; Rice, P. The Auditory Filterbank. In *SVOS Final Report. Part A*: MRC Applied Psychology Unit: Cambridge, UK, 1988.
21. Qi, J.; Wang, D.; Jiang, Y.; Liu, R. Auditory features based on Gammatone filters for robust speech recognition. In Proceedings of the IEEE International Symposium on Circuits and Systems (ISCAS), Beijing, China, 19–23 May 2013; pp. 305–308. [CrossRef]
22. Cai, X.; Ko, S. Development of Parametric Filter Banks for Sound Feature Extraction. *IEEE Access* **2023**, *11*, 109856–109867. [CrossRef]
23. Jacome, K.G.R.; Grijalva, F.L.; Masiero, B.S. Sound Events Localization and Detection Using Bio-Inspired Gammatone Filters and Temporal Convolutional Neural Networks. *IEEE/ACM Trans. Audio Speech Lang. Process.* **2023**, *31*, 2314–2324. [CrossRef]
24. Sharan, R.V.; Moir, T.J. Subband Time-Frequency Image Texture Features for Robust Audio Surveillance. *IEEE Trans. Inf. Secur.* **2015**, *10*, 2605–2615. [CrossRef]
25. Park, H.; Yoo, C.D. CNN-Based Learnable Gammatone Filterbank and Equal-Loudness Normalization for Environmental Sound Classification. *IEEE Signal Process. Lett.* **2020**, *27*, 411–415. [CrossRef]
26. Salehi, H.; Suelzle, D.; Folkeard, P.; Parsa, V. Learning-Based Reference-Free Speech Quality Measures for Hearing Aid Applications. *IEEE/ACM Trans. Audio Speech Lang. Process.* **2018**, *26*, 2277–2288. [CrossRef]
27. Zhao, X.; Shao, Y.; Wang, D. CASA-Based Robust Speaker Identification. *IEEE Trans. Audio Speech Lang. Process.* **2012**, *20*, 1608–1616. [CrossRef]
28. Cosentino, S.; Falk, T.H.; McAlpine, D.; Marquardt, T. Cochlear Implant Filterbank Design and Optimization: A Simulation Study. *IEEE/ACM Trans. Audio Speech Lang. Process.* **2014**, *22*, 347–353. [CrossRef]
29. Darling, A.M. Properties and Implementation of Gammatone Filters: A Tutorial. Available online: https://www.phon.ucl.ac.uk/home/shl5/Darling1991-GammatoneFilter.pdf (accessed on 4 March 2023).
30. Flanagan, J.L. Models for approximating basilar membrane displacement. *Bell Syst. Tech. J.* **1960**, *39*, 1163–1191. [CrossRef]
31. Boer, E.D. On the Principle of Specific Coding—A System Analysis of the Inner Ear Mechanism. In Proceedings of the International Federation of Automatic Control, Genova, Italy, 4–8 June 1973; Volume 6, pp. 187–194. [CrossRef]
32. Aertsen, A.M.H.J.; Johannesma, P.I.M.; Hermes, D.J. Spectro-temporal receptive fields of auditory neurons in the grass frog. *Biol. Cybern.* **1980**, *38*, 235–248. [CrossRef]
33. Dau, T.; Püschel, D.; Kohlrausch, A. A quantitative model of the effective signal processing in the auditory system. I. Model structure. *J. Acoust. Soc. Am.* **1996**, *99*, 3615–3622. [CrossRef]
34. Zeng, F.G. Trends in cochlear implants. *Trends Amplif.* **2004**, *8*, 1–34. [CrossRef]
35. Loizou, P.C. Signal-processing techniques for cochlear implants. *IEEE Eng. Med. Biol. Mag.* **1999**, *18*, 34–46. [CrossRef] [PubMed]
36. Rubinstein, J.T. How cochlear implants encode speech. *Curr. Opin. Otolaryngol. Head Neck Surg.* **2004**, *12*, 444–448. [CrossRef] [PubMed]
37. Ay, S.U.; Zeng, F.G.; Sheu, B.J. Hearing with bionic ears [cochlear implant devices]. *IEEE Circuits Devices Mag.* **1997**, *13*, 18–23. [CrossRef]
38. Loeb, G. Cochlear prosthetics. *Annu. Rev. Neurosci.* **1990**, *13*, 357–371. [CrossRef] [PubMed]
39. Millar, J.; Tong, Y.; Clark, G. Speech processing for cochlear implant prostheses. *J. Speech Hear. Res.* **1984**, *27*, 280–296. [CrossRef] [PubMed]
40. Parkins, C.; Anderson, S. *Cochlear Prostheses: An International Symposium*; New York Academy of Sciences: New York, NY, USA, 1983.
41. Loizau, P.C. Mimicking the Human Ear. *IEEE Signal Process. Mag.* **1998**, *15*, 101–130. [CrossRef]
42. Schindler, R.; Icessler, D. Preliminary results with the Clarion cochlear implant. *Laryngoscope* **1992**, *102*, 1006–1013. [CrossRef]
43. Kessler, D.; Schindler, R. Progress with a multi-strategy cochlear implant system: The Clarion. In *Advances in Cochlear Implants*; Hochmair-Desoyer, I., Hochmair, E., Eds.; Manz: Vienna, Austria, 1994; pp. 354–362.
44. House, W. A personal perspective on cochlear implants. In *Cochlear Implants*; Schindler, R., Merzenich, M., Eds.; Raven Press: New York, NY, USA, 1985; pp. 13–16.

45. House, W.; Urban, J. Long-term results of electrode implantation and electronic stimulation of the cochlea in man. *Ann. Otol. Rhinol. Laryngol.* **1973**, *82*, 504–517. [CrossRef] [PubMed]
46. House, W.; Berliner, K. Cochlear implants: Progress and perspectives. *Ann. Otol. Rhinol. Laryngol.* **1982**, *295* (Suppl. 91), 1–124.
47. Loizou, P.C.; Dorman, M.; Tu, Z. On the number of channels needed to understand speech. *J. Acoust. Soc. Am.* **1999**, *106*, 2097–2103. [CrossRef] [PubMed]
48. Bäckström, T. Introduction to Speech Processing: Pre-Emphasis. Available online: https://speechprocessingbook.aalto.fi/Preprocessing/Pre-emphasis.html (accessed on 26 January 2024).
49. Oppenheim, A.V.; Schafer, R.W. Digital Filter Design Techniques. In *Digital Signal Processing*; Prentice Hall: Upper Saddle River, NJ, USA, 1975; pp. 239–250.
50. Dau, T.; Püschel, D.; Kohlrausch, A. A quantitative model of the effective signal processing in the auditory system. II. Simulations and measurements. *J. Acoust. Soc. Am.* **1996**, *99*, 3623–3631. [CrossRef] [PubMed]
51. Patterson, R. Auditory images: How complex sounds are represented in the auditory system. *Acoust. Sci. Technol.* **2000**, *21*, 183–190. [CrossRef]
52. Cooke, M. A glimpsing model of speech perception in noise. *J. Acoust. Soc. Am.* **2006**, *119*, 1562–1573. [CrossRef] [PubMed]
53. Kubin, G.; Kleijn, W.B. Multiple-description coding (MDC) of speech with an invertible auditory model. In Proceedings of the IEEE Workshop on Speech Coding Proceedings, Model, Coders, and Error Criteria (Cat. No.99EX351), Porvoo, Finland, 20–23 June 1999; pp. 81–83. [CrossRef]
54. Kubin, G.; Kleijn, W.B. On speech coding in a perceptual domain. In Proceedings of the IEEE International Conference on Acoustics, Speech, and Signal Processing, Phoenix, AZ, USA, 15–19 March 1999; pp. 205–208. [CrossRef]
55. Patterson, R.D.; Holdsworth, J.A. A functional model of neural activity patterns and auditory image. *Adv. Speech Hear. Lang. Process.* **2004**, *3*, 547–563.
56. Unoki, M.; Irino, T.; Glasberg, B.; Moore, B.C.; Patterson, R.D. Comparison of the roex and gammachirp filters as representations of the auditory filter. *J. Acoust. Soc. Am.* **2006**, *120*, 1474–1492. [CrossRef]
57. Schofield, D. *Visualizations of the Speech Based on a Model of the Peripheral Auditory System*; NPL Report DITC 62/85; National Physical Laboratory: Teddington, UK, 1985.
58. Zhang, F.; Underwood, G.; McGuire, K.; Liang, C.; Moore, D.R.; Fu, Q.-J. Frequency Change Detection and Speech Perception in Cochlear Implant Users. *Hear. Res.* **2019**, *379*, 12–20. [CrossRef]
59. Medscape General Medicine. Hearing Loss: Does Gender Play a Role? Available online: https://www.medscape.com/viewarticle/719262_6?form=fpf (accessed on 21 January 2024).
60. Reich, R.D. Instrument Identification through a Simulated Cochlear Implant Processing System. Master's Thesis, Massachusetts Institute of Technology, Cambridge, MA, USA, 2012.

Disclaimer/Publisher's Note: The statements, opinions and data contained in all publications are solely those of the individual author(s) and contributor(s) and not of MDPI and/or the editor(s). MDPI and/or the editor(s) disclaim responsibility for any injury to people or property resulting from any ideas, methods, instructions or products referred to in the content.

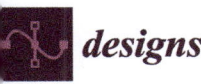 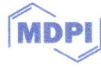

Article

Attention-Based DenseNet for Lung Cancer Classification Using CT Scan and Histopathological Images

Jia Uddin

AI and Big Data Department, Endicott College, Woosong University, Daejeon 3400, Republic of Korea; jia.uddin@wsu.ac.kr

Abstract: Lung cancer is identified by the uncontrolled proliferation of cells in lung tissues. The timely detection of malignant cells in the lungs, crucial for processes such as oxygen provision and carbon dioxide elimination in the human body, is imperative. The application of deep learning for discerning lymph node involvement in CT scans and histopathological images has garnered widespread attention due to its potential impact on patient diagnosis and treatment. This paper suggests employing DenseNet for lung cancer detection, leveraging its ability to transmit learned features backward through each layer continuously. This characteristic not only reduces model parameters but also enhances the learning of local features, facilitating a better comprehension of the structural complexity and uneven distribution in CT scans and histopathological cancer images. Furthermore, DenseNet accompanied by an attention mechanism (ATT-DenseNet) allows the model to focus on specific parts of an image, giving more weight to relevant regions. Compared to existing algorithms, the ATT-DenseNet demonstrates a remarkable enhancement in accuracy, precision, recall, and the F1-Score. It achieves an average improvement of 20% in accuracy, 19.66% in precision, 24.33% in recall, and 22.33% in the F1-Score across these metrics. The motivation behind the research is to leverage deep learning technologies to enhance the precision and reliability of lung cancer diagnostics, thus addressing the gap in early detection and treatment. This pursuit is driven by the potential of deep learning models, like DenseNet, to provide significant improvements in analyzing complex medical images for better clinical outcomes.

Keywords: lung cancer detection; DenseNet; attention mechanism; CT scans; histopathological images

Citation: Uddin, J. Attention-Based DenseNet for Lung Cancer Classification Using CT Scan and Histopathological Images. *Designs* **2024**, *8*, 27. https://doi.org/10.3390/designs8020027

Academic Editor: Richard Drevet and Hicham Benhayoune

Received: 9 January 2024
Revised: 11 March 2024
Accepted: 13 March 2024
Published: 18 March 2024

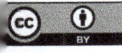

Copyright: © 2024 by the author. Licensee MDPI, Basel, Switzerland. This article is an open access article distributed under the terms and conditions of the Creative Commons Attribution (CC BY) license (https://creativecommons.org/licenses/by/4.0/).

1. Introduction

Cancer has long been acknowledged as a perilous disease with the potential for fatal outcomes. Lung cancer, a prevalent malignancy globally, stands out as a significant contributor to cancer-related mortality in both developed and developing nations. The majority of cases involve non-small-cell lung cancer (NSCLC), boasting a modest 5-year mortality rate of only 18%. Despite notable advancements in medical science leading to increased overall cancer survival rates, such progress is less pronounced in lung cancer due to the prevalence of advanced-stage cases among patients [1]. Cancer cells typically migrate from the lungs to the lymph glands and then enter the bloodstream, with natural lymph flow directing the spread toward the chest's center. Timely identification becomes crucial to preventing metastasis if the cancer spreads to other organs. Late-stage lesions are commonly treated with nonsurgical approaches like radiation, chemotherapy, surgical intervention, or monoclonal antibodies. This underscores the pivotal role of follow-up radiography in monitoring treatment response and tracking temporal changes in tumor radiography [2]. Cancer analysis is usually conducted in a pathological laboratory using various methods. Microscopic examinations, including biopsies, and electronic modalities such as CT scans, ultrasound, and others are employed to examine cancerous tissue. Among these, the CT scan is the most commonly utilized pathological test and is highly favored for diagnosis. This imaging technique captures high-resolution, high-contrast images of the lungs from different perspectives, offering a three-dimensional assessment of the lesion.

Recent studies have introduced predictive algorithms that leverage the differential expression of genes to categorize lung cancer patients according to different health outcomes, including the likelihood of relapse and overall survival rates. Previous research has underscored the importance of biomarkers in treating non-small-cell lung cancer (NSCLC). The emergence of artificial intelligence (AI) has facilitated the quantitative evaluation of radiographic tumor features, an approach referred to as "radiomics" [3]. Evidence from numerous studies suggests that non-invasive characterization of tumor features through radiomics offers enhanced predictive accuracy over traditional clinical evaluations.

Since the mid-19th century, pathologists have depended on traditional microscopy and glass slides to make precise diagnoses. This standard method requires pathologists to examine numerous glass slides by hand, a process that is both slow and requires significant effort. The advent of slide-scanning technology, which creates digital slides, has ushered classical pathology into a digital era, presenting various advantages for histopathology [4]. A key benefit is the use of computer simulations, like automated image analysis, which aids medical professionals in examining and quantitatively evaluating slides. This advancement aims to reduce the duration of manual examinations and improve the accuracy, consistency, and efficiency of pathologists' workflows. The employment of deep learning techniques for diagnostic support has recently sparked significant interest in histopathology.

In a clinical context, lung cancer CT scan images and normal lung images exhibit distinct characteristics that are crucial for accurate diagnosis. Radiologists analyze these images to identify potential abnormalities and distinguish between healthy and diseased lung tissue. For example, in CT scans, tumors or masses associated with lung cancer typically appear as areas of increased density on CT scans. They may be present as irregular, solid nodules or masses with varying degrees of density. However, normal lung tissue appears as a relatively homogenous pattern of lower density on CT scans. The texture is generally uniform, with no significant irregularities or masses.

For the effective classification of cancer and the selection of appropriate treatment options, a detailed analysis of lymph glands is crucial. Assessing multiple levels of lymph nodes is key for accurate prognosis and staging, which requires a thorough evaluation of lymph node condition [5]. Recently, histopathological images have been identified as reliable indicators of various treatment biomarkers. However, the manual review of numerous slides is a demanding and time-consuming task for pathologists, who are prone to errors due to the challenge of remembering which sections have already been reviewed. Various solutions introduced in this field have been shown to outperform pathologists in terms of identifying micro-metastases with greater accuracy, especially under the pressure of a busy schedule. Similarly, in lung cancer, the presence of primary tumor metastases plays a crucial role in determining the stage of cancer, treatment possibilities, and patient outcomes, just as it does in breast cancer [6].

DenseNet (Densely Connected Convolutional Networks) is a deep learning architecture [7] that has demonstrated effectiveness in various image-related tasks, including medical image analysis. Its unique structure and characteristics contribute to its success in handling medical CT scans and histopathology images for cancer detection. The combination of DenseNet architecture with a Squeeze-and-Excitation (SE) block [8], particularly for channel attention, enhances the model's capabilities for medical image analysis. The SE block enhances DenseNet by introducing channel-wise attention. This allows the model to assign different levels of importance to different channels (features) in the intermediate representations. In medical images, where certain features or channels are more informative for detecting specific patterns associated with cancer, channel attention helps to focus on relevant information. Based on this idea, to surpass the accuracy levels of the existing deep-learning-based lung cancer detection methods, we propose an attention-based DenseNet (ATT-DenseNet) for lung cancer detection using CT scan images and histopathological images. We consider three baseline deep learning algorithms. First, we compare the performance of the proposed method with DenseNet having no attention mechanism. Then, we compare it with AlexNet [9] followed by SqueezeNet [10]. ATT-DenseNet outperforms these two baseline deep learning architectures by achieving increased accuracy and an increased F1-score. The novelty of this work as inspired by [11] is summarized as follows:

- We introduce the SE feature channel attention block into DenseNet architecture. This strategic incorporation aims to accentuate cancer-relevant information within the feature map. By dynamically recalibrating feature responses, our enhancement ensures greater emphasis on regions pertinent to cancer, thereby amplifying their significance in the overall analysis.
- The network's ability is enhanced to focus on crucial features by substituting average pooling with max pooling in the third transition layer. This modification strategically places additional emphasis on important regions during the analysis, improving the model's capacity to capture relevant patterns associated with lung cancer.
- Drawing inspiration from [11], we implement an efficient method to prevent neuron deaths during model training. By addressing this challenge proactively, our methodology ensures the stability and robustness of the deep learning framework, leading to improved performance in lung cancer detection tasks.
- Sophisticated data augmentation techniques are employed, including rotation, scaling, and horizontal flipping, to preprocess both CT scan images [12] and histopathological images [13]. Furthermore, normalization of the dataset is performed to maintain appropriate pixel value ranges, thereby preventing potential distortions caused by excessively high or low values. These preprocessing steps are crucial for enhancing the model's ability to generalize across diverse datasets and improve overall performance.
- In contrast with other algorithms, the ATT-DenseNet shows a notable boost in accuracy, precision, recall, and the F1-Score. It attains an average increase of 20% in accuracy, 19.66% in precision, 24.33% in recall, and 22.33% in the F1-Score across these performance measures.

In summary, the methodology represents a comprehensive and innovative approach to lung cancer detection, incorporating cutting-edge techniques in deep learning, strategic architectural enhancements, and meticulous data preprocessing strategies. By addressing key challenges and leveraging the latest advancements in the field, we aim to significantly improve the accuracy and reliability of lung cancer diagnosis, ultimately contributing to advancements in healthcare and patient outcomes.

The structure of the remainder of this paper is organized as follows: Section 2 delves into related works, offering a concise review of current methodologies for detecting lung cancer. Following this, Section 3 thoroughly describes the methodology employed, including details of the dataset used, the DenseNet architecture, and the implementation of the attention block. Section 4 presents the experimental outcomes, showcasing a performance comparison with leading deep learning architectures currently considered state of the art. Finally, Section 5 concludes the paper.

2. Related Works

Machine learning algorithms have changed the research paradigm in the whole community of researchers starting from image processing [14] and network optimization [15,16] to healthcare applications. Lung cancer refers to the formation of malignant cells in the lungs, leading to an overall rise in mortality rates for both men and women due to the increasing incidence of cancer. The disease involves the rapid multiplication of cells in the lungs. While lung cancer cannot be completely eliminated, it can be mitigated [17]. The incidence of lung cancer is directly proportional to the number of individuals who engage in continuous smoking. Various classification approaches, including Naive Bayes, SVM, decision tree, and logistic regression, have been employed to assess the treatment of lung cancer.

2.1. Lung Cancer Detection Using CT Scan Images

Pradhan et al. [18] conducted a comprehensive evaluation of various machine learning approaches for the detection of lung cancer via IoT devices. This study included an extensive review of around 65 publications that applied machine learning algorithms for the prediction of different diseases. The objective was to investigate a variety of machine learning strategies for diagnosing a wide range of diseases, particularly focusing on uncovering existing deficiencies in lung cancer detection when integrated with medical IoT technology.

Bhatia et al. [19] utilized deep residual learning for lung cancer detection from CT scans, implementing a series of preprocessing techniques with the help of UNet and ResNet algorithms. These techniques were designed to accentuate areas within the lungs that are susceptible to cancer and to extract pertinent features from the scans. The features thus extracted were fed into several classifiers, such as Adaboost and Random Forest, to make individual predictions. These predictions from the classifiers were then aggregated to determine the probability of a CT scan showing signs of cancer.

Shin et al. [20] applied deep learning methods to study the properties of cell exosomes and to find parallels in human plasma extracellular vesicles. Their deep learning classifier, tested on exosome Surface-Enhanced Raman Scattering (SERS) data from both normal and lung cancer cell lines, attained a classification accuracy of 95%. Across a sample of 43 patients, this algorithm found that 90.7% of the plasma exosomes from patients were more similar to those of lung cancer cells than to those from healthy controls. This sample included individuals diagnosed with stage I and II lung cancer.

A model for detecting lung cancer that utilizes image analysis and machine learning has been crafted to discern the presence of lung cancer via CT scans and blood tests [21]. Although CT scan results are generally more effective than mammograms in identifying lung cancer, patient CT images are often classified simply into normal and abnormal categories [22,23]. It is important to note that among patients with non-small-cell lung cancer (NSCLC) who are at the same stage of tumor development, there is a significant variability in clinical outcomes and performance.

Lakshmanaprabhu et al. [24] presented a groundbreaking automatic diagnosis categorization system specifically designed for lung CT scans in their study. This system processes lung CT images utilizing a combination of the Optimal Deep Neural Network (ODNN) and Linear Discriminant Analysis (LDA) techniques.

2.2. Lung Cancer Detection Using Histopathological Images

A deep learning network, integrated with a tumor cell and metastatic staging system, was used to evaluate the reliability of personalized treatment recommendations generated by the deep learning preservation neural network. The effectiveness of the model was assessed using C statistics. The longevity predictions and treatment strategies produced by the computational intelligence survival neural network model were made accessible through the development of a user interface [25].

Ardila et al. [26] introduced a novel system aimed at predicting the risk of lung cancer by analyzing both historical and current computerized tomography (CT) dimensions of a patient.

The primary inspiration for our research comes from [27], where the authors introduced a classification method for cancer detection based on Convolutional Neural Networks (CNNs). However, we contend that employing a more sophisticated deep learning architecture, which includes an attention block, can more effectively discern image features, thereby enhancing the accuracy of cancer detection. Consequently, we introduce ATT-DenseNet as a novel approach for detecting cancer using CT scans and histopathological images, with this achieving superior accuracy compared to the CNN baselines previously considered.

Saric et al. introduce an entirely automated technique for detecting lung cancer in comprehensive slide images of lung tissue samples [28]. The classification process operates at the image patch level, employing CNNs. The study involves training two CNN architectures, namely VGG and ResNet, and subsequently comparing their performance. The findings indicate that the CNN-based methodology exhibits promise in supporting pathologists during lung cancer diagnosis.

Shahid et al. utilized a large dataset of lung and colon histopathology images, equally divided into five classes, for training and validation [29]. They fine-tuned a pretrained AlexNet by modifying four layers and achieved an initial accuracy of 89%. To enhance accuracy while maintaining computational efficiency, they applied a contrast enhancement technique to images in the underperforming class. This improved overall accuracy to 98.4%.

Yang et al. explore deep learning models' potential in identifying lung cancer subtypes and mimics from digital whole slide images (WSIs) [30]. A novel threshold-based approach is proposed for label inference of WSIs with complex tissue components.

3. Materials and Methods

In this section, we first talk about the datasets that we use for lung cancer detection, consisting of chest CT scan images and histopathological images. Next, we discuss some details about the channel attention squeeze and excitation block, which we refer to as an SE block throughout this paper. Lastly, details regarding the DenseNet architecture are presented at the end of this section.

3.1. Dataset Description

The dataset contains 15,000 histopathological images, each with dimensions of 768 × 768 pixels and stored in a JPEG format. These images come from a source that is compliant with HIPAA regulations and has been validated for accuracy. Initially, the collection included 750 images of lung tissue, which was equally divided among 250 images of benign lung tissue, 250 images of lung adenocarcinomas, and 250 images of lung squamous cell carcinomas.

- Lung benign tissue;
- Lung adenocarcinoma;
- Lung squamous cell carcinoma.

Figure 1 presents samples associated with these three classes.

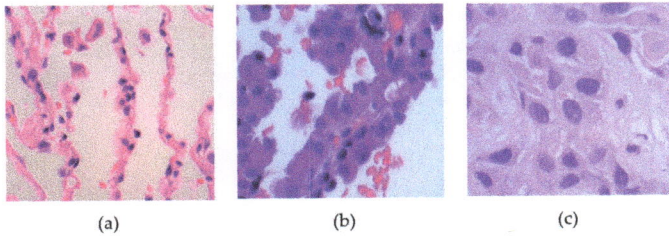

(a)   (b)   (c)

Figure 1. Histopathological images for lung cancer detection: (**a**) lung benign tissue, (**b**) adenocarcinoma, (**c**) squamous cell carcinoma.

For the chest CT scan images, we consider three classes of cancer and a normal class. Among the cancer classes, there are three types: adenocarcinoma, large-cell carcinoma, and squamous cell carcinoma. A total of 340 images for each class including the normal class have been used for training and testing. Figure 2 presents sample images from these classes.

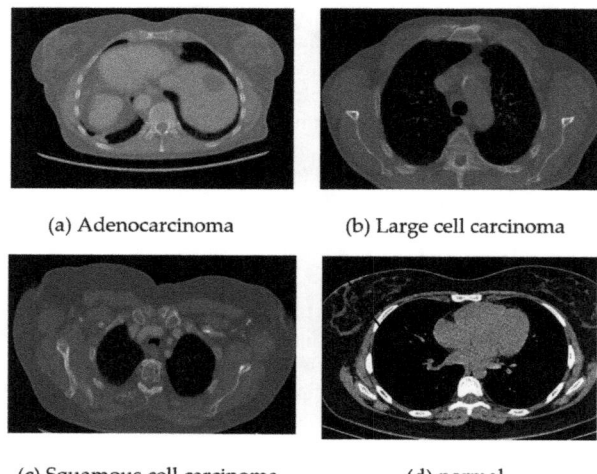

Figure 2. CT scans for lung cancer detection: (**a**) adenocarcinoma, (**b**) large-cell carcinoma, (**c**) squamous cell carcinoma, (**d**) normal.

3.2. DenseNet

DenseNet addresses significant challenges such as vanishing gradients and the inefficient use of parameters that are common in deep learning models [31]. Its standout feature is the implementation of dense connectivity, ensuring that each layer is directly linked to every other layer in a feedforward fashion. This structure promotes the seamless flow of information and gradients across the network, enhancing learning efficiency and stability. The fundamental component of DenseNet is the dense block, which consists of a series of layers where each layer receives input from all preceding layers and, in turn, passes its feature maps forward. This pattern of dense connections fosters substantial feature reuse across the network, effectively leveraging and amalgamating learned representations from various depths. Moreover, DenseNet mitigates the issue of vanishing gradients by introducing shortcut connections that facilitate a more straightforward flow of gradients during the training process, thereby improving the model's training efficiency and performance.

To manage the model's complexity and computational cost, DenseNet incorporates transition layers between dense blocks. These transition layers typically include a combination of convolutional and pooling operations, serving to reduce the number of channels and downsample spatial dimensions. The growth rate, a hyperparameter, determines the number of additional channels introduced by each layer in the dense block, influencing the network's capacity to learn and represent features.

In addition to dense connectivity, DenseNet often employs bottleneck layers within each dense block. These bottleneck layers consist of a 1×1 convolution followed by a 3×3 convolution, enhancing computational efficiency. The architecture typically concludes with a global average pooling layer, reducing spatial dimensions to a 1×1 grid, and a final classification layer.

The advantages of DenseNet include its ability to effectively utilize parameters, resulting in models with fewer parameters compared to traditional architectures. This efficient parameter usage, combined with dense connectivity, contributes to improved accuracy and training efficiency. DenseNet has proven particularly effective in image classification tasks and is widely adopted in the field of computer vision. A simplified representation of DenseNet is presented as follows:

- Dense block: Assuming that input for the dense block is X_l (output of the *l*th layer), H_l is a set of convolutional operations. Next, a function is needed for concatenating input

with the output of H_l. The output of the lth layer is the concatenation of all previous layer outputs and the output of the H_l operation.
- Transition layer: Input, X_l (output of the lth dense block). $θ_l$ is the compression factor that reduces the number of channels. Next, convolution and average pooling operations are performed. The output of the transition layer can be represented as follows:

$$X_{l+1} = Conv(AvgPool(X_l)θ_l). \qquad (1)$$

The transition layer is used to reduce the number of channels and spatial dimensions, aiding in parameter efficiency.
- Overall DenseNet Structure: If we assume X_0 as an input image, and $H_1, H_2, \ldots, H_L$ are dense blocks, $θ_1, θ_2, \ldots, θ_L$ are compression factors for each transition layer. k is the growth rate (number of additional channels added by each layer)

The overall structure is a sequence of dense blocks connected by transition layers, forming a dense and interconnected network. The DenseNet architecture for detecting lung cancer using chest CT scans and histopathological images is presented in Figure 3.

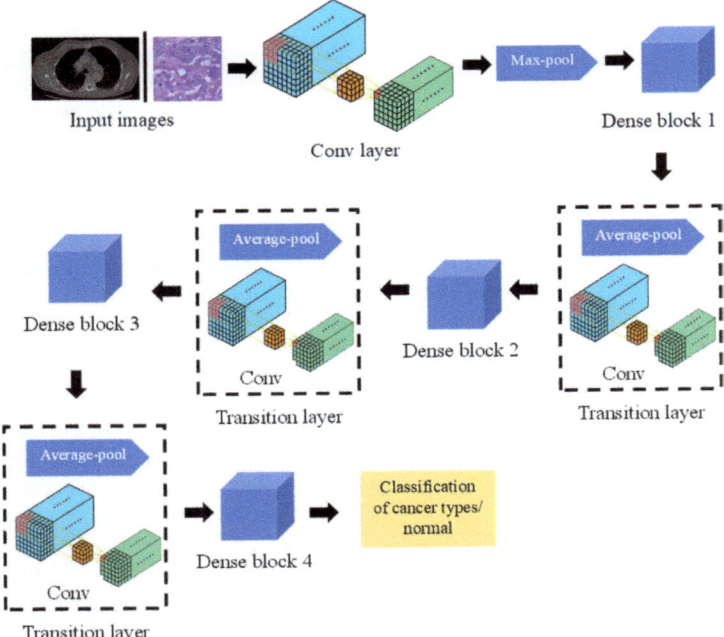

Figure 3. DenseNet architecture for lung cancer classification.

3.3. SE Block

The attention mechanism functions as a mechanism for resource allocation and can be categorized into various types, including channel attention, pixel attention, multistage attention, and others. In this study, we focus on the channel attention SE block, as introduced in [32]. The fundamental concept of this block is to determine feature weights based on the loss, assigning greater weight to effective feature maps. The SE block consists primarily of two components: squeeze and excitation.

The squeeze operation in neural network architectures compresses features along the spatial dimensions, effectively transforming each two-dimensional feature map into a single real number. This compression process generates a global receptive field, allowing the network to capture and respond to global information present in the input data. On the other hand, the excitation step is akin to the gating mechanism found in Recurrent Neural Networks (RNNs). This mechanism involves selectively amplifying or dampening specific features based on their relevance to the task at hand, enabling the network to focus on the most informative parts of the input data. Together, squeeze and excitation operations allow a neural network to dynamically adjust the importance of different channels, enhancing its ability to learn complex patterns and relationships in the data. It generates weights for each feature channel using parameters and learns these weights to explicitly model the correlation between feature channels. The graphical representation of the SE block is depicted in Figure 4. For any given transformation F_{tr}, mapping the input $X\left(X \in R^{H' \times W' \times C'}\right)$ to the feature map U where $U \in R^{H \times W \times C}$, we can construct a corresponding SE block to perform feature recalibration. The feature U first passes through a squeeze operation F_{sq}, which compresses U into a $1 \times 1 \times C$ feature. Next, through excitation operation F_{ex}, the feature from F_{sq} is excited. Lastly, through F_{scale}, the recalibration feature is achieved, where F_{scale} implies that the weights assigned to the excitation output are individually applied to each preceding feature channel through multiplication. Through this process, the original characteristics in the channel dimension are recalibrated, achieving a fine-tuning of the importance of each feature channel.

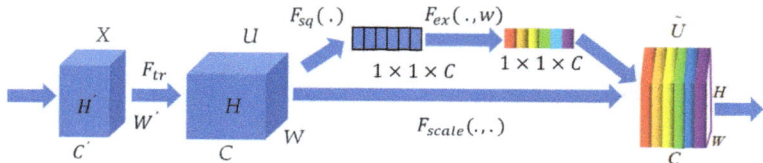

Figure 4. SE block structure.

The ATT-DenseNet model leverages a sophisticated attention mechanism, specifically the squeeze-and-excitation (SE) block, to improve its performance in lung cancer detection using CT and histopathological images. Here is a detailed explanation of how this attention mechanism is implemented and its impact on the model's performance:

3.3.1. Implementation of the SE Block

- Squeeze Operation: This component of the SE block compresses the spatial dimensions of the feature maps. Each two-dimensional feature map is aggregated into a single real number, effectively summarizing the spatial information into a channel descriptor. This operation creates a global receptive field for each channel, capturing global spatial information succinctly.
- Excitation Operation: The excitation step follows the squeezing of feature maps. It uses a fully connected layer to learn a set of weights for each channel. These weights are learned during training and are used to model the interdependencies between the channels. The operation is similar to a gating mechanism in recurrent neural networks (RNNs), allowing the model to assign adaptive importance to each channel based on the current input.
- Feature Recalibration: The output from the excitation step, which consists of weights for each channel, is used to recalibrate the original feature maps. This is achieved by scaling each channel of the feature map by its corresponding learned weight. The recalibrated feature maps emphasize informative features while suppressing less useful ones, enhancing the representational power of the network.

3.3.2. Impact on Model Performance

- Enhanced Feature Representation: By dynamically recalibrating the feature channels based on their relevance to the task at hand, ATT-DenseNet can focus more on important features while ignoring irrelevant ones. This results in a more discriminative feature representation, improving the model's accuracy in detecting lung cancer.

- Improved Model Generalization: The ability to adaptively adjust the importance of features based on the input allows ATT-DenseNet to generalize better across different datasets and imaging conditions. This adaptability is crucial in medical imaging, where variability across images is common.
- Efficient Use of Model Parameters: Despite the added complexity of the attention mechanism, the SE block's efficient design ensures that the increase in computational cost and parameters is minimal. This efficiency is particularly important in medical applications, where model deployment may need to be resource-conscious.

In summary, the attention mechanism used in ATT-DenseNet, embodied by the SE block, plays a critical role in enhancing the model's ability to detect lung cancer from CT and histopathological images. By focusing on relevant features and suppressing irrelevant ones, the model achieves improved performance metrics, including accuracy, precision, recall, and the F1-score, making it a powerful tool for early and accurate lung cancer detection.

The SE block significantly enhances the functionality of the ATT-DenseNet model by introducing a novel approach to feature recalibration within deep learning architectures. In its functionality, the SE block first executes a squeeze phase, which aggregates spatial information across the feature maps by compressing the spatial dimensions of each channel into a single value. This process captures global contextual information from each feature map, providing a comprehensive summary of the spatial attributes. Following this, the excitation phase employs a fully connected layer to learn weights for each channel, effectively determining the importance of each feature based on the aggregated global information. This mechanism enables the model to understand the intricate relationships between channels and to assign more weight to those features deemed crucial for the task at hand. The culmination of the SE block's process is the feature recalibration stage, wherein the original feature maps are scaled by the learned channel-specific weights. This recalibration allows the model to enhance or suppress features based on their learned importance, optimizing the network's focus and resource allocation towards the most informative features for the specific task of lung cancer detection.

The role of the SE block in emphasizing cancer-related information within the feature maps is pivotal for the enhanced performance of the ATT-DenseNet model in detecting lung cancer. By dynamically adjusting the emphasis on different features, the SE block enables the model to concentrate more effectively on the characteristics indicative of cancerous tissues, such as abnormal growth patterns and irregular tissue structures, while diminishing the focus on less relevant features. This selective attention to cancer-related features allows the model to be more sensitive and accurate in identifying potential cancerous lesions within CT and histopathological images. The ability to discern and prioritize critical cancer-related information over normal tissue characteristics significantly improves the model's diagnostic precision, enabling it to detect lung cancer with greater accuracy, precision, recall, and F1-score. Through the implementation of the SE block, ATT-DenseNet advances the field of medical imaging analysis by providing a more effective tool for the early detection and diagnosis of lung cancer, potentially leading to better patient outcomes through timely and accurate treatment planning.

3.4. Neuron Death Avoidance

PReLU (Parametric Rectified Linear Unit) is a variation of the popular ReLU (Rectified Linear Unit) activation function commonly used in neural networks [33]. While ReLU sets all negative values to zero, PReLU allows for a small negative slope, which is learned during training. Neuron death, or dying ReLU problem, can occur when the ReLU units always output zero for a particular input during training, leading to those units no longer updating their weights. This can happen when the input to a ReLU neuron is consistently negative, causing the gradient to be zero and thus preventing the weights from being updated. By allowing for a small negative slope in PReLU, even for negative inputs, it helps to alleviate this issue by providing a non-zero gradient for those inputs. This encourages the flow of gradients during backpropagation, preventing neurons from becoming inactive during training.

3.5. Pseudocode of the Proposed Method

The pseudocode describes a step-by-step method to analyze medical images for lung cancer using a special computer program. It starts by preparing the images in a consistent way. Then, for each image, it goes through several layers that automatically extract important features. A special attention mechanism then focuses on the most relevant features, making them more prominent for the final decision-making process. Finally, the program decides whether the image shows signs of lung cancer. The effectiveness of this process is checked by seeing how accurate and reliable the decisions are.

1. Input: CT Scan and Histopathological Images;
2. Preprocessing: Normalize images to the same scale;
3. For each image in the dataset:
    a. Pass image through DenseNet layers:
        - Convolutional layers: Extract features from the image;
        - Pooling layers: Reduce spatial dimensions of the feature maps;
        - Dense blocks: Enhance feature extraction through densely connected layers;
    b. Integrate Attention Mechanism:
        - Compute attention scores for feature maps generated by DenseNet;
        - Multiply attention scores with corresponding DenseNet feature maps;
    c. Classification Layer:
        - Flatten the attended feature maps;
        - Pass through fully connected layers to obtain the final classification;
4. Output: Lung cancer diagnosis (Cancerous or Non-Cancerous);
5. Evaluation:
    - Use metrics such as accuracy, precision, recall, and the F1-Score to evaluate model.

The problem statement in this paper focuses on the challenge of detecting lung cancer accurately and efficiently using CT and histopathological images. Despite advances in medical imaging, accurately diagnosing lung cancer early remains difficult due to the complex nature of tumor appearances and variations in imaging. This paper introduces the ATT-DenseNet model as a solution to improve diagnostic performance by leveraging deep learning and attention mechanisms to enhance the model's ability to focus on relevant features within the images, aiming to increase the accuracy, precision, recall, and F1-score of lung cancer detection. In the medical industry, this model could significantly impact early lung cancer diagnosis, treatment planning, and patient outcomes. It could be integrated into diagnostic imaging systems in healthcare facilities to assist radiologists and pathologists, enhancing the precision of lung cancer detection and enabling more personalized treatment strategies, ultimately leading to better patient care and survival rates.

4. Results

4.1. Parameter Settings and Implementation Details

For all the experimental results conducted, we used AMD Ryzen 7-5800HS CPU, having 40 GB of randomly accessible memory. NVIDIA GeForce RTX 4060 GPU was used for simulation. Furthermore, we used Tensorflow 2.15.0 and Python 3.10.12 for all the results acquired. Implementation details of the proposed ATT-DenseNet are described in Table 1. We used 70% of the data for training, and rest of the 30% data were used for validation.

Table 1. Hyper parameters associated with the model.

Parameters	Values
Number of filters (channels)	32
Growth rate	32
Dropout rate	0.2
Number of dense blocks	4
Learning rate	0.001
Batch size	64
Weight decay	0.0005
Optimizer	Adam

4.2. Histopathological Images

First, we present the results associated with cancer detection for histopathological images. In the context of evaluating the performance of classification models within machine learning, the confusion matrix stands out as a pivotal tool. This matrix provides a detailed breakdown of the predictions made by a model, allowing for a nuanced assessment of its performance in terms of accurately predicting different classes. The confusion matrix is structured as a table, categorizing predictions into four fundamental types: True Positives (TP), True Negatives (TN), False Positives (FP), and False Negatives (FN). TPs and TNs represent instances where the model has correctly predicted the positive and negative classes, respectively. By contrast, FPs and FNs reflect the errors in prediction, where the model incorrectly identifies the positive and negative classes.

Derived from the confusion matrix, several key performance metrics that offer insights into different aspects of the model's predictive accuracy are accuracy, precision, recall, and F1 score. These metrics, derived from the confusion matrix, are instrumental in comprehensively understanding the performance of a classification model. They highlight not only the model's accuracy but also the nature and extent of any prediction errors, thereby guiding further model refinement and optimization.

We had 750 images in total representing three different classes and an even distribution of 250 images for each class. We reserved 15% of the data for validation, and the results presented are based on this validation data performance. Figure 5 presents the confusion matrix for ATT-DenseNet implementation along with two other baselines, namely AlexNet and SqueezeNet.

Figure 6 presents a performance comparison of DenseNet, Alexnet, and SqueezeNet. The performance metrics considered are average accuracy, precision, recall and the F1-score.

As we can see from the presented confusion matrices in Figure 5, very few samples have been misclassified by the DenseNet compared to the baselines. Figure 6 provides a figure showing the performance of DenseNet against AlexNet and SqueezeNet in terms of accuracy, precision, recall, and F1 score. For all the performance metrics, DenseNet performs better. DenseNet's architecture allows for each layer to have direct access to the gradients from the loss function and the original input signal, leading to more efficient training and feature reuse. This is particularly useful in histopathological image analysis, where subtle features and patterns are crucial for accurate classification. Furthermore, in DenseNet, each layer receives a "collective knowledge" from all preceding layers, which improves the flow of gradients throughout the network. This leads to better learning and performance, as each layer can learn more complex features based on all previous layers. To further improve the performance, as presented in Section 3, we adopt ATT-DenseNet, which is our proposed method. We achieved the following performance (Figure 7), which surpasses the traditional DenseNet, AlexNet and SqueezeNet.

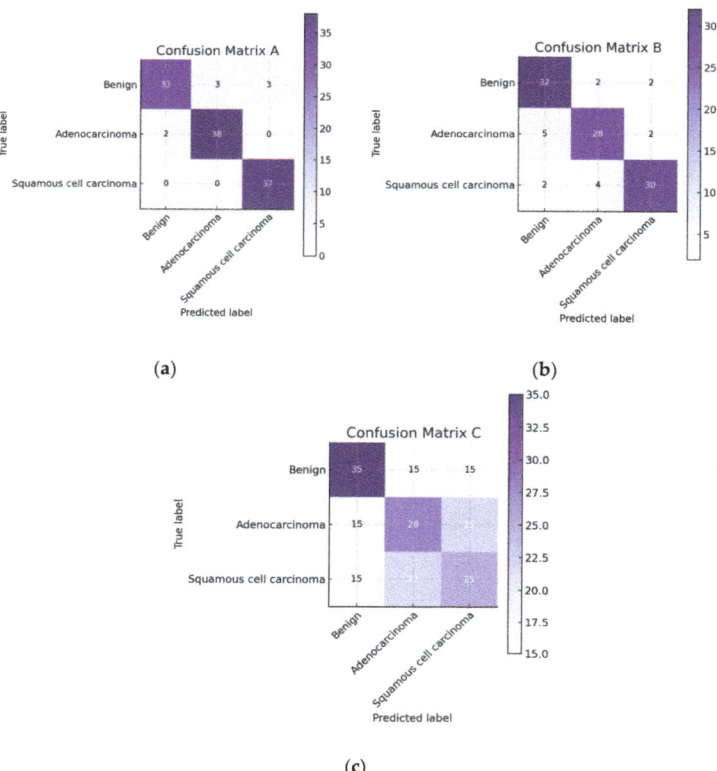

Figure 5. Confusion matrix for validation data (histopathological images): (**a**) DenseNet, (**b**) AlexNet, (**c**) SqueezeNet.

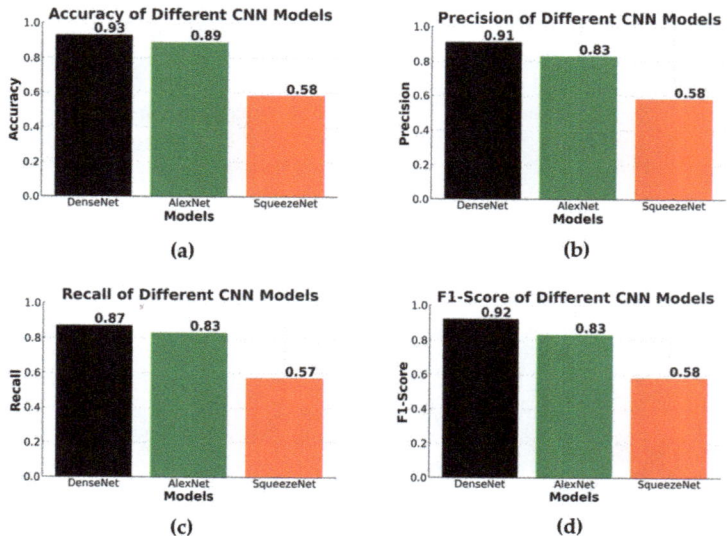

Figure 6. Performance analysis (histopathological images) of DenseNet, AlexNet, and SqueezeNet: (**a**) accuracy, (**b**) precision, (**c**) recall, and (**d**) the F1-score.

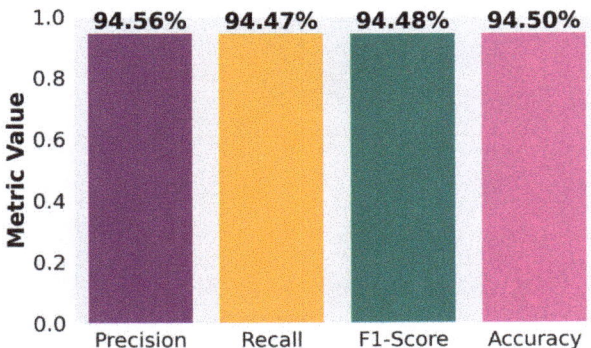

Figure 7. Performance analysis (histopathological images) of the ATT-DenseNet.

Finally, to show the better performance of ATT-DenseNet in a more vivid way, Figure 8 presents a comparison of the accuracy curves over 1000 epochs. As we can see from the figure, it outsmarts the baselines by significant margins, achieving an average accuracy of 0.954 (95.4 in percentage).

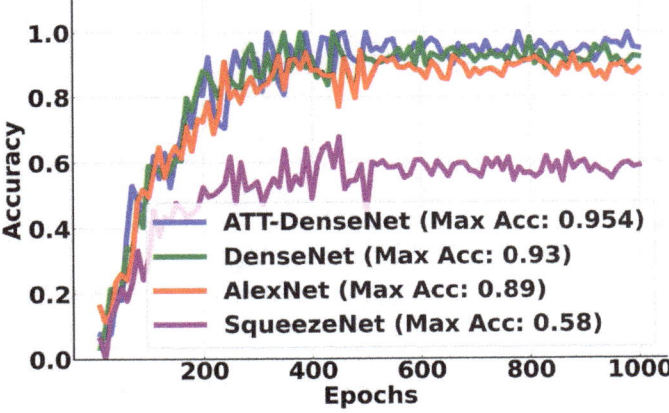

Figure 8. Performance analysis of ATT-DenseNet against all the other CNN baselines in terms of accuracy.

4.3. CT Scan Images

As mentioned in previous sections, the CT scan images used for cancer detection have four classes. The confusion matrix for the classification using ATT-DenseNet is presented in Figure 9. We do not extensively present the confusion matrices as we did before for histopathological images in order to avoid repetition. Furthermore, Figure 10 presents an accuracy curve comparison.

We can see from Figure 10 that the proposed ATT-DenseNet achieves higher accuracy compared to all the baselines by achieving 94% average accuracy on the test set of the data. Similarly, as presented in terms of histopathological images, the F1-score of ATT-DenseNet is found to be higher than all the other baselines for CT scan images. Finally, we compare the proposed method with RestNet in terms of accuracy and the F1-score and see that the proposed method performs better as well.

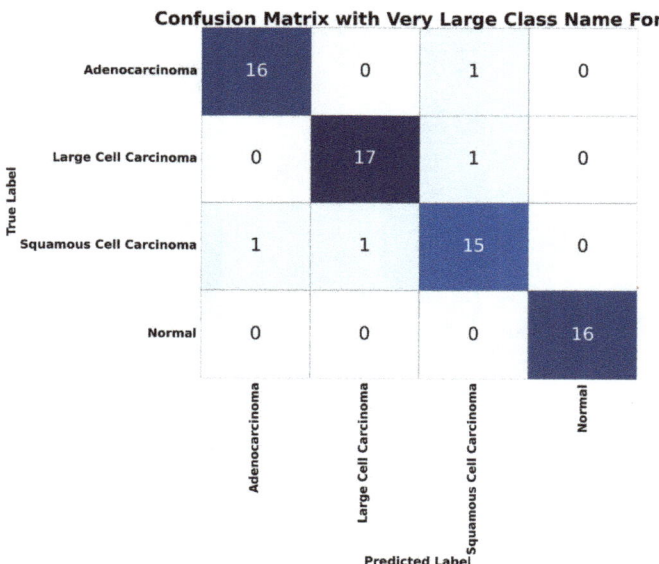

Figure 9. Confusion matrix for ATT-DenseNet for lung cancer classification using CT scan images.

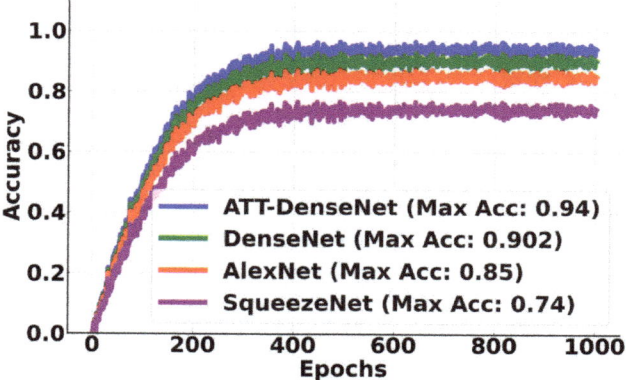

Figure 10. Performance analysis of ATT-DenseNet against all the other CNN baselines in terms of accuracy (CT images).

The proposed ATT-DenseNet mechanism adaptively recalibrates feature responses by explicitly modeling interdependencies between channels. This means that the method can dynamically emphasize informative features while suppressing irrelevant ones. By contrast, DenseNet without attention, SqueezeNet, and AlexNet lack such mechanisms to focus on the most relevant features, potentially leading to suboptimal feature utilization. Furthermore, the proposed ATT-DenseNet facilitates better discrimination of features by learning channel-wise relationships. By selectively emphasizing important features, the method can potentially enhance the discriminative power of the network, leading to improved classification performance. DenseNet without attention, SqueezeNet, and AlexNet do not have the capability to learn such discriminative features effectively. The adaptive nature of ATT-DenseNet allows the method to dynamically adjust feature importance based on the input, leading to improved generalization across the datasets and scenarios. This adaptability enables our model to capture complex patterns in the data more effectively compared to the fixed feature mappings of DenseNet without attention, SqueezeNet, and AlexNet. DenseNet's dense connectivity pattern enables feature reuse throughout the network, leading to parameter efficiency. This means DenseNet requires fewer parameters compared to ResNet or traditional architectures to achieve similar or better performance. With fewer parameters, DenseNet models can be trained faster and require less memory. DenseNet's dense connections facilitate a direct gradient flow from the later layers to the earlier layers during backpropagation. This helps alleviate the vanishing gradient problem, making it easier to train very deep networks. That is why, as presented in Figures 8, 10 and 11, we achieved better accuracy for the proposed ATT-DenseNet.

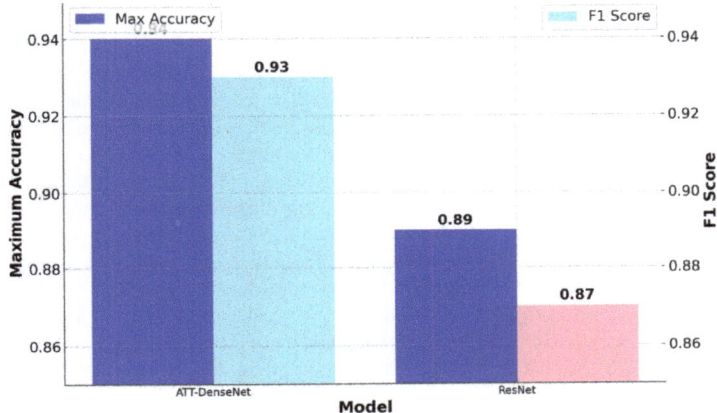

Figure 11. Performance analysis of ATT-DenseNet against all the other CNN baselines in terms of accuracy (CT images).

4.4. Computational Complexity and Reproducibility

DenseNet typically has a higher computational cost compared to SqueezeNet due to its larger number of parameters, with DenseNet often ranging from 20–30 million parameters, SqueezeNet usually having around 0.7–1.3 million parameters, and AlexNet falling in between, with approximately 60–70 million parameters. This higher parameter count in DenseNet leads to increased memory usage during training and inference, as well as longer training times, especially on datasets with a large number of samples. However, DenseNet's parameter efficiency and dense connectivity may offer better feature reuse and representation learning, potentially leading to higher accuracy and more robust models, particularly in scenarios with abundant computational resources. This is particularly beneficial in medical applications such as lung cancer classification, where accuracy is paramount and where even marginal improvements can have significant clinical implications. The intricate and nuanced patterns present in medical images require models capable of capturing fine-grained details, which DenseNet's dense connectivity facilitates. While the computational cost may be higher, the potential for improved accuracy and better performance in medical diagnosis justifies the investment in computational resources. Therefore, despite the higher computational cost, DenseNet is preferred for medical applications where accuracy and reliability are critical, even if it requires more computational resources compared to alternative architectures like SqueezeNet. The results in this section support this statement since ATT-DenseNet, the proposed method, outperforms the other two baselines with higher rates of accuracy.

We tested the reproducibility of the results multiple times with different sets of input extracted from the dataset. In particular, there were 15,000 images in total in the dataset. We took different batches of 750 images to perform the classification to see whether we obtained similar results.

4.5. Clinical Implications and Limitations

The ATT-DenseNet model, designed for lung cancer detection using CT and histopathological images, has significant clinical implications and potential impacts on patient diagnosis and treatment. The model's innovative approach, which emphasizes relevant image regions and utilizes advanced data preprocessing techniques, sets a new standard in the field. By achieving impressive average accuracies of 95.4% for histopathological images and 94% for CT scan images, ATT-DenseNet not only demonstrates superiority over traditional models like DenseNet, AlexNet, and SqueezeNet but also highlights its potential as a transformative tool in medical diagnostics. This enhanced accuracy and precision in detecting lung cancer could lead to earlier and more accurate diagnoses, enabling timely and personalized treatment plans for patients. Early detection is critical in improving survival rates for lung cancer patients, as it allows for interventions at a stage when the disease is more treatable. Furthermore, the ability of ATT-DenseNet to precisely identify cancerous tissues within images can assist in planning targeted therapies, reducing the need for invasive diagnostic procedures, and ultimately contributing to better patient outcomes. The model's emphasis on relevant regions within the images ensures that clinicians receive focused and significant diagnostic information, potentially streamlining the decision-making process in clinical settings and improving the efficiency of lung cancer screening programs.

The proposed method showcases significant improvements in detection metrics. However, it faces limitations in generalizability and class imbalance. The model's performance on diverse datasets is uncertain due to variations in imaging protocols and patient demographics, highlighting the need for models that adapt to different data characteristics. Additionally, the prevalent issue of class imbalance, where non-cancerous images outnumber cancerous ones, can skew the model towards predicting the majority class, potentially reducing its sensitivity to cancerous cases. Addressing these challenges requires further research into robust model design, advanced data augmentation, and balancing techniques to ensure the model's effectiveness across varied datasets and improved detection of cancerous images. We also want to include some formal methods for AI-based technique verification [34,35].

5. Conclusions

In this paper, we successfully developed the ATT-DenseNet model, which notably improved the accuracy, precision, recall, and the F1-score for lung cancer detection using CT and histopathological images. This model's innovative approach, which emphasizes relevant image regions and utilizes advanced data preprocessing techniques, sets a new standard in the field. The results, with an impressive average accuracy of 95.4% for histopathological images and 94% for CT scan images, not only demonstrate the superiority of ATT-DenseNet over traditional models like DenseNet, AlexNet, and SqueezeNet but also highlight its potential as a transformative tool in medical diagnostics, offering new possibilities for the early and accurate detection of lung cancer. Future research directions could explore further enhancements to the ATT-DenseNet model for even greater rates of accuracy and efficiency in lung cancer detection. Further research could also focus on reducing the model's computational requirements to facilitate its deployment in resource-limited settings, ensuring wider accessibility and use.

Funding: This research is funded by Woosong University Academic Research 2024.

Data Availability Statement: Data used in this research are publicly available.

Conflicts of Interest: The author declares no conflicts of interest.

References

1. Xu, Y.; Hosny, A.; Zeleznik, R.; Parmar, C.; Coroller, T.; Franco, I.; Mak, R.H.; Aerts, H.J.W.L. Deep Learning Predicts Lung Cancer Treatment Response from Serial Medical Imaging. *Clin. Cancer Res.* **2019**, *25*, 3266–3275. [CrossRef] [PubMed]
2. Faisal, M.I.; Bashir, S.; Khan, Z.S.; Hassan Khan, F. An Evaluation of Machine Learning Classifiers and Ensembles for Early Stage Prediction of Lung Cancer. In Proceedings of the 2018 3rd International Conference on Emerging Trends in Engineering, Sciences and Technology (ICEEST), Karachi, Pakistan, 21–22 December 2018; pp. 1–4.
3. Coudray, N.; Ocampo, P.S.; Sakellaropoulos, T.; Narula, N.; Snuderl, M.; Fenyö, D.; Moreira, A.L.; Razavian, N.; Tsirigos, A. Classification and Mutation Prediction from Non–Small Cell Lung Cancer Histopathology Images Using Deep Learning. *Nat. Med.* **2018**, *24*, 1559–1567. [CrossRef] [PubMed]
4. Ibrahim, D.M.; Elshennawy, N.M.; Sarhan, A.M. Deep-Chest: Multi-Classification Deep Learning Model for Diagnosing COVID-19, Pneumonia, and Lung Cancer Chest Diseases. *Comput. Biol. Med.* **2021**, *132*, 104348. [CrossRef] [PubMed]
5. Avanzo, M.; Stancanello, J.; Pirrone, G.; Sartor, G. Radiomics and Deep Learning in Lung Cancer. *Strahlenther. Onkol.* **2020**, *196*, 879–887. [CrossRef] [PubMed]
6. Lin, Y.; Xu, J.; Lan, H. Tumor-associated macrophages in tumor metastasis: Biological roles and clinical therapeutic applications. *J. Hematol. Oncol.* **2019**, *12*, 76. [CrossRef] [PubMed]
7. Zhong, Z.; Zheng, M.; Mai, H.; Zhao, J.; Liu, X. Cancer image classification based on DenseNet model. *J. Phys. Conf. Ser.* **2020**, *1651*, 012143. [CrossRef]
8. Hu, J.; Shen, L.; Albanie, S.; Sun, G.; Wu, E. Squeeze-and-Excitation Networks. *arXiv* **2019**, arXiv:1709.01507.
9. Tang, W.; Sun, J.; Wang, S.; Zhang, Y. Review of AlexNet for Medical Image Classification. *arXiv* **2023**, arXiv:2311.08655. [CrossRef]
10. Iandola, F.N.; Moskewicz, M.W.; Ashraf, K.; Han, S.; Dally, W.J.; Keutzer, K. SqueezeNet: AlexNet-Level Accuracy with 50x Fewer Parameters and <1MB Model Size. *arXiv* **2016**, arXiv:1602.07360.
11. Wang, K.; Jiang, P.; Meng, J.; Jiang, X. Attention-Based DenseNet for Pneumonia Classification. *IRBM* **2022**, *43*, 479–485. [CrossRef]
12. Clark, K.; Vendt, B.; Smith, K.; Freymann, J.; Kirby, J.; Koppel, P.; Moore, S.; Phillips, S.; Maffitt, D.; Pringle, M.; et al. The Cancer Imaging Archive (TCIA): Maintaining and Operating a Public Information Repository. *J. Digit. Imaging* **2013**, *26*, 1045–1057. [CrossRef]
13. Sethy, P.K.; Geetha Devi, A.; Padhan, B.; Behera, S.K.; Sreedhar, S.; Das, K. Lung Cancer Histopathological Image Classification Using Wavelets and AlexNet. *J. X-ray Sci. Technol.* **2023**, *31*, 211–221. [CrossRef] [PubMed]
14. Habib, M.A.; Hasan, M.J.; Kim, J.-M. A Lightweight Deep Learning-Based Approach for Concrete Crack Characterization Using Acoustic Emission Signals. *IEEE Access* **2021**, *9*, 104029–104050. [CrossRef]
15. Habib, M.A.; Zhou, H.; Iturria-Rivera, P.E.; Elsayed, M.; Bavand, M.; Gaigalas, R.; Ozcan, Y.; Erol-Kantarci, M. Hierarchical Reinforcement Learning Based Traffic Steering in Multi-RAT 5G Deployments. In Proceedings of the ICC 2023-IEEE International Conference on Communications, Rome, Italy, 28 May–1 June 2023; pp. 100–105.
16. Habib, M.A.; Zhou, H.; Iturria-Rivera, P.E.; Elsayed, M.; Bavand, M.; Gaigalas, R.; Furr, S.; Erol-Kantarci, M. Traffic Steering for 5G Multi-RAT Deployments Using Deep Reinforcement Learning. In Proceedings of the 2023 IEEE 20th Consumer Communications & Networking Conference (CCNC), Las Vegas, NV, USA, 8–11 January 2023; pp. 164–169.
17. Radhika, P.R.; Rakhi, A.S.N.; Veena, G. A Comparative Study of Lung Cancer Detection Using Machine Learning Algorithms. In Proceedings of the 2019 IEEE International Conference on Electrical, Computer and Communication Technologies (ICECCT), Coimbatore, India, 20–22 February 2019; pp. 1–4.
18. Pradhan, K.; Chawla, P. Medical Internet of Things Using Machine Learning Algorithms for Lung Cancer Detection. *J. Manag. Anal.* **2020**, *7*, 591–623. [CrossRef]
19. Bhatia, S.; Sinha, Y.; Goel, L. Lung Cancer Detection: A Deep Learning Approach. In *Soft Computing for Problem Solving*; Bansal, J.C., Das, K.N., Nagar, A., Deep, K., Ojha, A.K., Eds.; Springer: Singapore, 2019; pp. 699–705.
20. Shin, H.; Oh, S.; Hong, S.; Kang, M.; Kang, D.; Ji, Y.; Choi, B.H.; Kang, K.-W.; Jeong, H.; Park, Y.; et al. Early-Stage Lung Cancer Diagnosis by Deep Learning-Based Spectroscopic Analysis of Circulating Exosomes. *ACS Nano* **2020**, *14*, 5435–5444. [CrossRef] [PubMed]
21. Hyun, S.H.; Ahn, M.S.; Koh, Y.W.; Lee, S.J. A Machine-Learning Approach Using PET-Based Radiomics to Predict the Histological Subtypes of Lung Cancer. *Clin. Nucl. Med.* **2019**, *44*, 956–960. [CrossRef] [PubMed]
22. Rahane, W.; Dalvi, H.; Magar, Y.; Kalane, A.; Jondhale, S. Lung Cancer Detection Using Image Processing and Machine Learning HealthCare. In Proceedings of the 2018 International Conference on Current Trends towards Converging Technologies (ICCTCT), Coimbatore, India, 1–3 March 2018; pp. 1–5.
23. Rajasekar, V.; Krishnamoorthi, S.; Saračević, M.; Pepic, D.; Zajmovic, M.; Zogic, H. Ensemble Machine Learning Methods to Predict the Balancing of Ayurvedic Constituents in the Human Body: Ensemble Machine Learning Methods to Predict. *Comput. Sci.* **2022**, 117–132. [CrossRef]
24. Lakshmanaprabu, S.K.; Mohanty, S.N.; Shankar, K.; Arunkumar, N.; Ramirez, G. Optimal Deep Learning Model for Classification of Lung Cancer on CT Images. *Future Gener. Comput. Syst.* **2019**, *92*, 374–382.
25. Hosny, A.; Parmar, C.; Coroller, T.P.; Grossmann, P.; Zeleznik, R.; Kumar, A.; Bussink, J.; Gillies, R.J.; Mak, R.H.; Aerts, H.J.W.L. Deep Learning for Lung Cancer Prognostication: A Retrospective Multi-Cohort Radiomics Study. *PLoS Med.* **2018**, *15*, e1002711. [CrossRef]

26. She, Y.; Jin, Z.; Wu, J.; Deng, J.; Zhang, L.; Su, H.; Jiang, G.; Liu, H.; Xie, D.; Cao, N.; et al. Development and Validation of a Deep Learning Model for Non–Small Cell Lung Cancer Survival. *JAMA Netw. Open* **2020**, *3*, e205842. [CrossRef]
27. Rajasekar, V.; Vaishnnave, M.P.; Premkumar, S.; Sarveshwaran, V.; Rangaraaj, V. Lung Cancer Disease Prediction with CT Scan and Histopathological Images Feature Analysis Using Deep Learning Techniques. *Results Eng.* **2023**, *18*, 101111. [CrossRef]
28. Saric, M.; Russo, M.; Stella, M.; Sikora, M. CNN-based method for lung cancer detection in whole slide histopathology images. In Proceedings of the 2019 4th International Conference on Smart and Sustainable Technologies (SpliTech), Split, Croatia, 18–21 June 2019.
29. Mehmood, S.; Ghazal, T.M.; Khan, M.A.; Zubair, M.; Naseem, M.T.; Faiz, T.; Ahmad, M. Malignancy detection in lung and colon histopathology images using transfer learning with class selective image processing. *IEEE Access* **2022**, *10*, 25657–25668. [CrossRef]
30. Yang, H.; Chen, L.; Cheng, Z.; Yang, M.; Wang, J.; Lin, C.; Wang, Y.; Huang, L.; Chen, Y.; Peng, S.; et al. Deep learning-based six-type classifier for lung cancer and mimics from histopathological whole slide images: A retrospective study. *BMC Med.* **2021**, *19*, 80. [CrossRef] [PubMed]
31. Huang, G.; Liu, Z.; Van Der Maaten, L.; Weinberger, K.Q. Densely Connected Convolutional Networks. In Proceedings of the 2017 IEEE Conference on Computer Vision and Pattern Recognition (CVPR), Honolulu, HI, USA, 21–26 July 2017; pp. 2261–2269.
32. Jin, X.; Xie, Y.; Wei, X.-S.; Zhao, B.-R.; Chen, Z.-M.; Tan, X. Delving deep into spatial pooling for squeeze-and-excitation networks. *Pattern Recognit.* **2022**, *121*, 108159. [CrossRef]
33. He, K.; Zhang, X.; Ren, S.; Sun, J. Delving deep into rectifiers: Surpassing human-level performance on ImageNet Classification. In Proceedings of the 2015 IEEE International Conference on Computer Vision (ICCV), Santiago, Chile, 7–13 December 2015.
34. Krichen, M.; Mihoub, A.; Alzahrani, M.Y.; Adoni, W.Y.; Nahhal, T. Are formal methods applicable to machine learning and Artificial Intelligence? In Proceedings of the 2022 2nd International Conference of Smart Systems and Emerging Technologies (SMARTTECH), Riyadh, Saudi Arabia, 9–11 May 2022.
35. Raman, R.; Gupta, N.; Jeppu, Y. Framework for formal verification of machine learning based complex system-of-Systems. *Insight* **2023**, *26*, 91–102. [CrossRef]

Disclaimer/Publisher's Note: The statements, opinions and data contained in all publications are solely those of the individual author(s) and contributor(s) and not of MDPI and/or the editor(s). MDPI and/or the editor(s) disclaim responsibility for any injury to people or property resulting from any ideas, methods, instructions or products referred to in the content.

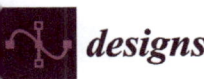

Article

The Biomechanical Analysis of Tibial Implants Using Meshless Methods: Stress and Bone Tissue Remodeling Analysis

Ana Pais [1,2,†], Catarina Moreira [3] and Jorge Belinha [2,3,*,†]

1 FEUP—Faculty of Engineering, University of Porto, Rua Dr. Roberto Frias, s/n, 4200-465 Porto, Portugal; anapais@fe.up.pt
2 INEGI—Institute of Science and Innovation in Mechanical and Industrial Engineering, Rua Dr. Roberto Frias, s/n, 4200-465 Porto, Portugal
3 ISEP—School of Engineering, Polytechnic University of Porto, Rua Dr. António Bernardino de Almeida, 431, 4249-015 Porto, Portugal; 1171151@isep.ipp.pt
* Correspondence: job@isep.ipp.pt
† These authors contributed equally to this work.

Abstract: Total knee arthroplasty (TKA) stands out as one of the most widely employed surgical procedures, establishing itself as the preferred method for addressing advanced osteoarthritis of the knee. However, current knee prostheses require refined design solutions. This research work focuses on a computational analysis of both the mechanical behavior of a knee joint implant and the bone remodeling process in the tibia following implantation. This research study delves into how specific design parameters, particularly the stem geometry, impact the prosthesis's performance. Utilizing a computed tomography scan of a tibia, various TKA configurations were simulated to conduct analyses employing advanced discretization techniques, such as the finite element method (FEM) and the radial point interpolation method (RPIM). The findings reveal that the introduction of the implant leads to a marginal increase in the stress values within the tibia, accompanied by a reduction in the displacement field values. The insertion of the longest tested implant increased the maximum stress from 5.0705 MPa to 6.1584 MPa, leading to a displacement reduction from 0.016 mm to 0.0142 mm. Finally, by combining the FEM with a bone remodeling algorithm, the bone remodeling process of the tibia due to an implant insertion was simulated.

Keywords: total knee arthroplasty; tibia bone; finite element method; meshless methods; bone remodeling

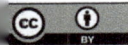

1. Introduction

Total knee arthroplasty (TKA) stands as one of the frequently conducted surgical interventions in the field of Orthopedics, offering the promise of enhancing functionality, alleviating pain, and reinstating the quality of life for patients [1]. It is estimated that in the USA, the growth in surgical requests from 2005 to 2030 will be around 673% (3.48 million) [1]. The main objective of a TKA is to reduce knee pain, based on the replacement of most of the damaged components of the joint with an implant, and the success of the surgery is estimated by the absence of pain and functional recovery of the knee in a short period [2]. TKA can encompass the surface of up to three bones: the femur, the patella, and the tibia; however, the latter is the area where most injuries leading to this surgical procedure occur [2]. In certain cases, for enhanced implant fixation and stability, a cylindrical extension known as the tibial stem is incorporated at the distal end of the tibial metal component whose primary function is to increase implant stability, particularly in challenging cases, by minimizing micromovements at the bone–implant interface, thereby mitigating the risk of aseptic loosening [3]. These tibial extensions come in various lengths and widths and can be secured through different methods, including total cementation, proximal cementation only, or a press-fit approach without the use of cement [3]. The existence and design of the tibial extension, including its size and method of fixation, can induce a phenomenon referred to as stress shielding, resulting in bone loss in the regions most affected, which may weaken the implant fixation, requiring the placement of a new prosthesis [4–7]. Stems are fundamental in most TKAs in aiding the transfer of loads from the damaged articular and metaphyseal bone to the tibial cortical limit and in distributing the increased stress of a specific joint [8]. Stems, at the cost of stress shielding, improve mechanical stability through shearing resistance, reduction in lift-off, and a decrease in micromovement [8]. In cases where the available bone reserve is inadequate to sustain the prosthesis, the incorporation of stems is generally advised [9]. When addressing substantial volume defects through bone grafting, the use of a stem becomes essential to shield the graft from excessive loads, since the knee joint bears loads several times the body weight and a failure in load transfer by the stem can subject the remaining trabecular bone to a load surpassing its maximum strength, resulting in a compromise in the fixation of the component [9]. While there is today a large consensus about the necessity of a stem for enhancing both the initial mechanical stability and the ultimate longevity of the component, the recommended lengths and diameters and fixation methods continue to be subjects of controversy [8]. It is noteworthy that it is highly unlikely that an ideal length, for example, will ever be determined, due to a huge heterogeneity in the anatomical characteristics of patients [8,10].

In cemented arthroplasty, the oldest fixation method, the cement ensures the union between the implant and the bone tissue, providing a uniform load distribution throughout the extent of the bone–implant interface [11]. However, the cement, usually composed of polymethyl methacrylate (PMMA), does not provide adhesive properties; it only fills the gaps located between the bone and the prosthesis [11]. Many studies have indicated that cemented fixation shows better short- and medium-term results, as it reduces patient pain and increases mobility and, consequently, their quality of life [11]. This method is mainly employed in cases of extensive bone damage and a significantly compromised internal cortex, particularly observed in individuals diagnosed with advanced osteoporosis [8]. However, some incidents with the use of cement have also been reported, as it degrades over time, causing the release of debris that leads to inflammation of the surrounding bone [12]. Another point to consider is the surgical intervention of revision, recurrent in younger patients, since the removal of the cement-fixed prosthesis is quite complicated, and therefore, this technique is then recommended only for patients over 65 years of age or patients with poor bone condition, in order to ensure a strong primary fixation [12,13]. The adversities and complexity related to cemented arthroplasty have encouraged the search for new fixation methodologies.

Unlike cemented arthroplasty, which results from the mechanical fixation of the cement, uncemented arthroplasty is based not only on mechanical fixation but also on the biological junction of the implant to the bone tissue [14]. This new technique aims to improve, in the long term, the success of implants in young patients, who demonstrate good bone quality. The main drawback of this approach is the pain in the lower limbs, which is a consequence of the poor fixation of the implant to the bone tissue [12].

Computational tools such as the FEM have been very useful for researchers in the field of arthroplasty. Studies using these tools focus on the implant geometry and materials as well as surgical techniques. With these studies, issues such as the minimization of stress shielding or micromotions, which can heavily hinder the success of the treatment, are dealt with. Completo et al. [15] conducted a study using the finite element method, which evaluated the distribution of loads and stability at the cement-bone interface for two fixation techniques, cemented and press-fit. The findings revealed that the load transmitted from the cemented stem to the bone was fourfold higher [15]. Quevedo González et al. [16] used a computational approach to study the effect on tibial stress of using a smaller tibial baseplate in order to prevent excessive rotation, having concluded that the consequences of this undersizing are minimal. Quevedo Gonzalez et al. [17] used a computational approach to determine that adding an anterior spike to the tibial baseplate would help to decrease the micromotions between the bone and the implant. Other approaches addressing implant geometry include the work of Liu et al. [18], who used a topology-optimization approach to improve the design of the metal plate, through a porous design, used to treat defects in the proximal tibia with TKA. Liu et al. [19] compared two techniques used in TKA, namely, the cement screw and the metal block, and concluded that the use of a metal block is more suitable for larger defects. Regarding the study of the most suitable materials, studies such as those of Bhandarkar and Dhatrak [20] and Apostolopoulos et al. [21] deal with the cushion material and tibial insert, respectively. In the first study, it is concluded that using a UHMWPE cushion leads to lower stresses in the inserts, and in the second work, an all-polyethylene TKA is compared to a metal-backed TKA and it is stated that the all-polyethylene one is cheaper and yields similar results to the metal one, with the disadvantage of requiring cement and having less flexibility. Finally, some studies concerning the arthroplasty of the ankle can also be mentioned, such as that of Jyoti and Ghosh [22] concerning the optimal resection length, which concluded that stress shielding and micromotion increase with resection depth, and thus, that this should be kept to a minimum; and the work of Jyoti et al. [23] concerning the interface of the implant, in which it is proposed that both the friction coefficient between the implant and the bone, and the implant design, along with the bone quality, heavily influence micromotion, while stress distribution is less influenced by the friction coefficient and more by the design of the implant and the quality of the bone.

The present computational approach aims at complementing experimental studies and international standards such as ISO DIS 22926 [24] and ISO/CD 5092:2023 [25]. Furthermore, this research employs meshless methods to achieve higher accuracy in obtaining solutions, thereby enhancing the quality of computational studies on implant biomechanics. Moreover, it incorporates a bone remodeling approach to assess if the implant could cause considerable bone loss as a result of stress shielding.

2. Numerical Formulation

2.1. Meshless Methods Formulation

Generally, in meshless methods the process initiates with the discretizaton of the problem's physical domain with a nodal distribution. Although, as in other discretization techniques, regular nodal distributions allow more accurate and stable results to be achieved, in meshless methods nodes can be irregularly distributed over the problem domain. Geometry features such as cracks and holes can have a higher nodal density to anticipate the stress concentration that may occur. Usually, a very dense nodal distribution will lead to more accurate results, with the consequence of presenting a much higher computational cost [26].

Next, to integrate the integro-differential equations governing the physical phenomenon under study, it is necessary to create a background integration mesh. Commonly, background integration cells are created and then filled with integration points representing volume portions. Most meshless methods requiring integration apply the Gauss–Legendre integration scheme to the integration cells [26].

The previous stage is followed by the imposition of nodal connectivity through influence domains. Thus, each integration point searches for a certain number of nodes within its vicinity (generally, following a radial search). The nodes within its vicinity form the influence-domain of the integration point. The literature shows that the size of the influence domain significantly affects the performance of the method.

Then, using the nodes forming the corresponding influence domain, the shape functions (and their partial derivatives) of a given integration point are built, and matrix B, from Equation (18), can be established.

Taking the example of the displacement field u, the displacement at an integration point x_I can be interpolated using the displacement values of the nodes within the influence domain of x_I,

$$u(x_I) = \sum_{i=1}^{n_d} \varphi_i(x_I) u(x_i) \qquad (1)$$

where the number of nodes inside the influence domain of x_I is represented as n_d, the displacement values of each node i belonging to the influence domain of x_I is indicated as $u(x_i)$, and $\varphi_i(x_I)$ is the value on node i of the shape functions of x_I.

For each integration point x_I, a local stiffness matrix is established, K_I, Equation (22). Then, all local stiffness matrices are assembled into a global stiffness matrix, allowing the final discrete system of equations $Ku = F$ to be obtained, which can be solved to obtain the displacement field $u = K^{-1}F$.

2.1.1. Influence Domains

The RPIM uses the concept of influence domains, which is shown schematically in Figure 1. The influence domain consists of the set of nodes in the vicinity of the interest point. The nodes within the spatial vicinity of integration point x_I constitute the influence domain of x_I. Influence domains can all have the same number of nodes or instead present different sizes and different numbers of nodes. Moreover, the shape of the influence domain can be any. In Figure 1a, the influence domains present the same size ($r_1 = r_2$), which leads to a different number of nodes in each influence domain, while in Figure 1b the number of nodes inside each influence domain is the same due to their different sizes: ($r_1 \neq r_2$).

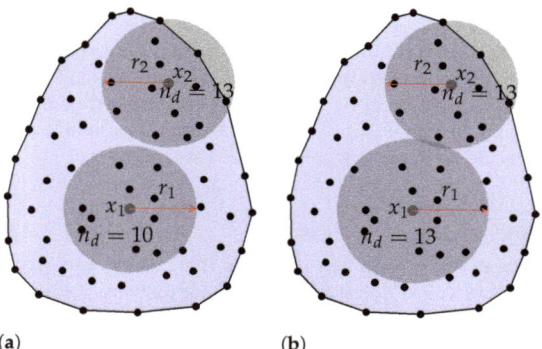

Figure 1. Influence domains: (**a**) fixed size; (**b**) variable size.

2.1.2. Shape Functions

Consider the integration point $x_I \in \mathbb{R}^3$ and its influence domain: $X_I = \{x_1, x_2, \ldots x_n\} \in \mathbb{R}^3$ with n being the total number of nodes within the influence domain of x_I. The shape function of x_I is calculated using only the n nodes belonging to its influence domain. Thus, the variable field $u(x_I)$ can be interpolated at x_I using

$$u(x_I) = r(x_I)^T a(x_I) + p(x_I)^T b(x_I) = \{r(x_I)^T \; p(x_I)^T\} \begin{Bmatrix} a(x_I) \\ b(x_I) \end{Bmatrix} \quad (2)$$

where $a(x_I)$ and $b(x_I)$ are non-constant coefficients of the radial basis function (RBF), $r(x_I)$, and of the polynomial basis function (PBF), $p(x_I)$, respectively. Although the literature describes several distinct RBFs [27], generally, radial point interpolation techniques apply the multi-quadrics RBF (MQ-RBF) [28]:

$$r_i(x_I) = (d_{iI}^2 + (\gamma d_c)^2)^p \quad (3)$$

The parameter d_c is the size coefficient, directly correlated with the numerical weight w_I of the integration point x_I, and the parameter d_{iI} is the Euclidean distance between the integration point x_I and the node x_i inside the influence domain of x_I. The parameters p and γ are shape parameters and, according to [27], these should present values so that γd_a is almost null and p is almost unity, which maximizes the method's performance.

The PBF possesses m terms (the monomials), which can be established using Pascal's triangle.

$$p(x_I) = \{p_1(x_I) \; p_2(x_I) \; \cdots \; p_m(x_I)\}^T \tag{4}$$

In radial point interpolation formulations, the constant PBF $p(x) = \{1\}$ or the linear PBF $p(x) = \{1 \; x \; y \; z\}^T$ is generally used.

The number of unknowns in the system $Ra(x_I) + Pb(x_I) = u_s$ is $n + m$. Therefore, to build a system of equations it is necessary to include a new set of equations. The literature shows that it is necessary to impose $P^T a(x_I) = 0$ to achieve a unique solution [27]. This leads to the following system of equations:

$$\begin{bmatrix} R & P \\ P^T & 0 \end{bmatrix} \begin{Bmatrix} a(x_I) \\ b(x_I) \end{Bmatrix} = M_T \begin{Bmatrix} a(x_I) \\ b(x_I) \end{Bmatrix} = \begin{Bmatrix} u_s \\ 0 \end{Bmatrix} \Rightarrow \begin{Bmatrix} a(x_I) \\ b(x_I) \end{Bmatrix} = M_T^{-1} \begin{Bmatrix} u_s \\ 0 \end{Bmatrix} \tag{5}$$

where $R \; [n \times n]$ is the radial moment matrix (Equation (6)), $P \; [n \times m]$ is the polynomial moment matrix, (Equation (7)), and u_s is a vector with the field function nodal parameters $[n \times 1]$.

$$R = \begin{bmatrix} (d_{11}^2 + (\gamma d_c)^2)^p & (d_{12}^2 + (\gamma d_c)^2)^p & \cdots & (d_{1n}^2 + (\gamma d_c)^2)^p \\ (d_{21}^2 + (\gamma d_c)^2)^p & (d_{22}^2 + (\gamma d_c)^2)^p & \cdots & (d_{2n}^2 + (\gamma d_c)^2)^p \\ \vdots & \vdots & \ddots & \vdots \\ (d_{n1}^2 + (\gamma d_c)^2)^p & (d_{n2}^2 + (\gamma d_c)^2)^p & \cdots & (d_{nn}^2 + (\gamma d_c)^2)^p \end{bmatrix} \tag{6}$$

$$P = \begin{bmatrix} p_1(x_1) & p_2(x_1) & \cdots & p_m(x_1) \\ p_1(x_2) & p_2(x_2) & \cdots & p_m(x_2) \\ \vdots & \vdots & \ddots & \vdots \\ p_1(x_n) & p_2(x_n) & \cdots & p_m(x_n) \end{bmatrix} \tag{7}$$

By back-substitution in Equation (2), it is possible to obtain

$$u_h = \{r(x_I)^T \; p(x_I)^T\} M_T^{-1} \begin{Bmatrix} u_s \\ 0 \end{Bmatrix} = \{\varphi(x_I)^T \; \psi(x_I)^T\} \begin{Bmatrix} u_s \\ 0 \end{Bmatrix} \tag{8}$$

In which $\phi(x_I)^T$ represents the RPI shape function vector, and $\psi(x_I)^T$ is a neglectable vector, a by-product of the additional set of equations: $P^T a(x_I) = 0$.

$$\varphi(x_I) = \{\varphi_1(x_I) \; \varphi_2(x_I) \; \cdots \; \varphi_n(x_I)\} \tag{9}$$

Finally, the RPI shape functions verify the Kronecker delta property, which allows for the direct imposition of boundary conditions, as they pass through all the nodes in the influence domain:

$$\varphi_i(x_j) = \delta_{ij} \begin{cases} 1 & (i = j) \\ 0 & (i \neq j) \end{cases} \tag{10}$$

as well as satisfying the partition of unity:

$$\sum_{i=1}^{n} \varphi_i(x_i) = 1 \tag{11}$$

2.2. Weak Form and Discrete System of Equations

Assuming well-known essential boundaries and the initial and final time conditions (i.e., the compatibility conditions), the energy principle dictates that out of all possible displacement configurations satisfying such compatibility conditions, the unique final solution is the one minimizing the Lagrangian functional. The minimization of the Lagrangian functional for a solid with domain Ω and boundary Γ can be represented as

$$\delta \int_{t_1}^{t_2} \left[\frac{1}{2} \int_\Omega \rho \dot{u}^T \dot{u} d\Omega - \frac{1}{2} \int_\Omega \varepsilon^T \sigma d\Omega + \int_\Omega u^T b d\Omega + \int_{\Gamma_t} u^T \bar{t} d\Gamma \right] = 0 \tag{12}$$

where ρ is the solid-mass density, $\dot{u}$ is the velocity, ε is the strain tensor, σ is the stress tensor, u is the displacement vector, b are the body forces, and $\bar{t}$ are the traction forces applied to the boundary $\Gamma \in \Omega$. The first term of (12) refers to the kinetic energy and is, therefore, discarded in static problems. The second term is referent to the strain energy and the last two terms are referent to the work produced by the external forces. The variational operand can be moved inside the integral and the second integral in (12) is rearranged. Thus, for Equation (12) to be valid for the compatibility conditions, its integrand must be equal to zero. Such an equality results in the Galerkin weak form.

$$\int_\Omega \delta\varepsilon^T \sigma d\Omega = \int_\Omega \delta u^T b d\Omega + \int_{\Gamma_t} \delta u^T \bar{t} d\Gamma \tag{13}$$

where $\delta\varepsilon$ is the virtual strain tensor and δu is the virtual displacement.

The principle of virtual work states that if a solid body is in equilibrium, the virtual work produced by the inner stresses and the body applied external forces are null when the body experiments a virtual displacement.

The energy conservation principle states that if the work produced by the inner stresses is equal to the work produced by the applied external forces, then the body is in equilibrium. If the work produced by the applied external forces is calculated with a virtual displacement field and the work produced by the inner stresses is calculated using a virtual strain field resultant from the same virtual displacement field, then the principle of virtual work is obtained. Thus, knowing that stresses and strains are related through the generalized Hooke's law equation, Equation (14),

$$\sigma = D\varepsilon \tag{14}$$

and strains are linearly related to displacements, Equation (15),

$$\varepsilon = Lu \tag{15}$$

the weak form Equation (13) can be re-written in terms of displacement as follows:

$$\int_\Omega \delta u^T B^T D B u d\Omega = \int_\Omega \delta u^T H b d\Omega + \int_\Gamma \delta u^T H \bar{t} d\Gamma \tag{16}$$

Inverting the material compliance matrix C, it is possible to obtain the constitutive material matrix $D = C^{-1}$. Assuming the Voigt notation, the material compliance matrix C can be presented as

$$C = \begin{bmatrix} c_1 & c_3 & c_3 & 0 & 0 & 0 \\ c_3 & c_1 & c_3 & 0 & 0 & 0 \\ c_3 & c_3 & c_1 & 0 & 0 & 0 \\ 0 & 0 & 0 & c_2 & 0 & 0 \\ 0 & 0 & 0 & 0 & c_2 & 0 \\ 0 & 0 & 0 & 0 & 0 & c_2 \end{bmatrix} \tag{17}$$

where $c_1 = 1/E$ and $c_3 = -\nu/E$, being that E and ν are the Young's modulus and the Poisson ratio of the material, respectively. In Equation (16), B is the deformation matrix:

$$B(x_I) = \sum_{i=1}^n L\varphi_i(x_I) = \begin{bmatrix} \frac{\partial \varphi_i}{\partial x} & 0 & 0 \\ 0 & \frac{\partial \varphi_i}{\partial y} & 0 \\ 0 & 0 & \frac{\partial \varphi_i}{\partial z} \\ \frac{\partial \varphi_i}{\partial y} & \frac{\partial \varphi_i}{\partial x} & 0 \\ 0 & \frac{\partial \varphi_i}{\partial y} & \frac{\partial \varphi_i}{\partial z} \\ \frac{\partial \varphi_i}{\partial z} & 0 & \frac{\partial \varphi_i}{\partial x} \end{bmatrix} \tag{18}$$

so that the strain and displacement relation is

$$\varepsilon(x_I) = B(x_I)u \qquad (19)$$

for any integration point x_I. H is a diagonal matrix containing the shape functions $\varphi(x_I)$. The virtual displacement can be removed from (16),

$$\int_\Omega B^T DB d\Omega u = \int_\Omega Hb d\Omega + \int_\Gamma H\bar{t} d\Gamma \qquad (20)$$

obtaining the discrete system of equations. Equation (20) can be written in the matrix form as

$$K^e u^e = F^e \qquad (21)$$

where the elemental stiffness matrix K^e is

$$K^e = \int_\Omega B^T DB d\Omega \qquad (22)$$

and the force vector F^e is given by

$$F^e = \int_\Omega Hb d\Omega + \int_\Gamma H\bar{t} d\Gamma \qquad (23)$$

Finally, the global system of equations is assembled from the element matrices so that the displacement field can be solved.

2.3. Bone Tissue Remodeling Algorithm

Bone remodeling is a vital process for bone health and maintenance, allowing bones to develop, repair, and renew throughout life. This process is complex and highly coordinated, involving the removal and replacement of deteriorated bone tissue through the activity of various cellular components. These components ensure mineral homeostasis and structural integrity [29]. The cellular groups that sequentially carry out the process of bone resorption and formation compose the bone remodeling unit, which has been termed the basic multicellular unit (BMU) [30]. Initially, a BMU is formed by osteoclasts responsible for bone resorption. Subsequently, the bone surface is covered by reversal cells and prepared for bone replacement. In the next step, osteoblasts release and deposit osteoid, the unmineralized bone matrix [29].

The bone remodeling cycle includes five sequential phases: activation, resorption, reversal, formation, and termination [29].

Several studies [31–34] affirm the correlation between the mechanical properties of bones and their apparent density. Additionally, various bone tissue models [35–38] in the literature delineate the evolution of trabecular architecture based on mechanical stimuli, employing diverse formulations and assumptions.

The apparent density of bone is given by

$$\rho_{app} = \frac{w_{sample}}{V_{sample}} \qquad (24)$$

where ρ_{app} corresponds to the apparent density, w_{sample} represents the wet mineralized mass of a given sample, and V_{sample} represents the volume of the same sample. Alternatively, it is also possible to represent this property as a function of its porosity p:

$$\rho_{app} = \rho_0(1-p) \qquad (25)$$

where ρ_0 corresponds to the density of compact bone, approximately 2.1 g/cm^3, and porosity p is calculated from V_{holes}/V_{sample}, where V_{holes} is the total volume of holes.

The apparent density holds significance in its connection to the mechanical attributes of bone tissue, specifically the elasticity modulus and ultimate stress. Belinha [26] employed polynomial laws to establish a relationship between the mechanical properties of bone tissue and apparent density, incorporating a transition density of 1.3 g/cm³ to differentiate between trabecular and cortical bone.

Thus, in this work the following phenomenological law was considered [26]:

$$E^{bone}_{cortical}[\text{MPa}] = 68{,}357.14\rho^3_{app} - 276{,}771.43\rho^2_{app} + 386{,}136.43\rho_{app} - 177{,}644.29 \qquad (26)$$

$$E^{bone}_{trabecular}[\text{MPa}] = 805.86\rho^2_{app} + 721.61\rho_{app} \qquad (27)$$

$$\sigma^{bone}_{c}[\text{MPa}] = 20.3508\rho^3_{app} + 26.7984\rho^2_{app} \qquad (28)$$

In Equations (26) to (28), $E^{bone}_{cortical}$ corresponds to the elastic modulus of cortical bone, $E^{bone}_{trabecular}$ corresponds to the elastic modulus of trabecular bone, and σ^{bone}_{c} corresponds to the ultimate compressive stress.

In the bone remodeling process, there is strong evidence of the correlation between the loads (stress or strain) that the area is subject to, and the shape that the bone takes. This has led to the requirement to develop some semi-empirical laws in order to model how the bone will functionally adapt to the load case it is subject to. These laws are the basis for computational tools which aim at predicting bone adaptation under stress or strain states or changes in stiffness [26]. The model employed in this study [39–43] assumes that, regardless of the material law applied, the induced stress serves as an optimization tool. It aims to maximize structural integrity while minimizing mass. This perspective is analogous to viewing induced stress as an optimization tool, where the objective function is minimized, as discussed by Belinha [26].

Figure 2 summarizes the bone remodeling iterative algorithm.

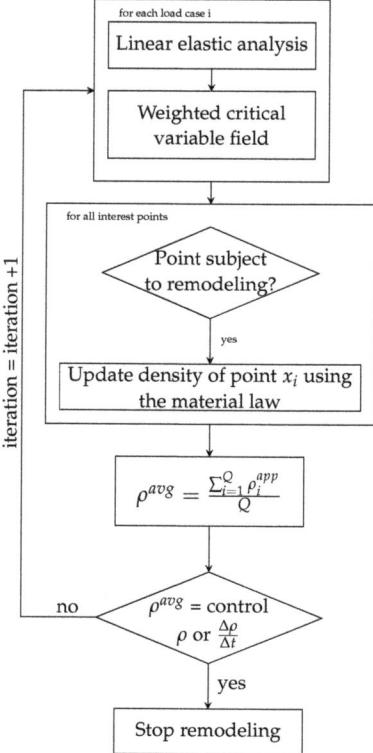

Figure 2. Flowchart for the bone remodeling algorithm.

The bone remodeling nonlinear equation is presented as a differential Equation (29) in which a temporal–spatial based functional, $\rho_{app}(x,t)$, is minimized with respect to time, and where $\rho_{app}(x,t) : \mathbb{R}^{(d+1)} \mapsto \mathbb{R}$ is defined for the one temporal dimension and the d spatial dimensions.

$$\frac{\partial \rho_{app}(x,t)}{\partial t} \cong \frac{\Delta \rho_{app}(x,t)}{\Delta t} = \left(\rho_{app}^{model}\right)_{t_j} - \left(\rho_{app}^{model}\right)_{t_{j+1}} = 0 \qquad (29)$$

It is assumed that the d-dimensional domain is discretized in N nodes, $X = \{x_1, x_2, \ldots x_N\} \in \Omega$, leading to Q integration points, where $Q = \{x_1, x_2, \ldots x_Q\} \in \Omega$, being that $x_i \in \mathbb{R}^d$. The temporal domain is discretized in iterative fictitious time steps $t_j \in \mathbb{R}$, where $j \in \mathbb{N}$. Within the same iterative time step t_j, the average apparent density of the iteration point x_I is defined by $\rho_I = g(\sigma_I)$:

$$\rho_{app}^{model} = Q^{-1} \sum_{i=1}^{Q} (\rho_{app})_I \qquad (30)$$

Then, $g(\sigma_I) : \mathbb{R}^3 \mapsto \mathbb{R}$ is defined as in (31).

$$g(\sigma_I) = max\left(\{\sigma_1^{-1}(\rho_I)\ \sigma_2^{-1}(\rho_I)\ \sigma_3^{-1}(\rho_I)\}\right) \qquad (31)$$

Here, σ_j are the principal stresses obtained for integration point x_I and $\sigma_j^{-1}(\rho_I)$ are the inverse functions of $\sigma_j(\rho_I)$, defined with the material law.

The inverse equation of stress as a function of apparent density (28) is then applied to the integration points with von Mises stress values inside the following interval, where $\sigma_m^{VM} = min(\sigma^{VM})$ and $\sigma_M^{VM} = max(\sigma^{VM})$:

$$\sigma^{VM}(x_I) \in \left[\sigma_m^{VM}, \sigma_m^{VM} + \alpha \cdot \Delta \sigma^{VM}\right] \cup \left]\sigma_M^{VM} - \beta \cdot \Delta \sigma^{VM}, \sigma_M^{VM}\right] \qquad (32)$$

The parameters α and β define the growth rate and the decay rate of the apparent density. The remodeling equilibrium is achieved when Equation (33) is verified, where α, β and $\rho_{app}^{control}$ depend on the analyzed problem.

$$\frac{\Delta \rho}{\Delta t} = 0 \wedge \left(\rho_{app}^{model}\right)_{t_j} = \rho_{app}^{control} \qquad (33)$$

In summary, at each iteration the linear elastic analysis is run on the model. The elastic properties of the bone material are obtained from the density at each point using (26) and (27). With the obtained variable fields, the critical values for the variables are determined. The points with higher values of stress will have their density increased and the points with lower stress will have their density decreased, being that the new density value is determined through (28).

3. Tibia and Implant Numerical Models

In this section, the construction of 3D models for the numerical applications analyzed in this study is presented. Note that all the calculations were performed using an original code developed by the authors using the Matlab© (Natick, MA, USA: The MathWorks Inc.) environment. All the routines and images produced were programmed by the authors without using any toolbox of Matlab©. Nevertheless, the 3D models were created in Autodesk Fusion© (San Francisco, CA, USA: Autodesk) and the 3D discretizatons were produced with ABAQUS© (Johnston, RI, USA: Dassault Systemes Simulia Corp).

The stress and displacement analysis of the proximal tibia was run in three-dimensional models discretized into 4-node tetrahedral elements. The analysis of osteointegration to the implant was run on a two-dimensional model in order to allow for a finer mesh and, consequently, a finer trabecular arrangement. The two-dimensional model was discretized into 3-node plane-stress elements. Table 1 summarizes the number of nodes and elements used for each model.

Table 1. Mesh information for each model.

Implant Length	Element Type	Nodes	Elements
0	4-node tetrahedral	2083	9522
12 mm	4-node tetrahedral	5273	1171
30 mm	4-node tetrahedral	6908	1487
40 mm	3-node plane stress	1901	3630
40 mm	4-node tetrahedral	6299	1360

The knee joint is subjected to loads that vary significantly with the activity the individual performs. The loads applied in the model took into account another study, which analyzed the gait of an individual, where it was concluded that the average peak force was 1645 N [18]. According to the literature, the axial force is considered the primary point of evaluation of the model's response, since it was previously determined as an indicator of injury risk. Thus, it was found that the axial load was 987 N and 658 N for the medial and lateral platforms of the tibia, respectively, since the load ratio between the medial and lateral platforms is 60%:40% [18,44]. It is important to note that the applied loads do not take into account the forces of the ligaments, muscles, and tendons. The tibia is kept in balance by the surrounding tissues and other bones of the lower limbs. The difficulty in representing this system in a finite element model leads to simplifications in terms of boundary conditions. Therefore, the nodes located at the most distal part of the model were fixed, effectively constraining any rigid-body movement.

Figure 3a shows the boundary conditions applied to the three-dimensional model without the implant. Equivalent boundary conditions were applied to the implant model as well. The loads labeled as F1 and F2 were distributed among the nodes in the vicinity of the positions indicated in Figure 3a, with moduli of 658 N and 987 N, respectively. For the remodeling analysis, the same two forces were considered. However, in order to more accurately emulate the shear loading which occurs during locomotion, these two loads were applied considering a 10° angle, as shown in Figure 3b.

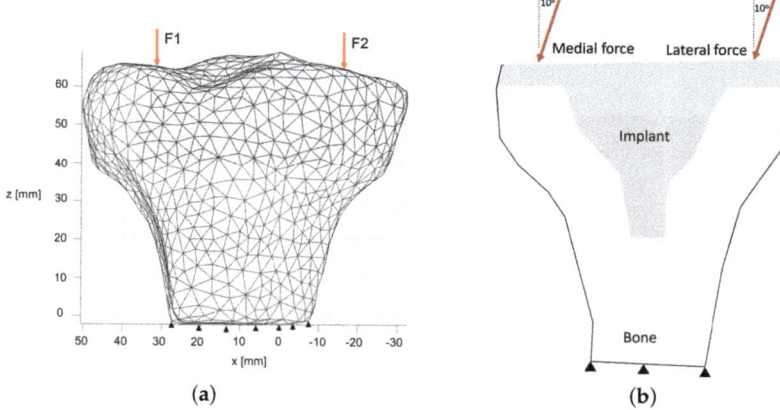

Figure 3. Schematic representation of the essential and natural boundary conditions applied to (**a**) the three-dimensional model and (**b**) the two-dimensional implant model.

Concerning the models featuring an implant, these were developed by converting the mesh model into a spline model, enabling the precise modeling of the implant's shape. When the implant comprised three components, as depicted in Figure 4a, the model was transformed into a spline model as illustrated in Figure 4b. This simplification resulted in a unified structure with distinct material properties assigned to the bone and implant areas, as visible in Figure 4c.

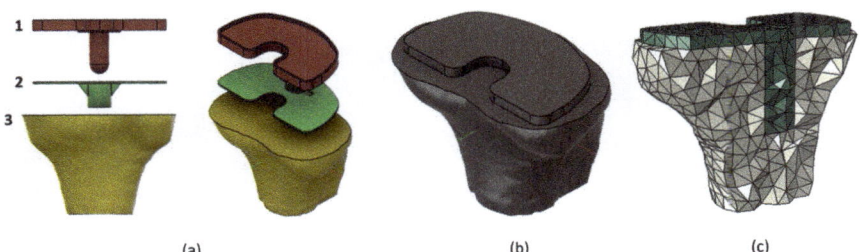

Figure 4. Implant model. (**a**) 1—tibial plate, 2—cement, 3—tibia; (**b**) simplified assembled model; (**c**) simplified model representation showing the implant and surrounding bone.

Healthy cortical bone has an elastic modulus of 17 GPa; however, in this study, this property was varied (Table 2) in order to check the impact of this change on the distribution of the effective von Mises stress, as well as on the displacement field. The implant was considered to be Ti-6Al-4V.

The initial implant model shown in Figure 4a was modeled based on the the commercial implant by DePuy Synthes®.

Table 2. Mechanical properties of the implant material and cortical bone.

	Young's Modulus [GPa]	Poisson's Ratio
Implant—Ti-6Al-4V	110	0.34
Low-stiffness bone	5	0.33
Healthy cortical bone	17	0.33
High-stiffness bone	25	0.33

4. Results and Discussion

4.1. Structural Analysis of the Proximal Tibia

The Von Mises stress does not depend on the Young's modulus of the material but it will differ between numerical methods. Thus, Figure 5 shows a set of points to evaluate the von Mises stress and the respective results.

The displacements, however, will depend on the mechanical properties. Figure 6 shows the displacement field results for the three conditions and both methods. Because the results for both methods are very similar, only one of them is shown.

Additionally, the displacement was analyzed at two points in the proximal part of the tibia, labeled in Figure 5a as point A and B. For the three materials and both methods, the displacement values are shown in Table 3.

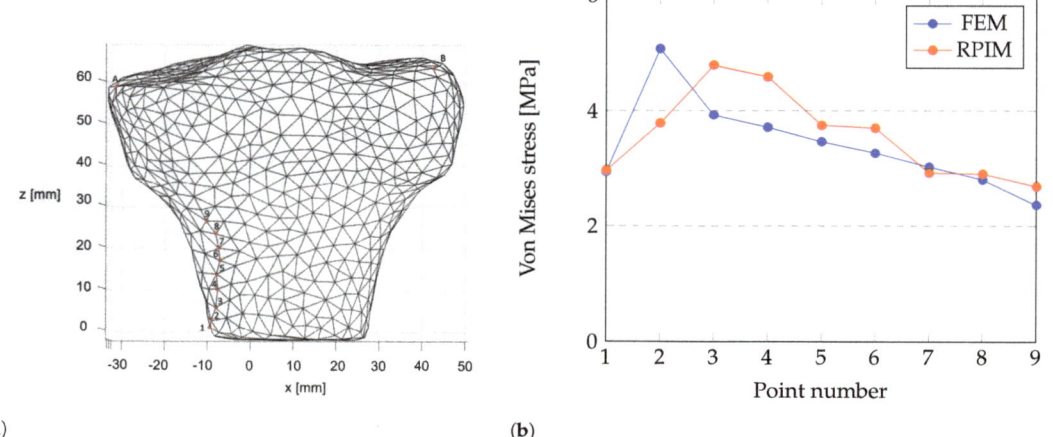

Figure 5. Von Mises stress results: (**a**) selected points in the model (A and B are two representative points of load application and, therefore, are used to evaluate the displacement and points 1 to 9 are the points selected to evaluate stress since each point is further from the fixed ending); (**b**) von Mises stress at each point calculated with the FEM and the RPIM.

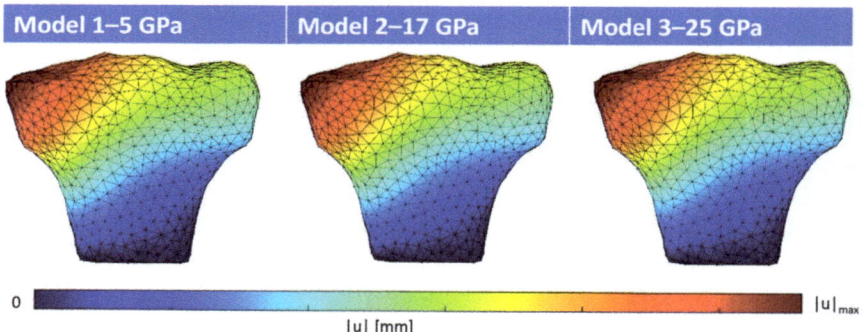

Figure 6. Displacement field for each material, where the maximum displacements $|u|_{max}$ are 0.050, 0.016, and 0.010 for model 1, model 2, and model 3, respectively.

Table 3. Displacement at two points calculated with the FEM and RPIM for all tested materials.

Method	Young's Modulus	Point	u_x [mm]	u_y [mm]	u_z [mm]	$|u|$ [mm]
FEM	5 GPa	A	−0.0281	−0.0158	−0.0451	0.0555
		B	−0.0241	−0.0193	−0.0035	0.031
	17 GPa	A	−0.0082	−0.0046	−0.0132	0.0163
		B	−0.007	−0.0056	−0.001	0.0091
	25 GPa	A	−0.0056	−0.0031	−0.009	0.0111
		B	−0.0048	−0.0038	−0.0007	0.0062
RPIM	5 GPa	A	−0.0286	−0.0161	−0.0471	0.0575
		B	−0.0246	−0.0203	−0.004	0.0322
	17 GPa	A	−0.0084	−0.0047	−0.0138	0.0169
		B	−0.0072	−0.0059	−0.0011	0.0094
	25 GPa	A	−0.0057	−0.0032	−0.0094	0.0115
		B	−0.0049	−0.004	−0.0008	0.0064

4.2. Structural Analysis of the Implant and Influence of Implant Length

The Von Mises stress fields for all the implant lengths considering healthy bone only are shown in Figure 7.

Concerning the stress analysis of the model without the implant, the FEM analysis concluded that the highest stress value occurs for point 2 while the RPIM analysis concluded that the highest stress value occurs for point 3. This phenomenon is due to the fact that the stress field is a field that has been extrapolated to the nodes, which means that the stress value is being smoothed at the nodes. By increasing the number of nodes in the mesh, this effect starts to diminish, and the maximum stress begins to approach the base of the fixture.

The maximum stress values verified after the insertion of the implant, between 5.0568 and 5.9497 MPa for the FEM and between 4.4690 and 6.1584 for the RPIM, are similar to the values verified at the unimplanted model of 5.0705 MPa for the FEM and 4.7880 MPa for the RPIM model, which indicate that stress shielding would not occur. The maximum stress values occur at similar locations for the implanted and unimplanted models.

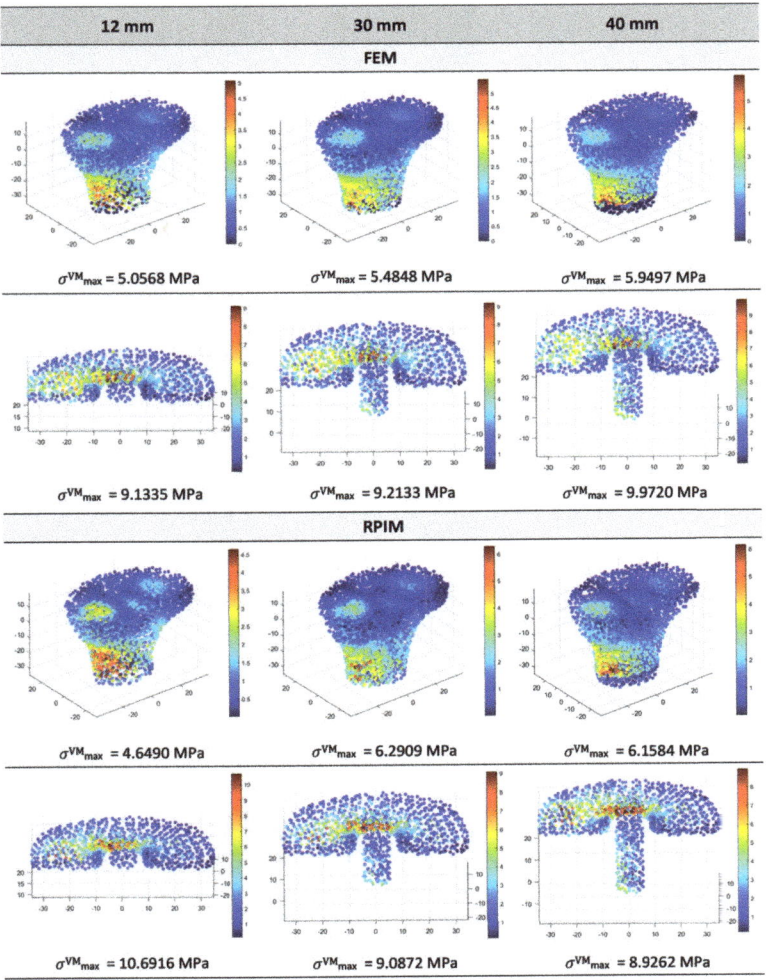

Figure 7. Von Mises stress field at the nodes for the tested implants.

Stress is an important measure to evaluate the occurrence of stress shielding (SS) as it indicates whether adequate loading is being applied to the bone. It can be quantified as the stress change before and after implant insertion [45] (34):

$$SS = \frac{\sigma_{bone} - \sigma_{implanted-bone}}{\sigma_{bone}} \quad (34)$$

where σ_{bone} and $\sigma_{implantedbone}$ denote the Von Mises stress of the bone without and with the implant, respectively. Considering the maximum Von Mises stress verified at all stem lengths, the occurrence of SS can be discarded since the stress value increases after insertion.

The displacement fields for all implant lengths are shown in Figure 8.

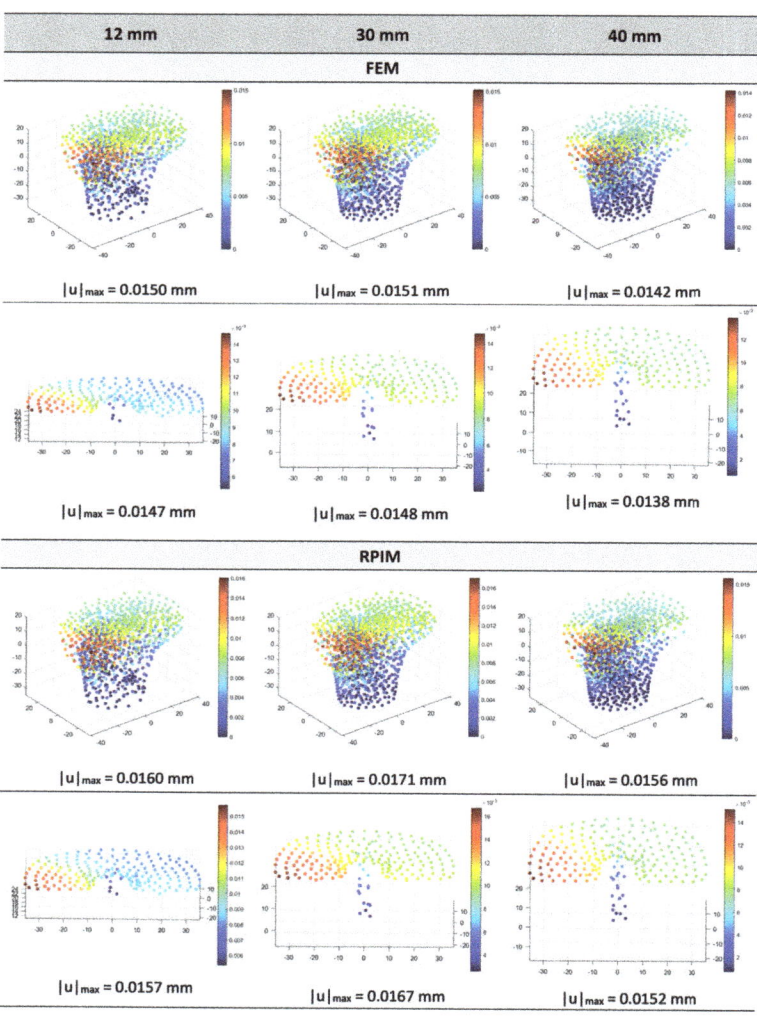

Figure 8. Displacement field at the nodes for the tested implants.

The maximum displacement, which occurs at the medial side, is similar with and without the implant. The unimplanted model, taking into consideration the healthy bone, is 0.016 mm, while for the FEM this value ranges between 0.0142 and 0.0151 mm and 0.0156 and 0.0171 mm for the RPIM. It should be noted that the mesh model for the tibia varies with each implant length, which could account for some of the discrepancies observed between the two methods as the essential and natural boundary conditions were not being applied to the exact same nodal coordinates. Thus, excluding the RPIM analysis of the 30 mm length implant, the stress verified at the tibia would increase with implant length.

The greater the stiffness of the implant, the less load will be transferred to the bone from the deformation suffered by the stem [45]. The evaluation of displacements suffered by the implant is, therefore, an important measure of stress shielding. Since it was verified that the implant displacements are in the range of the displacements of the intact bone, similar stiffness values were achieved.

The measured displacements with the RPIM are higher than the FEM while the stress values are lower. It is expected that the results obtained through RPIM will be closer to the actual results, after conducting a convergence study (which helps to ensure that the results are more accurate), or if a denser mesh is generated, as was the case in the study developed by Marques et al. [46].

In conclusion, the tested stem sizes for an implant in the selected material are not likely to induce stress shielding. Nevertheless, this study does not consider bone heterogeneities, which alter the mechanical properties and consequently the structural response.

4.3. Bone Remodeling Analysis

Regarding the osteointegration evaluation, two analyses were considered. First, the medial and lateral forces were considered as two separate forces acting at two different moments, and for the second case, those forces acted simultaneously. Figure 9a shows the apparent density maps for the two tested load combinations. Only a finite element analysis was considered for this stage.

Concerning the bone remodeling analysis, there is no significant difference between the imposition of the medial and lateral loads simultaneously or as different loads. Regarding the trabecular arrangement, there are three major bone resorption areas, as indicated by the numbers in Figure 9b. Additionally the main trabecula formed by the algorithm is aligned with the load angle as expected, since the algorithm states that higher stress areas are subject to having their density increased and lower stress areas are subject to having their density decreased, leading to alignment of the density map with the stress map.

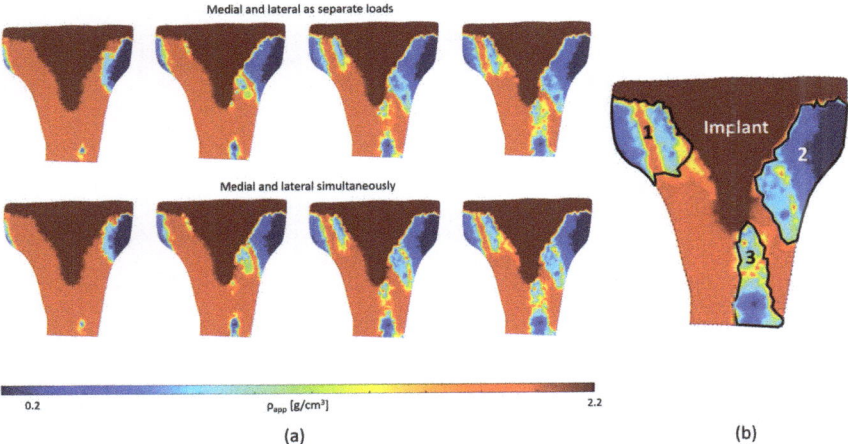

Figure 9. (**a**) Evaluation of osteointegration using the FEM along the iterations; (**b**) indication of the main resorption (indicated by numbers 1 to 3) and growth areas after implant insertion.

5. Conclusions

Utilizing computational approaches enhances the study of implant design and surgical techniques alongside clinical and experimental research. In summary, longer stem lengths, such as 40 mm, result in higher maximum stress in the proximal tibia but lead to lower displacements compared to shorter lengths. However, the 30 mm model stood out as an outlier in the maximum displacement due to the use of different models for testing each length. Additionally, bone remodeling analysis confirmed the expected anatomical structures, including areas of bone resorption and the diaphysis, through the observed density distribution.

Author Contributions: Conceptualization, A.P. and J.B.; methodology, A.P. and J.B.; software, A.P. and J.B.; validation, C.M.; formal analysis, C.M.; investigation, C.M., A.P. and J.B.; resources, C.M., A.P. and J.B.; data curation, C.M.; writing—original draft preparation, A.P.; writing—review and editing, A.P. and J.B.; visualization, A.P. and J.B.; supervision, A.P. and J.B.; project administration, J.B.; funding acquisition, J.B. All authors have read and agreed to the published version of the manuscript.

Funding: The authors truly acknowledge the funding provided by LAETA, under project UIDB/50022/2020 and the doctoral grant SFRH/BD/151362/2021 financed by the Portuguese Foundation for Science and Technology (FCT), Ministério da Ciência, Tecnologia e Ensino Superior (MCTES), Portugal, with funds from the State Budget (OE), European Social Fund (ESF) and PorNorte, under the MIT Portugal Program.

Data Availability Statement: Data are contained within the article.

Conflicts of Interest: The authors declare no conflicts of interest.

References

1. Fernandes, D.A.; Poeta, L.S.; Martins, C.A.d.Q.; Lima, F.d.; Rosa Neto, F. Balance and quality of life after total knee arthroplasty. *Rev. Bras. Ortop. (Engl. Ed.)* **2018**, *53*, 747–753. [CrossRef]
2. Yueh, S.; Noori, M.; Mahadev, S.; Noori, N.B. Finite Element Analysis of Total Knee Arthroplasty. *Am. J. Biomed. Sci. Res.* **2021**, *14*, 6–15. [CrossRef]
3. Filip, A.C.; Cuculici, S.A.; Cristea, S.; Filip, V.; Negrea, A.D.; Mihai, S.; Pantu, C.M. Tibial Stem Extension versus Standard Configuration in Total Knee Arthroplasty: A Biomechanical Assessment According to Bone Properties. *Medicina* **2022**, *58*, 634. [CrossRef] [PubMed]
4. Peters, C.L.; Erickson, J.; Kloepper, R.G.; Mohr, R.A. Revision total knee arthroplasty with modular components inserted with metaphyseal cement and stems without cement. *J. Arthroplast.* **2005**, *20*, 302–308. [CrossRef]
5. Cintra, F.F.; Yepéz, A.K.; Rasga, M.G.S.; Abagge, M.; Alencar, P.G.C. Tibial Component in Revision of Total Knee Arthroplasty: Comparison Between Cemented and Hybrid Fixation. *Rev. Bras. Ortop. (Engl. Ed.)* **2011**, *46*, 585–590. [CrossRef]
6. Lonner, J.H.; Klotz, M.; Levitz, C.; Lotke, P.A. Changes in bone density after cemented total knee arthroplasty: Influence of stem design. *J. Arthroplast.* **2001**, *16*, 107–111. [CrossRef] [PubMed]
7. Shannon, B.D.; Klassen, J.F.; Rand, J.A.; Berry, D.J.; Trousdale, R.T. Revision total knee arthroplasty with cemented components and uncemented intramedullary stems. *J. Arthroplast.* **2003**, *18*, 27–32. [CrossRef] [PubMed]
8. Kang, S.G.; Park, C.H.; Song, S.J. Stem fixation in revision total knee arthroplasty: Indications, stem dimensions, and fixation methods. *Knee Surg. Relat. Res.* **2018**, *30*, 187–192. [CrossRef]
9. Crawford, D.A.; Berend, K.R.; Morris, M.J.; Adams, J.B.; Lombardi, A.V. Results of a Modular Revision System in Total Knee Arthroplasty. *J. Arthroplast.* **2017**, *32*, 2792–2798. [CrossRef]
10. Bottner, F.; Laskin, R.; Windsor, R.E.; Haas, S.B. Hybrid component fixation in revision total knee arthroplasty. *Clin. Orthop. Relat. Res.* **2006**, *446*, 127–131. [CrossRef]
11. Ni, G.X.; Lu, W.W.; Chiu, K.Y.; Fong, D.Y. Cemented or uncemented femoral component in primary total hip replacement? A review from a clinical and radiological perspective. *J. Orthop. Surg. (Hong Kong)* **2005**, *13*, 96–105. [CrossRef] [PubMed]
12. Kadir, M.R.A. *Computational Biomechanics of the Hip Joint*; Springer: Berlin/Heidelberg, Germany, 2013.
13. Dorr, L.D.; Wan, Z.; Gruen, T. Functional results in total hip replacement in patients 65 years and older. *Clin. Orthop. Relat. Res.* **1997**, *336*, 143–151. [CrossRef] [PubMed]
14. Kozelskaya, A.I.; Rutkowski, S.; Frueh, J.; Gogolev, A.S.; Chistyakov, S.G.; Gnedenkov, S.V.; Sinebryukhov, S.L.; Frueh, A.; Egorkin, V.S.; Choynzonov, E.L.; et al. Surface Modification of Additively Fabricated Titanium-Based Implants by Means of Bioactive Micro-Arc Oxidation Coatings for Bone Replacement. *J. Funct. Biomater.* **2022**, *13*, 285. [CrossRef] [PubMed]
15. Completo, A.; Simões, J.A.; Fonseca, F.; Oliveira, M. The influence of different tibial stem designs in load sharing and stability at the cement-bone interface in revision TKA. *Knee* **2008**, *15*, 227–232. [CrossRef] [PubMed]

16. Quevedo González, F.J.; Sculco, P.K.; Kahlenberg, C.A.; Mayman, D.J.; Lipman, J.D.; Wright, T.M.; Vigdorchik, J.M. Undersizing the Tibial Baseplate in Cementless Total Knee Arthroplasty has Only a Small Impact on Bone-Implant Interaction: A Finite Element Biomechanical Study. *J. Arthroplast.* **2023**, *38*, 757–762. [CrossRef] [PubMed]
17. Quevedo Gonzalez, F.J.; Lipman, J.D.; Sculco, P.K.; Sculco, T.P.; De Martino, I.; Wright, T.M. An Anterior Spike Decreases Bone-Implant Micromotion in Cementless Tibial Baseplates for Total Knee Arthroplasty: A Biomechanical Study. *J. Arthroplast.* **2023**, 4–8. [CrossRef] [PubMed]
18. Liu, Y.; Chen, B.; Wang, C.; Chen, H.; Zhang, A.; Yin, W.; Wu, N.; Han, Q.; Wang, J. Design of Porous Metal Block Augmentation to Treat Tibial Bone Defects in Total Knee Arthroplasty Based on Topology Optimization. *Front. Bioeng. Biotechnol.* **2021**, *9*, 765438. [CrossRef] [PubMed]
19. Liu, Y.; Zhang, A.; Wang, C.; Yin, W.; Wu, N.; Chen, H.; Chen, B.; Han, Q.; Wang, J. Biomechanical comparison between metal block and cement-screw techniques for the treatment of tibial bone defects in total knee arthroplasty based on finite element analysis. *Comput. Biol. Med.* **2020**, *125*, 104006. [CrossRef]
20. Bhandarkar, S.; Dhatrak, P. Optimization of a knee implant with different biomaterials using finite element analysis. *Mater. Today Proc.* **2022**, *59*, 459–467. [CrossRef]
21. Apostolopoulos, V.; Tomáš, T.; Boháč, P.; Marcián, P.; Mahdal, M.; Valoušek, T.; Janíček, P.; Nachtnebl, L. Biomechanical analysis of all-polyethylene total knee arthroplasty on periprosthetic tibia using the finite element method. *Comput. Methods Programs Biomed.* **2022**, *220*, 106834. [CrossRef]
22. Mondal, S.; Ghosh, R. The role of the depth of resection of the distal tibia on biomechanical performance of the tibial component for TAR: A finite element analysis with three implant designs. *Med Eng. Phys.* **2023**, *119*, 104034. [CrossRef]
23. Jyoti; Mondal, S.; Ghosh, R. Biomechanical analysis of three popular tibial designs for TAR with different implant-bone interfacial conditions and bone qualities: A finite element study. *Med Eng. Phys.* **2022**, *104*, 103812. [CrossRef]
24. ISO 22926:2023; Implants for Surgery Specification and Verification of Synthetic Anatomical Bone Models for Testing. ISO: Geneva, Switzerland, 2023.
25. ISO/CD 5092:2023; Additive Manufacturing for Medical. ISO: Geneva, Switzerland, 2023.
26. Belinha, J. *Meshless Methods in Biomechanics—Bone Tissue Remodelling Analysis*; Springer: Porto, Portugal, 2014.
27. Belinha, J. *Meshless Methods in Biomechanics: Bone Tissue Remodelling Analysis*; Lecture Notes in Computational Vision and Biomechanics; Springer International Publishing: Berlin/Heidelberg, Germany, 2014.
28. Hardy, R.L. Theory and applications of the multiquadric-biharmonic method 20 years of discovery 1968–1988. *Comput. Math. Appl.* **1990**, *19*, 163–208. [CrossRef]
29. Raggatt, L.J.; Partridge, N.C. Cellular and molecular mechanisms of bone remodeling. *J. Biol. Chem.* **2010**, *285*, 25103–25108. [CrossRef] [PubMed]
30. Sabet, F.A.; Najafi, A.R.; Hamed, E.; Jasiuk, I. Modelling of bone fracture and strength at different length scales: A review. *Interface Focus* **2016**, *6*, 20–30. [CrossRef] [PubMed]
31. Carter, D.R.; Hayes, W.C. The compressive behavior of bone as a two-phase porous structure. *J. Bone Jt. Surgery. Am. Vol.* **1977**, *59*, 954–962. [CrossRef]
32. Goldstein, S.A. The mechanical properties of trabecular bone: Dependence on anatomic location and function. *J. Biomech.* **1987**, *20*, 1055–1061. [CrossRef]
33. Rice, J.C.; Cowin, S.C.; Bowman, J.A. On the dependence of the elasticity and strength of cancellous bone on apparent density. *J. Biomech.* **1988**, *21*, 155–168. [CrossRef]
34. Martin, R.B. Determinants of the mechanical properties of bones. *J. Biomech.* **1991**, *24*, 79–88. [CrossRef]
35. Pauwels, F. *Gesammelte Abhandlungen zur Funktionellen Anatomie des Bewegungsapparates*; Springer: Berlin/Heidelberg, Germany, 2013.
36. Cowin, S.C.; Hegedus, D.H. Bone remodeling I: theory of adaptive elasticity. *J. Elast.* **1976**, *6*, 313–326. [CrossRef]
37. Cowin, S.C.; Sadegh, A.M.; Luo, G.M. An Evolutionary Wolff's Law for Trabecular Architecture. *J. Biomech. Eng.* **1992**, *114*, 129–136. [CrossRef] [PubMed]
38. Rodrigues, H.; Jacobs, C.; Guedes, J.M.; Bendsøe, M.P. Global and local material optimization models applied to anisotropic bone adaptation. In Proceedings of the IUTAM Symposium on Synthesis in Bio Solid Mechanics, Copenhagen, Denmark, 24–27 May 1998; Springer: Berlin/Heidelberg, Germany, 1999; pp. 209–220.
39. Carter, D.R.; Fyhrie, D.P.; Whalen, R.T. Trabecular bone density and loading history: Regulation of connective tissue biology by mechanical energy. *J. Biomech.* **1987**, *20*, 785–794. [CrossRef] [PubMed]
40. Whalen, R.T.; Carter, D.R.; Steele, C.R. Influence of physical activity on the regulation of bone density. *J. Biomech.* **1988**, *21*, 825–837. [CrossRef]
41. Carter, D.R.; Orr, T.E.; Fyhrie, D.P. Relationships between loading history and femoral cancellous bone architecture. *J. Biomech.* **1989**, *22*, 231–244. [CrossRef] [PubMed]
42. Belinha, J.; Natal Jorge, R.M.; Dinis, L.M. Bone tissue remodelling analysis considering a radial point interpolator meshless method. *Eng. Anal. Bound. Elem.* **2012**, *36*, 1660–1670. [CrossRef]
43. Belinha, J.; Jorge, R.M.N.; Dinis, L.M.J.S. A meshless microscale bone tissue trabecular remodelling analysis considering a new anisotropic bone tissue material law. *Comput. Methods Biomech. Biomed. Eng.* **2013**, *16*, 1170–1184. [CrossRef]

44. Taddei, F.; Pani, M.; Zovatto, L.; Tonti, E.; Viceconti, M. A new meshless approach for subject-specific strain prediction in long bones: Evaluation of accuracy. *Clin. Biomech.* **2008**, *23*, 1192–1199. [CrossRef] [PubMed]
45. Liu, B.; Wang, H.; Zhang, N.; Zhang, M.; Cheng, C.K. Femoral Stems With Porous Lattice Structures: A Review. *Front. Bioeng. Biotechnol.* **2021**, *9*, 772539. [CrossRef]
46. Marques, M.; Belinha, J.; Dinis, L.M.J.S.; Natal Jorge, R. A brain impact stress analysis using advanced discretization meshless techniques. *Proc. Inst. Mech. Eng. Part H J. Eng. Med.* **2018**, *232*, 257–270. [CrossRef]

Disclaimer/Publisher's Note: The statements, opinions and data contained in all publications are solely those of the individual author(s) and contributor(s) and not of MDPI and/or the editor(s). MDPI and/or the editor(s) disclaim responsibility for any injury to people or property resulting from any ideas, methods, instructions or products referred to in the content.

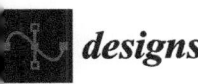

Article

Finite Element Analysis of Patient-Specific Cranial Implants under Different Design Parameters for Material Selection

Manuel Mejía Rodríguez [1], Octavio Andrés González-Estrada [2,*] and Diego Fernando Villegas-Bermúdez [2]

1 School of Mechanical Engineering, Universidad del Valle, Cali 760042, Colombia; manuel.mejia@correounivalle.edu.co
2 School of Mechanical Engineering, Universidad Industrial de Santander, Bucaramanga 680002, Colombia; dfvilleg@uis.edu.co
* Correspondence: agonzale@uis.edu.co

Abstract: This work presents the study of the thickness vs. stiffness relationship for different materials (PMMA and PEEK) in patient-specific cranial implants, as a criterion for the selection of biomaterials from a mechanical perspective. The geometry of the implant is constructed from the reconstruction of the cranial lesion using image segmentation obtained from computed axial tomography. Different design parameters such as thickness and perforations are considered to obtain displacement distributions under critical loading conditions using finite element analysis. The models consider quasi-static loads with linear elastic materials. The null hypothesis underlying this research asserts that both biomaterials exhibit the minimum mechanical characteristics necessary to withstand direct impact trauma at the implant center, effectively averting critical deformations higher than 2 mm. In this way, the use of PMMA cranioplasties is justified in most cases where a PEEK implant cannot be accessed.

Keywords: patient-specific implant; medical imaging; cranial implant; biomaterial; PMMA; PEEK; finite element analysis

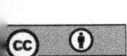

1. Introduction

Globally, cranioencephalic trauma affects an estimated 200 individuals out of 10,000, with a higher prevalence among men in a ratio of 3:2, particularly within the age range of 20 to 30, possibly due to increased engagement in sports and high-risk activities [1]. Industrialized nations report falls from one's own height as the leading cause (60% of cases), alongside traffic accidents and acts of violence, collectively contributing to a 3.4% mortality rate [2,3]. In Latin America, head trauma is predominantly linked to traffic accidents (motorcyclists and pedestrians) and violence (internal guerrilla conflicts) [4]. In Colombia, limited demographic studies focus on the incidence of mild or moderate traumatic brain injury, situations often requiring cranial implants. Research in Cali between 2003 and 2004 indicated that 52% and 30% of admitted traumatic brain injury cases were categorized as mild and moderate, respectively [5]. The mortality rate in Colombia for the period 2010–2017 was 10.7 per 100,000 inhabitants [6].

Biomechanics is a multidisciplinary field that plays a crucial role in addressing bone injuries and defects, particularly in the development of orthopedic implants. These implants, made from a variety of biomaterials, are essential for proper bone alignment and healing [7]. To enhance the interaction between these implants and bone tissue, bioinspired surface modifications are being explored, with the aim of creating next-generation implants [8]. The biomechanics of bone fractures and fixation, including the use of implants, is a key area of study in orthopedic trauma [9]. Orthopedic implant studies encompass design, new materials, and physiology [10,11]. To ensure the final product effectively restores the functionality of the missing biological structure, these disciplines must collaborate [12].

Engineering is vital in evaluating prototype designs, identifying flaws, refining implants, and assuring patients of improved quality of life.

For over 80 years, scientists have been investigating and evaluating various synthetic biomaterials to address cranial defects [12], and the exploration for new materials, including those with biodegradable features, continues [13]. Among them, we find PMMA, a polymethylmethacrylate ceramic mixed with a liquid monomer, which passes from a liquid system to a non-Newtonian one to end up solidifying, through an exothermic energetic release process, in the form desired by the orthopedist. PMMA is a durable, malleable, and relatively inexpensive biomaterial [14], very efficient in aesthetic terms for sealing asymmetric and extensive defects, with great properties for surgical use [15]. PMMA has demonstrated remarkable success rates exceeding 97% and boasts a notably low complication rate of less than 2.3% [16,17]. Inconveniences have also been reported due to the low porosity of PMMA implants, since it does not favor the cell growth of osteocytes, nor does it facilitate its vascularization, creating an inert material susceptible to infection, although the literature reports less than 5% of infections with this biomaterial [18]. Finally, low mechanical properties are attributed to it in terms of tensile strength (36 MPa), 4.7 times less than cortical bone (170 MPa) [19], which raises doubts in surgeons when assessing its mechanical strength and stiffness, especially considering that many of these patients may be at risk of experiencing significant impacts.

Currently, surgeons have put their interest in PEEK (Polyether Ether Ketone), a thermally stable biomaterial [20] with success rates exceeding 99% [21], as indicated by studies. This biomaterial boasts low post-surgical complication rates ranging from 0% to 9% [16,22], and infection-related complications are less than 6% [23,24]. Moreover, PEEK exhibits a tensile strength of 80 MPa, two times lower than cortical bone strength. These attributes position PEEK as a promising biomaterial for surgical applications, presenting a high success rate, low complication rates, and advantageous mechanical properties when compared to alternative materials like PMMA.

Both biomaterials exhibit comparable clinical success rates, low complication rates, low infection rates, and high aesthetic satisfaction reported by patients [22], making them seemingly suitable for shielding the brain from mechanical trauma. However, they diverge in mechanical properties and costs, with PMMA being approximately 55% more economical than PEEK (USD 2702 vs. USD 4684, approximate value for an implant in Colombia without osteosynthesis material). In [25], the authors proposed an integrative surgery management system for cranial reconstructions using patient-specific implants made of PMMA as an accessible and cost-effective solution for low-income countries. This cost differential underscores a significant economic consideration in choosing between the two materials for neurosurgical implants while maintaining comparable clinical effectiveness and patient satisfaction.

The digitization of medical implants and their subsequent analysis using computational mechanics, such as finite element (FE) analysis, has significantly advanced the exploration and investigation of implant design [26,27]. These tools allow engineers to evaluate various parameters, including thickness, geometrical features, thermal properties, materials, and applied boundary conditions. This enables the creation of more customized implants from a mechanical perspective, blending the most favorable attributes to ensure prolonged implant durability [28]. Computational modeling and simulation play a crucial role in the total product life cycle of implants, analyzing both surgical procedures and devices, taking into account the topics of both hard and soft tissue mechanics.

Research using FE analysis has been reported applied to cranial implants evaluating the variable thickness vs. type of material, where it has been concluded that the thickness factor is more relevant to stresses than the material used for its manufacture. However, the situation differs when it comes to deformation, and the elastic modulus of the material significantly affects the displacement field. In another set of experiments, researchers evaluated the stress–strain behavior of two types of cranial implants, titanium (Ti) and PEEK, under axial loading [29]. Special interest has been given to the geometric shape of the system of miniplates that hold the implant–skull interface and how these react to different types of loads [30,31]. In general, there has been a surge in research within the literature employing FE approaches to evaluate cranial implants [32–35], driven by a heightened interest in the subject. In [32], the authors employed finite element analysis to assess implant behavior under varied intracranial pressure conditions, considering the influence of fixation points, for different materials. The study in [33] models cranial implants with meshless methods, comparing solid and porous structures, for titanium alloy (Ti6Al4V) and PEEK, indicating titanium's overall superiority, while PEEK excels in weight and osseointegration. In [35], evaluation of von Mises stresses and deformations in a customized PMMA-based cranial implant with the fixation system demonstrated effective protection without physiological harm or anchoring failures.

This work presents the study of the thickness vs. stiffness relationship for different materials (PMMA and PEEK), as a criterion for the selection of biomaterials from a mechanical perspective. Our null hypothesis is that the two biomaterials offer the minimum mechanical characteristics to withstand a direct impact trauma in the geometric center of the implant, e.g., as a result of a ball impact, and avoid critical deformations greater than 2 mm. In this way, the use of PMMA cranioplasties is justified in most cases where a PEEK implant cannot be accessed. First, the subject for the study is presented. Leveraging a computed tomography (CT) scan, we extract essential spatial and topological data, forming the foundation for precise model identification. Next, we continue with the design of a patient-specific implant, tailoring the solution to the individual's unique anatomical characteristics. Finally, the structural integrity of the implant is assessed through finite element analysis, providing comprehensive insights into its performance under varying conditions, including material, topology, and thickness.

2. Materials and Methods

2.1. Model Identification

The subject of analysis in this study was the 3D reconstruction of a 32-year-old male patient's cranium, originally from Ibagué, Colombia, who experienced a fracture and subsequent loss of bone tissue. The spatial and topological characteristics of the cranial defect were derived from a computed tomography (CT) scan of the cranial bones, as depicted in Figure 1. The relevant data were encoded in a DICOM (Digital Imaging and Communications in Medicine) extension file, with spatial slices at 0.625 mm and a gap of 0.625 mm between cuts, with a Gantry at 0°. The CT scan utilized a General Electric Dual HiSpeed scanner (General Electric, Chicago, IL, USA) with 250 slices, a pixel size of 0.124 mm, and implemented the B70s algorithm. This comprehensive imaging approach provided detailed insights into the structural alterations resulting from the injury.

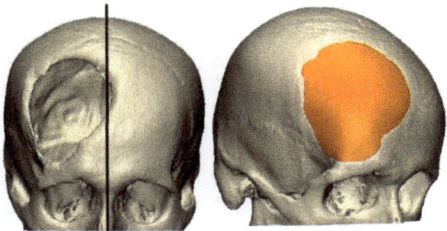

Figure 1. Midline used to reflect the right zone in the left zone (cranial defect).

2.2. Design of the Patient-Specific Implant (PSI)

For the personalized design of the implant based on the anatomy of the patient, a geometric and topological symmetry was assumed with respect to the sagittal axis, which was conveniently taken from the crista galli eminence and the anterior nasal spine of the patient [36]. Once this area was reflected on the defect, the thickness was calculated from the bone tables, and the customized implant was constructed using the CAD software

Mimics v13 (Materialise, Leuven, Belgium). We have checked that the edges of the implant had a smooth continuity with the edges of the bone defect and were consistent with the anatomy of the patient. Figure 1 shows part of the defect and the patient-specific implant solution.

2.3. Finite Element Model

To evaluate the deformations of the implant under loading conditions, we use a standard Galerkin finite element numerical model to solve the elasticity problem. This method has been commonly used to evaluate the mechanical response in biomechanical applications [35,37,38]. Using a variational formulation of the elasticity problem and the finite element approximation of displacements, the following system of equations is obtained:

$$\mathbf{KU} = \mathbf{f} \tag{1}$$

where **K** is the stiffness matrix, **U** is the vector of nodal displacements and **f** is the load vector. Finite element analysis involves defining analysis type, boundary conditions, material model, and mesh generation. Post-processing evaluates results, followed by an analysis of their implications. To ensure the reliability and accuracy of the analysis, a mesh independence test is conducted, verifying the convergence of displacement solutions, considering that our quantity of interest is the total deformation. This iterative process ensures the robustness of the finite element method and the consistency of results, providing a comprehensive understanding of the studied phenomena.

For the problem under consideration, a linear static structural analysis with a direct solver is suitable to evaluate the behavior of the bone tissue, under the imposed boundary conditions. In a compression test, the bone tissue experiences loading that is applied slowly or at a constant rate, and the response of the material is observed under this quasi-static condition. For a linear analysis, the displacements are solved under the following assumptions: The stiffness matrix **K** is essentially constant, such that the materials have linear elastic behavior and small deformations theory is used. The load vector **f** is statically applied, i.e., no time-varying forces are considered, and no inertial effects are included.

The geometry of both the cranial implant (CI) and the skull base were exported in an IGES format, to generate a 3D model that is discretized to represent the geometric characteristics of the patient. The modeling software used was Ansys Workbench 2023 R1 (ANSYS Inc., Canonsburg, PA, USA). This FE tool allows an approximation of the differential equations that govern the stress–strain behavior of the elasticity problem, providing in a non-invasive way results that closely resemble real-world scenarios [39].

The research methodology focused on a 2^k factorial design of experiments (DOE) with k factors corresponding to three key input variables of interest: (i) implant thickness, (ii) biomaterial, and (iii) uniformly distributed perforations. The choice of a 2^k factorial design is motivated by its efficiency in exploring the effects of multiple factors simultaneously while requiring a relatively small number of experimental runs. This design allows for the systematic investigation of main effects and interaction effects, providing a comprehensive understanding of variable relationships. The statistical simplicity of analysis, resource savings, and the ability to efficiently screen factors make the 2^k factorial design an advantageous choice. Table 1 provides details on the uncoded variables, where the design typically involves only two levels for each factor.

Table 1. Input variables for the factorial design of the experiment.

Factors	Coded Level	
	−1	+1
Implant thickness (A)	3 mm	5 mm
Biomaterial (B)	PEEK	PMMA
Perforations (C)	No	Yes

Source. Own elaboration.

In a 2^k factorial design of experiments with three factors, the effects represent the influence or impact of each factor and their interactions on the response variable. The general equation for calculating the main effects of each factor in a 2^k factorial design is as follows:

$$E_i = \frac{1}{2^{k-1}} \left(\sum_{j=1}^{2^{k-1}} Y_{i1} - \sum_{j=1}^{2^{k-1}} Y_{i2} \right) \qquad (2)$$

where E_i denotes the effect of the i-th factor, Y_{i1} and Y_{i2} are the average responses at the high and low levels of the i-th factor, respectively. Additionally, for interaction effects between two factors, the equation reads:

$$E_{ij} = \frac{1}{2^{k-2}} \left(\sum_{j=1}^{2^{k-2}} Y_{i1j1} + Y_{i2j2} - \sum_{j=1}^{2^{k-2}} Y_{i1j2} + Y_{i2j1} \right) \qquad (3)$$

where E_{ij} represents the interaction effect between the i-th and j-th factors, Y_{i1j1} are the average responses at the high levels of the i-th and j-th factors, Y_{i2j2} are the average responses at the low levels of the i-th and j-th factors, and the remaining terms represent the coupled responses.

The properties of bone and alloplastic material were assumed and modeled under a continuous homogeneous isotropic approach, with a linear elastic model governed by the elastic modulus and Poisson's ratio, which has shown a very good correlation for stress–strain analysis in human bones [40,41]. The mechanical properties of the linear elastic material models of the two biomaterials, PEEK and PMMA, are listed in Table 2, together with those of the cranial bone [42–44].

Table 2. Mechanical properties of the biomaterial PEEK, PMMA, and cranial bone.

Material	Elastic Modulus (MPa)	Poisson's Ratio
PEEK	4000	0.38
PMMA	3000	0.38
Cranial bone	15,000	0.3

Source. Own elaboration.

A load of 700 N was applied at the central apex of the implant as a remote force to avoid stress concentration effects, as previously used in [45], Figure 2. We did not consider the internal cranial hydrostatic pressure (15 mmHg) on the implant [45,46]. In the clinical procedure, patients are previously subjected to mechanical devices that regulate the intracranial pressure. Moreover, in [47], the authors measured the forces due to brain pulsation and indicated that they resulted in stresses one order of magnitude lower than the yield stress of the cranioplasty material. We measured the subarachnoid space in the CT scan for a maximum displacement of 2 mm, which is in agreement with values reported [48]. Cranial implants may incorporate holes or perforations to enable suturing for secure attachment to the skull, promote tissue integration and vascularization, facilitate drainage and fluid management, allow customization for individual patient needs, reduce weight for improved comfort, and provide diagnostic access or monitoring options when necessary. Thus, the implants were also drilled in a symmetrical pattern of 3 rows, with holes spaced at 1 cm and a diameter of 1.7 mm, as shown in Figure 3, since it was a factor to be evaluated.

A fixed boundary condition at the level of the flat edge of the cranial remnant was assumed, and the contact between the implant and the portion of the skull was defined as a non-separation condition, Figure 4. On the other hand, the center for the reference frame was located at the apex of the implant with a k-direction perpendicular to the surface at this point (Figure 2a). Convergence tests of the solution in displacements were performed to validate mesh independence using four meshes, with a final variation of 0.2% in the last mesh, as shown in Table 3, for a final element size of 1 mm, and a total of 1,521,702 elements. Skewness measure of the mesh was evaluated for element quality, with values below 0.95.

Finally, meshes of second-order tetrahedral elements, considering the parameters in Table 4, were produced for the bone tissue and the implants, as shown in Figure 5.

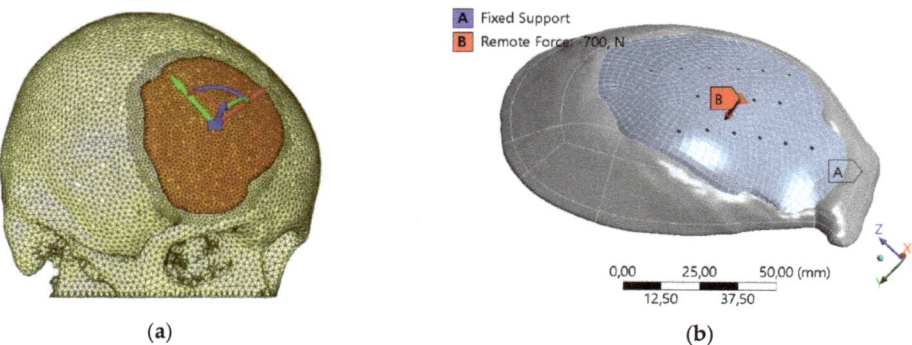

Figure 2. (**a**) Reference frame with *k*-direction perpendicular to the skull surface, (**b**) force vector perpendicular to the implant.

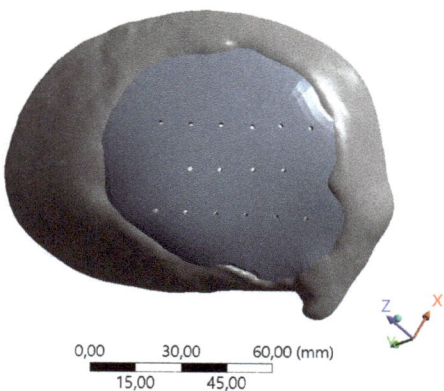

Figure 3. Drilled implant at the apex level.

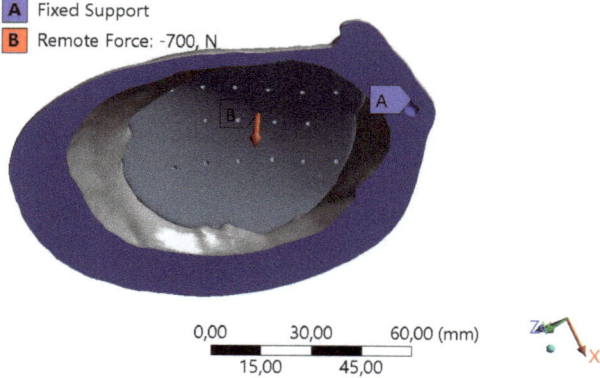

Figure 4. Boundary conditions. Load condition of 700 N on the implant apex in red, restriction of all degrees of freedom on the flat area of the cranial edge in blue.

Table 3. Mesh independence test for total normal displacement.

Number of Elements	Max. Total Displacement (mm)
224,302	0.28775632
399,475	0.29616231
761,202	0.29734957
1,521,702	0.29806294

Source. Own elaboration.

Table 4. Mesh parameters for the implant and bone solids.

Parameter	Implant	Bone
Edge length (mm)	1	1
Minimum edge length (mm)	0.5	1
Smooth transition	Yes	Yes
Bend angle	7.5°	
Number of elements	576,596	749,866
Tetrahedra	Yes	Yes

Source. Own elaboration.

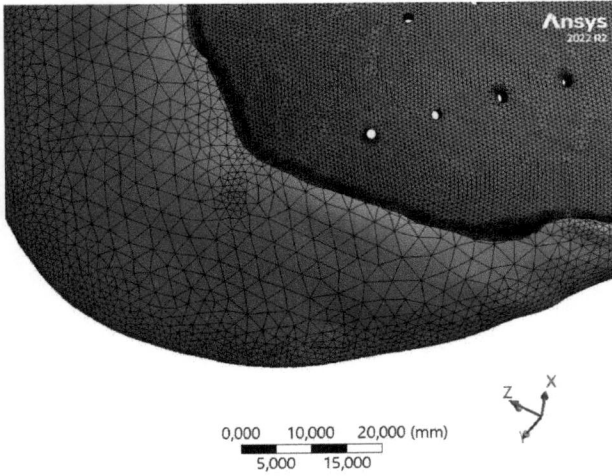

Figure 5. Meshing of the implant and bone solids.

Following this, the study assesses outcomes by modeling implants using both PEEK and PMMA biomaterials on cranial cortical bone. Under identical load conditions and constraints, the study aims to gauge the mechanical performance of both materials based on deformation parameters. This comparative analysis provides insights into how PEEK and PMMA perform in simulated conditions, aiding in the evaluation and selection of these biomaterials for cranial applications.

3. Results

In our study, a 2^3 factorial experiment was undertaken to examine the impacts of material type (PEEK and PMMA), implant thickness (3 mm and 5 mm), and the presence of perforations for suturing (with and without) on cranial implant performance. This design resulted in eight experimental runs, encompassing all possible combinations of these factors. The response variable, indicating the primary outcome (i.e., maximum displacement), was measured for each experimental run. Employing statistical analysis, we assessed the main effects and potential interactions among these factors, aiming to discern the influence of material choice, thickness variations, and the presence of perforations on the properties of cranial implants. The findings contribute valuable insights into optimizing cranial implant design based on these critical factors. The results of the eight experiments are presented in Table 5, which shows the maximum total displacements for different implant configurations.

Table 5. Average results of the 2^3 factorial experiment.

Experiment	A	B	C	Outlet (mm) ξ
1	−	−	−	0.787
2	−	−	+	0.811
3	−	+	−	1.089
4	−	+	+	1.125
5	+	−	−	0.225
6	+	−	+	0.237
7	+	+	−	0.300
8	+	+	+	0.316

Source. Own elaboration.

Figures 6 and 7 show the total displacements for the implants under a load of 700 N applied on the apex of the implant for two experiments of the different configurations of biomaterial, thickness, and perforations.

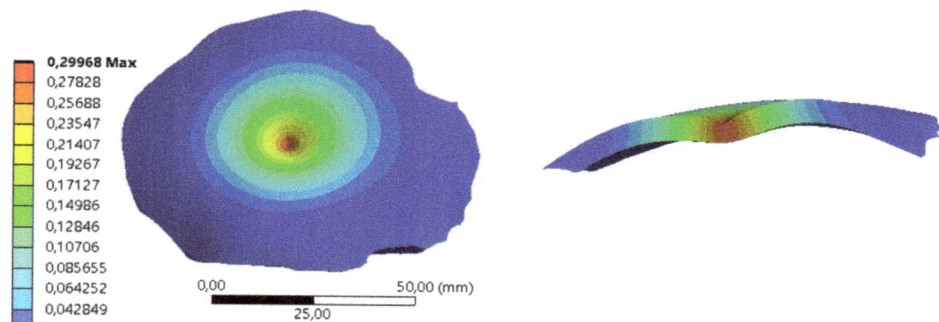

Figure 6. Total displacements (mm) of the 5 mm thickness PEEK implant.

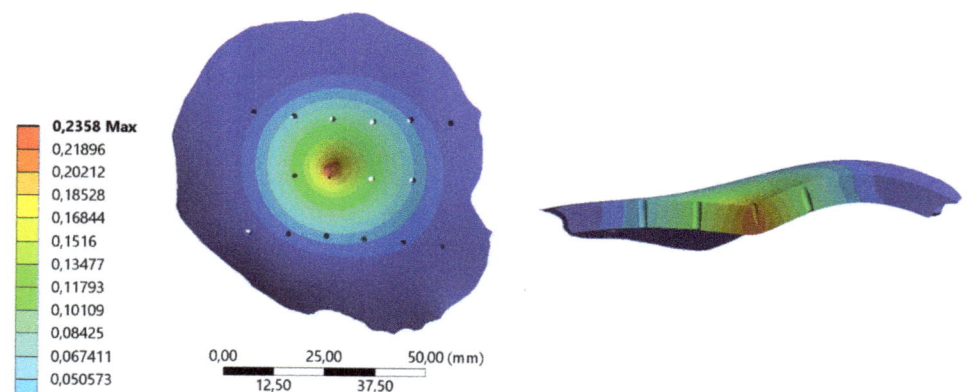

Figure 7. Total displacements (mm) of the 5 mm thickness PEEK implant with perforations.

The effect that each one of the factors studied has on the normal displacements of the surface is presented in Table 6. The results of our study revealed several key findings regarding the main effects and interactions of factors on our experimental outcome. Regarding the main effects, implant thickness exhibited a notable negative effect with a coefficient of -0.684 (± 0.01), indicating that increasing implant thickness was associated with a decrease in the observed outcome. Conversely, the choice of biomaterial showed a positive effect of 0.193 (± 0.01), suggesting that certain biomaterials, i.e., PMMA, were associated with higher outcomes. Perforations, as a main effect, had a minimal effect with a coefficient of 0.022 (± 0.01). In terms of two-factor interactions, the interaction between thickness and biomaterial showed a negative effect of -0.116 (± 0.01), suggesting that the combination of certain thicknesses and biomaterials led to a reduction in the outcome. The interactions between thickness and perforations (-0.008 ± 0.01) and biomaterial and perforations (0.004 ± 0.01) had relatively minor effects on the observed outcome. These results provide insights into the complex interplay between implant characteristics and their impact on our experimental outcome.

Table 6. Calculated effects and standard errors for the factorial design.

Main Effects	Effect	Standard Error
Thickness	-0.684	± 0.01
Biomaterial	0.193	± 0.01
Perforations	0.022	± 0.01
Two-factor interactions		
Thickness × Biomaterial	-0.116	± 0.01
Thickness × Perforations	-0.008	± 0.01
Biomaterial × Perforations	0.004	± 0.01

Source. Own elaboration.

The perforations or holes variable does not seem to have a noticeable influence on the deformations of the implant when the biomaterial is PMMA. Otherwise, when the biomaterial is PEEK, and the thickness is 3 mm, this combination seems to influence the displacements. In the configuration of change of thickness and biomaterial, it is observed that for thicknesses of 3 mm the biomaterial influences, but for thicknesses of 5 mm, it is not significant. The largest deformation was observed in the combination of 3 mm thickness, PMMA biomaterial, and holes with a displacement of 1.125 mm. In consideration of the influence of thickness, we have included data corresponding to thickness values of 4 mm and 6 mm. This addition is intended to facilitate a comprehensive understanding of the relationship between displacement and thickness increment. The influence of the thickness on the normal displacements to the surface in different combinations of biomaterials is presented in Figure 8. Comparing the displacement values between PMMA and PEEK implants at each thickness level, it appears that PEEK generally exhibits lower displacement values than PMMA, and the difference diminishes as we increase the thickness. The displacement decreases non-linearly with thickness for both materials, and when considering displacement as proportional to the elastic modulus, these findings align with the ratio of their respective elastic moduli. These findings can inform clinical decisions regarding the selection of implant materials and thicknesses based on desired mechanical performance and patient-specific factors such as bone quality and surgical requirements.

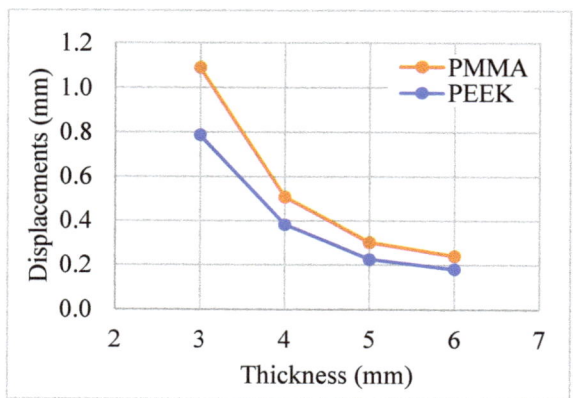

Figure 8. Effect of thickness on normal displacements for PEEK and PMMA for the implant without perforations.

4. Conclusions

In this study, we investigated the relationship between implant thickness and deformation, focusing on patient-specific cranial implants constructed from two different biomaterials, PMMA and PEEK. Our goal was to assess their mechanical performance under quasi-static loads, particularly in terms of maximum total deformation. While the paper explores readily accessible techniques, its main objective is to address the cost-benefit aspects of employing PMMA implants in clinical applications, particularly in comparison to more expensive alternatives, an aspect that has not been previously explored in the literature. Our experience indicates that this matter lacks clarity for practitioners, and its relevance is notably significant in developing countries. Achieving a comprehensive grasp of the materials and their mechanical performance is relevant in this context. The outcomes of this research shed light on several crucial aspects of implant design and selection. As expected, the choice of biomaterial significantly impacts the deformation characteristics of cranial implants. We observed that PMMA and PEEK exhibit different levels of normal displacements due to their different elastic moduli. Generally, biomaterials with higher elastic moduli experience less deformation under equivalent stress conditions.

Our study adds a practical dimension to existing research [49] by considering implant perforations as an important factor in surgical procedures. Moreover, we did not consider implants thinner than 3 mm because the fabrication of these implants, generally by the biomaterial injection technique, are difficult to perform for clinical use. In comparison to previous literature, our findings diverge in terms of deformation outcomes. Díaz et al. [38] report displacements of 0.3 mm in PEEK biomaterial for a cranioplasty in the upper part of the cranial vault, although the implant thickness is not reported. Ridwan-Pramana et al. [50] report displacements less than 0.03 mm in specific configurations of several plates and positive contact angles between implant and skull; we understand that the other configurations are idealized and do not represent, in many cases, the real topological conditions of these defects in surgery. Finally, it is known that the perpendicular distance between the cranial tissue and the bone plate is around 2 mm [48,51]. For this reason, a deformation of the material close to this length would be critical. This deformation is closely linked to the thickness and material of the implant [49]. Thus, it is necessary for future research to include geometric variables, such as the radius of curvature of the implant. This will allow for a more precise standardization of results, catering to specific implant geometries and providing a more comprehensive understanding of implant performance. The finite element models employed in this study recreated real-life implant conditions under direct impacts, although the osteosynthesis system was not included.

This research validates the null hypothesis that both PMMA and PEEK biomaterials are suitable for withstanding deformation in the normal direction. Furthermore, we found that by adjusting the thickness variable in PMMA biomaterial, deformation levels comparable to those of PEEK can be achieved. These results suggest the potential for PMMA implants, particularly 4 mm thick with perforations, to serve as an effective alternative to PEEK implants, offering a cost-effective solution while maintaining the desired mechanical performance in cranial implants. However, further research and validation are essential to confirm the feasibility and clinical implications of these findings.

While the study enhances understanding of cranial implant performance, limitations exist. Focusing on quasi-static loads excludes dynamic conditions, and implants thinner than 3 mm were omitted. Idealized assumptions about perforations may oversimplify surgical scenarios. Future research should explore geometric variables, incorporate dynamic conditions, explore thinner implants, and integrate osteosynthesis systems for a more realistic analysis. Clinical validation is crucial to confirm practical implications. Despite these limitations, the study suggests the potential of cost-effective PMMA implants as comparable alternatives to PEEK implants, emphasizing the need for further research and validation in clinical settings.

Author Contributions: Conceptualization, M.M.R., O.A.G.-E. and D.F.V.-B.; Data curation, M.M.R.; Formal analysis, M.M.R., O.A.G.-E. and D.F.V.-B.; Investigation, M.M.R., O.A.G.-E. and D.F.V.-B.; Methodology, M.M.R., O.A.G.-E. and D.F.V.-B.; Supervision, O.A.G.-E.; Validation, M.M.R. and O.A.G.-E.; Writing—original draft, M.M.R.; Writing—review and editing, O.A.G.-E. and D.F.V.-B. All authors have read and agreed to the published version of the manuscript.

Funding: This work was supported by Universidad Industrial de Santander (grant numbers VIE-2522 and 3716). The authors have no competing interests to declare that are relevant to the content of this article.

Institutional Review Board Statement: The study was conducted according to the guidelines of the Declaration of Helsinki, and approved by the Ethics Committee of Industrial University of Santander (Act 18, 18 October 2019).

Data Availability Statement: Data will be made available on request.

Conflicts of Interest: The authors declare that they have no known competing financial interests or personal relationships that could have appeared to influence the work reported in this paper.

References

1. Alted López, E.; Bermejo Aznárez, S.; Chico Fernández, M. Actualizaciones en el manejo del traumatismo craneoencefálico grave. *Med. Intensiv.* **2009**, *33*, 16–30. [CrossRef]
2. Majdan, M.; Mauritz, W. Unintentional fall-related mortality in the elderly: Comparing patterns in two countries with different demographic structure. *BMJ Open* **2015**, *5*, e008672. [CrossRef]
3. Faul, M.; Xu, L.; Wald, M.M.; Coronado, V.; Dellinger, A.M. Traumatic brain injury in the United States: National estimates of prevalence and incidence, 2002–2006. *Inj. Prev.* **2010**, *16*, A268. [CrossRef]
4. Peñaherrera Oviedo, C.; Soria Viteri, J. Pregunta de investigación y estrategia PICOT. *Medicina (B Aires)* **2015**, *19*, 66. [CrossRef]
5. Guzmán, F.; Moreno, M.C.; Montoya, A. Evolución de los pacientes con trauma craneoencefálico en el Hospital Universitario del Valle: Seguimiento a 12 meses. *Colomb. Med.* **2008**, *39*, 25–28. [CrossRef]
6. Umaña Laiton, L.E. *Características Sociodemográficas Relacionadas con la Mortalidad por Trauma Craneoencefálico en Adultos en Colombia. 2010–2017*; Universidad del Rosario: Bogotá, Colombia, 2021.
7. Kim, T.; See, C.W.; Li, X.; Zhu, D. Orthopedic implants and devices for bone fractures and defects: Past, present and perspective. *Eng. Regen.* **2020**, *1*, 6–18. [CrossRef]
8. González-Estrada, O.A.; Pertuz Comas, A.D.; Ospina, R. Characterization of hydroxyapatite coatings produced by pulsed-laser deposition on additive manufacturing Ti6Al4V ELI. *Thin Solid Films* **2022**, *763*, 139592. [CrossRef]
9. Altmann, M.; Cognet, J.-M.; Eschbach, L.; Gasser, B.; Richards, G.; Simon, P. Materiales utilizados en la osteosíntesis. *EMC-Técnicas Quirúrgicas-Ortop. y Traumatol.* **2009**, *1*, 1–8. [CrossRef]
10. Bonda, D.J.; Manjila, S.; Selman, W.R.; Dean, D. The Recent Revolution in the Design and Manufacture of Cranial Implants. *Neurosurgery* **2015**, *77*, 814–824. [CrossRef] [PubMed]
11. Corredor, E.; González-Estrada, O.A.; Ospina-Ospina, R. Deposición de láser pulsado de hidroxiapatita en Ti-6Al-4V producido por manufactura aditiva. *Rev. UIS Ing.* **2022**, *21*, 107–122. [CrossRef]

12. Aydin, S.; Kucukyuruk, B.; Abuzayed, B.; Aydin, S.; Sanus, G.Z. Cranioplasty: Review of materials and techniques. *J. Neurosci. Rural Pract.* **2011**, *2*, 162–167. [CrossRef] [PubMed]
13. Chmal-Fudali, E.; Basińska, D.; Kucharska-Jastrząbek, A.; Struszczyk, M.H.; Muzalewska, M.; Wyleżoł, M.; Wątrobiński, M.; Andrzejewski, J.; Tarzyńska, N.; Gzyra-Jagieła, K. Effect of the Advanced Cranial and Craniofacial Implant Fabrication on Their Degradation Affinity. *Materials* **2023**, *16*, 6070. [CrossRef] [PubMed]
14. Caro-Osorio, E.; De la Garza-Ramos, R.; Martínez-Sánchez, S.; Olazarán-Salinas, F. Cranioplasty with polymethylmethacrylate prostheses fabricated by hand using original bone flaps: Technical note and surgical outcomes. *Surg. Neurol. Int.* **2013**, *4*, 136. [CrossRef] [PubMed]
15. Webb, J.C.J.; Spencer, R.F. The role of polymethylmethacrylate bone cement in modern orthopaedic surgery. *J. Bone Jt. Surg.-Ser. B* **2007**, *89*, 851–857. [CrossRef] [PubMed]
16. Liang, E.S.; Tipper, G.; Hunt, L.; Gan, P.Y.C. Cranioplasty outcomes and associated complications: A single-centre observational study. *Br. J. Neurosurg.* **2016**, *30*, 122–127. [CrossRef] [PubMed]
17. Paredes, I.; Castaño-León, A.M.; Munarriz, P.M.; Martínez-Perez, R.; Cepeda, S.; Sanz, R.; Alén, J.F.; Lagares, A. Cranioplasty after decompressive craniectomy. A prospective series analyzing complications and clinical improvement. *Neurocirugia* **2015**, *26*, 115–125. [CrossRef]
18. Huang, G.J.; Zhong, S.; Susarla, S.M.; Swanson, E.W.; Huang, J.; Gordon, C.R. Craniofacial reconstruction with poly(methyl methacrylate) customized cranial implants. *J. Craniofac. Surg.* **2015**, *26*, 64–70. [CrossRef]
19. Cuppone, M.; Seedhom, B.B.; Berry, E.; Ostell, A.E. The Longitudinal Young's Modulus of Cortical Bone in the Midshaft of Human Femur and its Correlation with CT Scanning Data. *Calcif. Tissue Int.* **2004**, *74*, 302–309.
20. Fan, J.P.; Tsui, C.P.; Tang, C.Y.; Chow, C.L. Influence of interphase layer on the overall elasto-plastic behaviors of HA/PEEK biocomposite. *Biomaterials* **2004**, *25*, 5363–5373. [CrossRef]
21. Iaccarino, C.; Viaroli, E.; Fricia, M.; Serchi, E.; Poli, T.; Servadei, F. Preliminary Results of a Prospective Study on Methods of Cranial Reconstruction. *J. Oral Maxillofac. Surg.* **2015**, *73*, 2375–2378. [CrossRef]
22. Zhang, J.; Tian, W.; Chen, J.; Yu, J.; Zhang, J.; Chen, J. The application of polyetheretherketone (PEEK) implants in cranioplasty. *Brain Res. Bull.* **2019**, *153*, 143–149. [CrossRef]
23. Alonso-Rodriguez, E.; Cebrián, J.L.; Nieto, M.J.; Del Castillo, J.L.; Hernández-Godoy, J.; Burgueño, M. Polyetheretherketone custom-made implants for craniofacial defects: Report of 14 cases and review of the literature. *J. Cranio-Maxillofac. Surg.* **2015**, *43*, 1232–1238. [CrossRef] [PubMed]
24. Rosenthal, G.; Ng, I.; Moscovici, S.; Lee, K.K.; Lay, T.; Martin, C.; Manley, G.T. Polyetheretherketone implants for the repair of large cranial defects: A 3-center experience. *Neurosurgery* **2014**, *75*, 523–528. [CrossRef] [PubMed]
25. Ulmeanu, M.-E.; Mateș, I.M.; Doicin, C.-V.; Mitrică, M.; Chirteș, V.A.; Ciobotaru, G.; Semenescu, A. Bespoke Implants for Cranial Reconstructions: Preoperative to Postoperative Surgery Management System. *Bioengineering* **2023**, *10*, 544. [CrossRef] [PubMed]
26. Geng, J.P.; Ma, Q.S.; Xu, W.; Tan, K.B.C.C.; Liu, G.R.R. Finite element analysis of four thread-form configurations in a stepped screw implant. *J. Oral Rehabil.* **2004**, *31*, 233–239. [CrossRef]
27. Morrison, T.M.; Dreher, M.L.; Nagaraja, S.; Angelone, L.M.; Kainz, W. The Role of Computational Modeling and Simulation in the Total Product Life Cycle of Peripheral Vascular Devices. *J. Med. Device* **2017**, *11*, 024503. [CrossRef]
28. Moiduddin, K.; Mian, S.H.; Alkhalefah, H.; Ramalingam, S.; Sayeed, A. Customized Cost-Effective Cranioplasty for Large Asymmetrical Defects. *Processes* **2023**, *11*, 1760. [CrossRef]
29. Lethaus, B.; Safi, Y.; Ter Laak-Poort, M.; Kloss-Brandstätter, A.; Banki, F.; Robbenmenke, C.; Steinseifer, U.; Kessler, P. Cranioplasty with customized titanium and PEEK implants in a mechanical stress model. *J. Neurotrauma* **2012**, *29*, 1077–1083. [CrossRef]
30. Chamrad, J.; Marcián, P.; Narra, N.; Borák, L. Evaluating DifferentShapes of Cranial Fixation Mini-plates Using Finite Element Method. In *EMBEC & NBC 2017: Joint Conference of the European Medical and Biological Engineering Conference (EMBEC) and the Nordic-Baltic Conference on Biomedical Engineering and Medical Physics (NBC), Tampere, Finland, June 2017*; Springer: Singapore, 2018; pp. 747–750.
31. Santos, P.O.; Carmo, G.P.; Sousa, R.J.A.d.; Fernandes, F.A.O.; Ptak, M. Mechanical Strength Study of a Cranial Implant Using Computational Tools. *Appl. Sci.* **2022**, *12*, 878. [CrossRef]
32. Bogu, V.P.; Ravi Kumar, Y.; Khanara, A.K. Modelling and structural analysis of skull/cranial implant: Beyond mid-line deformities. *Acta Bioeng. Biomech.* **2017**, *19*, 125–131. [CrossRef]
33. Phanindra Bogu, V.; Ravi Kumar, Y.; Kumar Khanra, A. Homogenous scaffold-based cranial/skull implant modelling and structural analysis—Unit cell algorithm-meshless approach. *Med. Biol. Eng. Comput.* **2017**, *55*, 2053–2065. [CrossRef]
34. Mian, S.H.; Moiduddin, K.; Elseufy, S.M.; Alkhalefah, H. Adaptive Mechanism for Designing a Personalized Cranial Implant and Its 3D Printing Using PEEK. *Polymers* **2022**, *14*, 1266. [CrossRef]
35. Moncayo-Matute, F.P.; Torres-Jara, P.B.; Vázquez-Silva, E.; Peña-Tapia, P.G.; Moya-Loaiza, D.P.; Abad-Farfán, G. Finite element analysis of a customized implant in PMMA coupled with the cranial bone. *J. Mech. Behav. Biomed. Mater.* **2023**, *146*, 106046. [CrossRef]
36. Winder, J.; McKnight, W.; Golz, T.; Giese, A.; Busch, L. Comparison of Custom Cranial Implant Source Data: Manual, Mirrored and CAD generated skull surfaces. In *Medical Image Computing & Computer Assisted Intervention*; Medical Image Computing and Computer Assisted Intervention Society: Copenhagen, Denmark, 2006.

47. Maldonado, J.A.; Puentes, D.A.; Quintero, I.D.; González-Estrada, O.A.; Villegas, D.F. Image-Based Numerical Analysis for Isolated Type II SLAP Lesions in Shoulder Abduction and External Rotation. *Diagnostics* **2023**, *13*, 1819. [CrossRef]
48. Díaz, J.M.; González-Estrada, O.A.; López, C.I. Biomechanical analysis of a cranial patient specific implant on the interface with the bone using the finite element method. In Proceedings of the VII Latin American Congress on Biomedical Engineering CLAIB 2016, Bucaramanga, Santander, Colombia, 26–28 October 2016; Springer: Berlin/Heidelberg, Germany, 2017; Volume 60, pp. 405–408.
49. Tanaka, E.; Rodrigo, D.P.; Tanaka, M.; Kawaguchi, A.; Shibazaki, T.; Tanne, K. Stress analysis in the TMJ during jaw opening by use of a three-dimensional finite element model based on magnetic resonance images. *Int. J. Oral Maxillofac. Surg.* **2001**, *30*, 421–430. [CrossRef]
50. Koolstra, J.H.; Van Eijden, T.M.G.J. Combined finite-element and rigid-body analysis of human jaw joint dynamics. *J. Biomech.* **2005**, *38*, 2431–2439. [CrossRef] [PubMed]
51. Van Eijden, T.M.G.J.; Van Der Helm, P.N.; Van Ruijven, L.J.; Mulder, L. Structural and mechanical properties of mandibular condylar bone. *J. Dent. Res.* **2006**, *85*, 33–37. [CrossRef] [PubMed]
52. Reilly, D.T.; Burstein, A.H. The elastic and ultimate properties of compact bone tissue. *J. Biomech.* **1975**, *8*, 393–405. [CrossRef] [PubMed]
53. Chen, F.; Gatea, S.; Ou, H.; Lu, B.; Long, H. Fracture characteristics of PEEK at various stress triaxialities. *J. Mech. Behav. Biomed. Mater.* **2016**, *64*, 173–186. [CrossRef] [PubMed]
54. Preusser, T.; Rumpf, M.; Sauter, S.; Schwen, L.O. 3D composite finite elements for elliptic boundary value problems with discontinuous coefficients. *SIAM J. Sci. Comput.* **2011**, *33*, 2115–2143. [CrossRef]
55. Safi, Y.; Hohenberger, S.; Robbenmenke, C.; Banki, F.; Kessler, P.; Schmitz-rode, T.; Steinseifer, U. Investigation of the failure behavior of a cranial implant-skull model under different load conditions using FEM. *SIMULIA Cust. Conf.* **2010**, *1*, 16.
56. Czosnyka, M.; Pickard, J.D. Monitoring and interpretation of intracranial pressure. *J. Neurol. Neurosurg. Psychiatry* **2004**, *75*, 813–821. [CrossRef] [PubMed]
57. Goldberg, C.S.; Antonyshyn, O.; Midha, R.; Fialkov, J.A. Measuring Pulsatile Forces on the Human Cranium. *J. Craniofac. Surg.* **2005**, *16*, 134–139. [CrossRef] [PubMed]
58. Saboori, P.; Sadegh, A. Histology and Morphology of the Brain Subarachnoid Trabeculae. *Anat. Res. Int.* **2015**, *2015*, 279814. [CrossRef]
59. Marcián, P.; Narra, N.; Borák, L.; Chamrad, J.; Wolff, J. Biomechanical performance of cranial implants with different thicknesses and material properties: A finite element study. *Comput. Biol. Med.* **2019**, *109*, 43–52. [CrossRef]
60. Ridwan-Pramana, A.; Marcián, P.; Borák, L.; Narra, N.; Forouzanfar, T.; Wolff, J. Structural and mechanical implications of PMMA implant shape and interface geometry in cranioplasty—A finite element study. *J. Cranio-Maxillofac. Surg.* **2016**, *44*, 34–44. [CrossRef]
61. Martínez, F.; Mañana, G.; Panuncio, A.; Laza, S. Revisión anatomo-clínica de las meninges y espacios intracraneanos con especial referencia al hematoma subdural crónico. *Rev. Mex. Neurocienc.* **2008**, *9*, 47–60.

Disclaimer/Publisher's Note: The statements, opinions and data contained in all publications are solely those of the individual author(s) and contributor(s) and not of MDPI and/or the editor(s). MDPI and/or the editor(s) disclaim responsibility for any injury to people or property resulting from any ideas, methods, instructions or products referred to in the content.

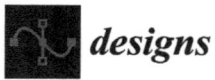

Article

Analysis of the Accuracy of CAD Modeling in Engineering and Medical Industries Based on Measurement Data Using Reverse Engineering Methods

Paweł Turek *, Wojciech Bezłada, Klaudia Cierpisz, Karol Dubiel, Adrian Frydrych and Jacek Misiura

Faculty of Mechanical Engineering and Aeronautics, Rzeszów University of Technology, 35-959 Rzeszów, Poland; 162873@stud.prz.edu.pl (W.B.); 166938@stud.prz.edu.pl (K.C.); 160019@stud.prz.edu.pl (K.D.); 166947@stud.prz.edu.pl (A.F.); jmisiura@prz.edu.pl (J.M.)
* Correspondence: pturek@prz.edu.pl

Abstract: The reverse engineering (RE) process is often necessary in today's engineering and medical industries. Expertise in measurement technology, data processing, and CAD modeling is required to ensure accurate reconstruction of an object's geometry. However, errors are generated at every stage of geometric reconstruction, affecting the dimensional and geometric accuracy of the final 3D-CAD model. In this article, the geometry of reconstructed models was measured using contact and optical methods. The measurement data representing 2D profiles, 3D point clouds, and 2D images acquired in the reconstruction process were saved to a stereolithography (STL) model. The reconstructed models were then subjected to a CAD modeling process, and the accuracy of the parametric modeling was evaluated by comparing the 3D-CAD model to the 3D-STL model. Based on the results, the model used for clamping and positioning parts to perform the machining process and the connecting rod provided the most accurate mapping errors. These models represented deviations within ±0.02 mm and ±0.05 mm. The accuracy of CAD modeling for the turbine blade model and the pelvis part was comparable, presenting deviations within ±0.1 mm. However, the helical gear and the femur models showed the highest deviations of about ±0.2 mm. The procedures presented in the article specify the methods and resolution of the measurement systems and suggest CAD modeling strategies to minimize reconstruction errors. These results can be used as a starting point for further tests to optimize CAD modeling procedures based on the obtained measurement data.

Keywords: reverse engineering; CAD modeling; accuracy; turbine blade; helical gear; anatomical model

Citation: Turek, P.; Bezłada, W.; Cierpisz, K.; Dubiel, K.; Frydrych, A.; Misiura, J. Analysis of the Accuracy of CAD Modeling in Engineering and Medical Industries Based on Measurement Data Using Reverse Engineering Methods. *Designs* **2024**, *8*, 50. https://doi.org/10.3390/designs8030050

Academic Editors: Richard Drevet and Hicham Benhayoune

Received: 22 April 2024
Revised: 12 May 2024
Accepted: 21 May 2024
Published: 24 May 2024

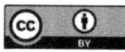

Copyright: © 2024 by the authors. Licensee MDPI, Basel, Switzerland. This article is an open access article distributed under the terms and conditions of the Creative Commons Attribution (CC BY) license (https://creativecommons.org/licenses/by/4.0/).

1. Introduction

The manual measurement of free surfaces is almost impossible due to the inability to obtain enough measurement data to describe a given feature of the measured geometry. However, the remarkable advancements in the computerization of measurement systems and their integration with computer-aided design (CAD) systems have resolved this issue [1–3]. This led to the development of coordinate measuring methods that allow the digitization of geometries optically [4,5] and via contact [6,7]. The results of these processes are digital data in the form of measurement points with coordinates usually expressed in the global coordinate system of the measuring machine. It is also possible to obtain digital data from 2D images obtained with computer tomography (CT) [8,9] or magnetic resonance imaging (MRI) [10]. The development of contact and optical coordinate measuring systems has contributed to optimizing production by reducing the time consumption of measurement procedures, increasing the accuracy and repeatability of measurements, and eliminating errors caused by human factors [11].

Coordinating measuring is also crucial in reverse engineering (RE) [12,13]. The task of RE is to convert an existing object into its digital form e.g., through a stereolithography

(STL) file, which in turn provides the basis for further work by designers and computer analysists using CAD systems [14]. Through RE methods, it is possible to reconstruct this information based on an existing object that does not have technological or construction documentation. The RE process is most often used in the automotive [15,16], aerospace [17,18], or archaeological [19,20] industries. It is also very often used in medicine, for example, in the process of developing the geometry of anatomical structures [21,22], designing surgical instruments [23–25], or implants [26]. However, errors arise at each stage of the geometric reconstruction process [12,27]. Thus, equations are created between the actual model and the digital model. It is necessary to develop procedures at each stage of the reconstruction process to minimize the resulting differences. One of the critical aspects is selecting an appropriate measurement system that will allow the acquisition of the necessary amount of measurement data, which will enable the reconstruction of the object's geometry in CAD at a later stage [28]. It is also essential to pay attention to the accuracy of the acquired measurement data. The accuracy of the reconstruction of the product geometry is influenced not only by the accuracy of the measurement system [5] but also by the adopted measurement strategy [6,28] and the quality of the measurement data processing [5,29,30]. The processing stage mainly involves filtering, combining, and positioning the measurement data [12,14]. The hybrid modeling process in the CAD system is also a crucial stage. It is most often associated with shape approximation involving spline curves and splaying of non-uniform rational B-spline (NURBS) surfaces, allowing a surface model to be obtained [22,29,31]. The last stage is usually a solid modeling process. The quality of the final 3D-CAD model obtained is mainly determined by the competence of the operator taking the measurements and the person processing the measurement data to obtain the 3D-CAD model. Researchers have conducted multiple studies to assess the accuracy of 3D-CAD model development based on acquired measurement data. These studies have mainly focused on testing the accuracy of measurement systems according to their relevant guidelines [32–34]. The tests have involved models created using additive and subtractive methods. Most often, the tests have been carried out on contact-based measurement systems such as coordinate measuring machines (CMMs) [35–37] and articulated-arm coordinate measuring machines (AACMMs) [38]. Additionally, research is being conducted on systems that use structured light [39–41] and laser light [42,43] to illuminate the model. In diagnostics, several studies have been carried out on tomographic measurement systems such as multi-detector computed tomography (MDCT) [44], cone beam computed tomography (CBCT) [45], and μCT [46,47].

However, there need to be more structured procedures that allow the reconstruction and development of a final 3D-CAD model using different methods and measurement data. Additionally, attention has yet to be given to the accuracy of the 3D-CAD modeling process based on the obtained measurement data. Considering this, this article analyzes a modeling process for 3D-STL models, whose geometries were obtained from measurements acquired using various coordinate measuring methods. This study selected models that are often used in the machining, aviation, and medical industries. Based on the developed 3D-CAD model, the process of evaluating the accuracy of CAD modeling was carried out. Knowledge of the errors in the obtained CAD modeling can, in the future, improve the reconstruction of geometries from data obtained using coordinate measurement systems.

2. Materials and Methods

One of the main steps in the RE process is obtaining information about the object's geometric dimensions. These are obtained using contact or optical coordinate measuring systems. The presented research addresses the process of geometric reconstruction to develop 3D-CAD models for the following:

- a pulley based on measured 2D profiles;
- a model for clamping and positioning parts therein to perform the machining process, and a connecting rod based on a 3D point cloud obtained from a laser light scanner;

- a bevel gear and a turbine blade feather based on a three-dimensional point cloud obtained from a structured light scanner;
- the anatomical structures of the hip joint (femur and pelvic fragment) based on collected data represented as 2D images.

2.1. Geometric Reconstruction Based on Data Obtained Using the iNEXIV Optical System and MarSurf XC 20

The process of reconstructing the geometry based on the obtained 2D profiles was carried out using the pulley model as an example. Using an iNEXIVE optical microscope, the measurements of the hub bore, splineway dimensions, and outer diameter were taken (Figure 1a). In the measurement process, the first step was to clean the pulley of any debris. The software for the microscope was launched, and the measuring table was set up with the wheel in the appropriate position. A binarized video preview and sharpened edges of the model's geometric features were acquired to obtain accurate measurements. This was accomplished by adjusting the intensity of light incident on the object and the distance of the optical system from the measured geometry. The next step involved selecting three points on the hole's perimeter to define the measurement section along which the geometry profiles were measured. The measurement resolution was also established, set at 0.02 mm for the pulley geometry. The 2D profiles were generated based on the measurements and then saved in drawing exchange format (DXF). The MarSurf XC20 was used to measure the shape of the pulley groove (Figure 1b). This device features advanced contour measurement technology for efficient and accurate profile measurement. The system consists of a measuring table and a tripod equipped with an arm and a measuring head. The measuring probe was selected based on the size and shape of the object to be measured, and moved along the measuring section in one plane, with the length of the section defined by the operator. The movements were controlled through special software on a computer. To perform the measurement, a dialog box defined the measurement segment and resolution, which in this case was 0.001 mm. The results were saved in 2D profiles in text (TXT) format.

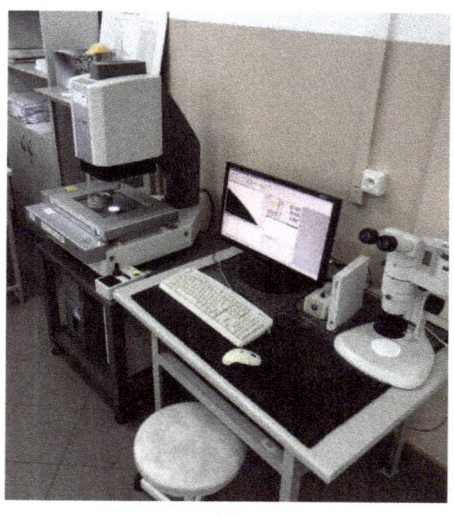
(a)

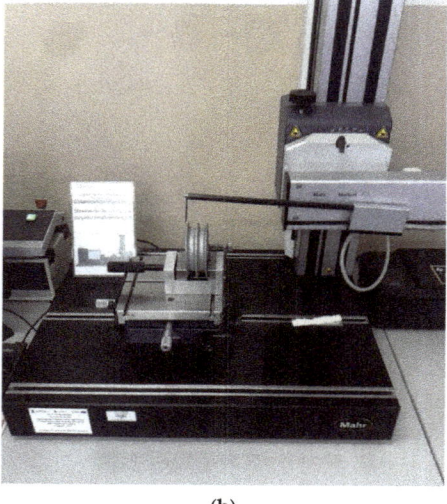
(b)

Figure 1. Measurement of pulley geometry using: (**a**) an o iNEXIVE optical microscope; (**b**) MarSurf XC20.

Siemens NX software (version 2312) was used to reconstruct the pulley geometry. The first step was to load the measurement data obtained from an optical microscope.

The data analysis started with reconstructing the pulley's diameter using the *Fit Curve* function. For this, the *Fit Circle* option was selected from the dialog box, which fitted a circle to a set of points. The diameter of the pulley bore was reconstructed similarly. The dimensions of the splineway were parameterized using the *Fit Line* option. The *Fit Curve* and *Fit Line* functions were also used to develop the data collected on the MarSurf XC 20 system, allowing parameterization of the pulley and groove profiles. Once the profiles were developed, they were oriented to the corresponding planes in CAD system space and the traditional solid modeling process was carried out on them. The process involved extracting the sketches from measurements taken with an optical microscope using the *Extrude* function. Next, the previously created profile obtained with the MarSurf XC 20 was used to create the grooves of the pulley. The sketch was set on a plane passing through the center of the solid obtained in the previous step, and the *Revolve* function was used to create the grooves. A vector parallel to the axis of the pulley was selected as the vector of rotation, while the value of the angle of rotation was assumed to be $360°$. The Boolean option Subtract was used to subtract the profile from the solid. The *Mirror Feature* function was used to select the second part of the solid, with the plane of mirroring being the plane passing through the center of the pulley, which at the same time was parallel to the face. After performing all the operations, a solid 3D-CAD pulley model was obtained and then exported to standard for the exchange of product (STEP) format.

2.2. Geometric Reconstruction Based on Data Obtained Using the Articulated-Arm Coordinate Measuring Machine MCA II with a Laser Head MMD×100

In this study, the process of reconstructing the geometry of a model for clamping and positioning parts in a machining process and a connecting rod was carried out based on an obtained 3D point cloud. The data representing the geometry of the models were acquired using the MCA II measuring-arm system with a mounted MMD×100 head, which illuminated the object with laser light. Using a beam of laser light to illuminate an object is a well-known technique for measuring objects. In this method, a beam of laser light is deflected by a mirror towards the scanned model. The beam is then scattered on the object's surface, and the camera records its position. This method is suitable for short-range measurements because the accuracy of the measurement is inversely proportional to the distance of the laser from the scanned model. Before taking any measurements, the components were coated with an anti-reflective spray to prevent laser light from reflecting off their surfaces. The scanning process was carried out in various stages, each involving scanning the models for clamping and positioning parts for a machining process (Figure 2a) and a connecting rod (Figure 2b) from different angles to obtain comprehensive geometric information with the applied maximum resolution of point clouds set to 0.01 mm. The outcome of the measurement process was a three-dimensional point cloud that mapped out the models' geometry, which was saved in STL format. Next, any noise and software errors in the triangle mesh created during the measurement were removed. Lastly, the 3D-STL models underwent a CAD modeling process using Siemens NX software.

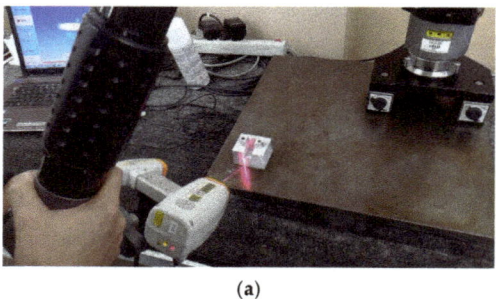 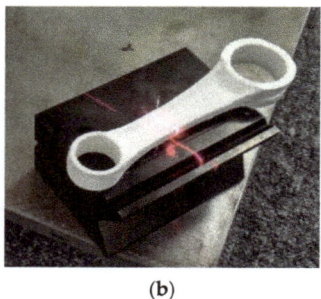

(a) (b)

Figure 2. Measurement using a laser scanner of: (**a**) a model for clamping and positioning parts in a machining process; (**b**) a connecting rod.

The process of CAD modeling of the geometry of the equipment used for clamping and positioning parts in the machining process consisted of several steps. In the first step, the *Section Curve* function was used. This allowed the generation of planes to intersect the model, onto which measurement points defining the basic dimensions of the geometry were then projected. With the obtained points, it was possible to create sketches. The next step was to extract the elaborated sketches using the *Extrude* function. Thus, the process of 3D-CAD geometric modeling began with the development of the basic geometric dimensions of the model based on the sketches developed, ending with a section of the model defining the clamping directly. The developed solid model was exported to STEP format in the final step.

In the CAD modeling of the geometry of the connecting rod model, in the first stopper based on the *Detect Primitives* option, the basic areas defining planar and cylindrical surfaces were assigned to selected parts of the triangle mesh. Next, a median plane was defined onto which points mapping the outline of the side surface of the connecting rod were dropped. Curves were created based on the *Fit Curve–Fit Spline* option and then extruded. Thus, the side surfaces were defined. Its profile was also developed to select the top surface based on the projection of points on the plane. Based on the obtained points, curves were created using the *Fit Spline* and *Fit Circle* options. With the sketch fully parameterized, the missing surfaces were created. Each created surface was sewn together to create a fully described surface model, which was then saved into a solid model. The final step was to perform filleting and chamfering on the model. The solid model obtained in the final phase of the reconstruction process was exported to STEP format.

2.3. Geometric Reconstruction Based on Data Obtained from GOM Scan 1 Structured Light Scanner

The process of geometric reconstruction based on the obtained three-dimensional point cloud was carried out using the examples of a model of a helical gear and a turbine blade. The data representing the three-dimensional point cloud were acquired using a GOM Scan 1 scanner (Figure 3). The system illuminated the object with a structured light to make measurements. It was equipped with a measurement head mounted on a tripod, allowing the head's appropriate height and angle to be set relative to the object on the rotary table. In the case of methods that illuminate the object with structured light, information about the entire surface of the measured object is obtained from measurements based on Gray's stripe projection. A specific raster is projected onto the surface of the measured object. A prerequisite for correct measurement is good visibility of the stripes on the surface of the workpiece. The non-contact coordinate measuring system works with a rotary table and GOM Inspect software (version 2021). In our study, first of all, the calibration process of the GOM Scan 1 measuring system was carried out. To carry out the measurements, it was necessary to check, among other things, the exposure time, the alignment of the measuring head in relation to the plane of the object to be measured, the number of markers on the geometry, and the reflectivity of the object surface. In addition, where a rotary table was used, it was also necessary to determine the number of its angular settings during geometric measurement. A matting agent was applied to the models' surfaces to prepare them for scanning and to minimize light reflection. Additionally, several reference points were attached to the models to define their initial position and orientation in space. This ensured greater repeatability, thus reducing the impact of systematic and random errors when digitizing the geometry. The measurement was carried out with the highest possible resolution, 0.01 mm. Finally, the measurement process resulted in a three-dimensional point cloud that mapped the geometry of the models, which was saved in STL format. The obtained triangle mesh underwent further processing, and CAD modeling was performed using Siemens NX software. First, a preliminary analysis of the triangle mesh was conducted. Based on this analysis, the noise created during the measurement process was removed.

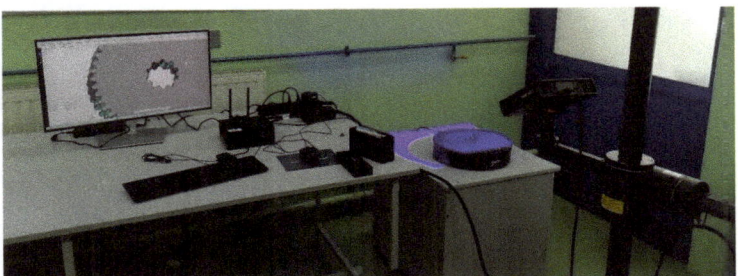

Figure 3. Measurement stand equipped with a structured light scanner.

The CAD modeling of the turbine blade geometry consisted of several steps. In the first step, it was necessary to define the plane using the *"Datum Plane"* tool. In the next step, sections were generated on the surface of the 3D-STL model using the *"Section Curve"* tool. The operation was duplicated, obtaining nine sections of the blade. Points were projected on the obtained section planes. The *"Fit Curve"* tool was used to join the points. Each parameterized profile consisted of four curves. The convex and concave parts of the blade, as well as the edge of attack and trailing edge, were modeled separately. The curves in the subsequent sections were created similarly. To avoid the phenomenon of surface waviness and to obtain a more accurate representation of the turbine blade, guide curves were created using the *"Studio Spline"* tool. Next, surface patches were spanned on the created curves. For this purpose, the *"Through Curve Mesh"* command was used. The surface model was converted into a solid model and exported to STEP format in the next step.

The CAD modeling of the helical gear geometry consisted of several steps. The first step was to reconstruct the contour of the functional surface and spline. In the NX environment, the *Section Curve* function was used. This function defines a curve that represents a cross-section through a three-dimensional object. The *Fit Curve* function in the program was used to create parameterized curves for a set of points. The vertices of the tooth heads were selected as the fit points, thus obtaining the first circle. Similarly, a second circle was created based on points at the teeth's feet. By approximating the sets of points, a tip diameter and a root diameter of the gear were obtained. With the *Extrude* function, a solid representation of the diameter was extruded. The *Fit Curve* function was again used to make teeth on the elaborated solid. Based on the *Fit Spline* option, curves were fitted to the acquired point cloud to develop a tooth space. Surfaces were spanned on the fitted curves to develop the side surface of the tooth using the *Fit Surface* option. The prepared sketches, surfaces, and vectors parallel to the edge of the plane were selected. The result was a ray that was the path of the notch drawing. The program selected the solid by default and cut the material from it to form the notch. The next step was to work out the rest of the teeth similarly. The solid model obtained in the last phase of the process reconstruction was exported to STEP format.

2.4. Geometric Reconstruction Based on Data Acquired with a Multi-Slice Computed Tomography (CT) Scanner

The first stage of reconstructing bone structures representing a fragment of the pelvis and the femur consisted of obtaining Digital Imaging and Communications in Medicine (DICOM) measurement data. The research was conducted on a patient scanned on a Siemens Somatom Definition AS+ multi-slice tomography scanner. A traditional scanning protocol for the hip joint area was used during the measurement process. The obtained volumetric data were characterized by an anisotropic voxel structure: 0.4 mm × 0.4 mm × 0.7 mm. The ITK-SNAP program performed the numerical processing of DICOM data and geometric reconstruction. Segmentation of bone structures in the hip joint area was performed using the thresholding method based on the collected DICOM data, which belongs to the area method group, involving selecting pixels with a similar shade and classifying them into one group defining a given tissue. In segmenting the bone structures of the pelvic fragment and the femur, a lower threshold value of 200 HU was selected. On the set of 2D contours created as a result of the segmentation process, the process of reconstructing the 3D geometry of the bone structures was carried out. The reconstruction process used the isosurface, which is a type of surface rendering method based on the marching cube algorithm. Due to the presence of disproportionate triangles in the resulting 3D-STL model, a surface editing process was carried out, which involved creating a triangle mesh consisting of more regular triangles. Models prepared this way were saved to STL format and loaded into NX Siemens software. In the second stage, the CAD modeling process began. The same functions were applied to the model of the pelvic fragment and the femur. First, a mesh model of curves intersecting at right angles was developed. The developed curves were then dropped, through selecting *Project Curve*, on the surfaces of the 3D-STL models of anatomical structures. In the next step, parameterized surfaces were spanned on the curves that were projected onto the surface of the 3D-STL model using *Rapid Surfacing*. Because some surfaces on the 3D-STL models could not be automatically generated, a manual surface-filling process was carried out in some places. This was possible through moving the nodal points that determined the course of each dropped curve. Finally, the creation of surface models ended with covering the polygonal mesh with elementary NURBS-type surface patches. Each lobe, in addition to determining its boundaries through the dropped curve, was further described by a certain number of control points, determining the quality of the lobe's fit to the corresponding section of the polygonal mesh. The surface model obtained in the last phase of the process was saved as a solid model and exported to STEP format.

3. Results

In the context of the information given in Section 2,

(a) a pulley a CAD modeling methodology was developed (Figure 4), and three deviation map (Figure 5)
(b) a model of parts used for clamping and positioning a CAD modeling methodology was developed (Figure 6), and three deviation map (Figure 7), and for a connecting rod a CAD modeling methodology was developed (Figure 8), and three deviation map (Figure 9)
(c) a turbine blade a CAD modeling methodology was developed (Figure 10), and three deviation map (Figure 11), and for a helical gear a CAD modeling methodology was developed (Figure 12), and three deviation map (Figure 13)
(d) a femur a CAD modeling methodology was developed (Figure 14), and three deviation map (Figure 15), and for a pelvic part a CAD modeling methodology was developed (Figure 16), and three deviation map (Figure 17)

The process of verifying the accuracy of implementing the CAD modeling process was carried out using Focus Inspection and GOM Inspect software. The fitting of the nominal

3D-STL model obtained at the measurement stage and the reference 3D-CAD model generated at the design stage was performed using the best-fit method. This method is an iterative process that minimizes the square of the distance between two models. During implementation, the accuracy of the alignment must be about 0.005 mm. If the parameter value is larger, the process continues until the value is smaller. In addition, statistical data were developed in Tables 1–7 to define the maximum and minimum deviation values, range, mean, and standard deviation values.

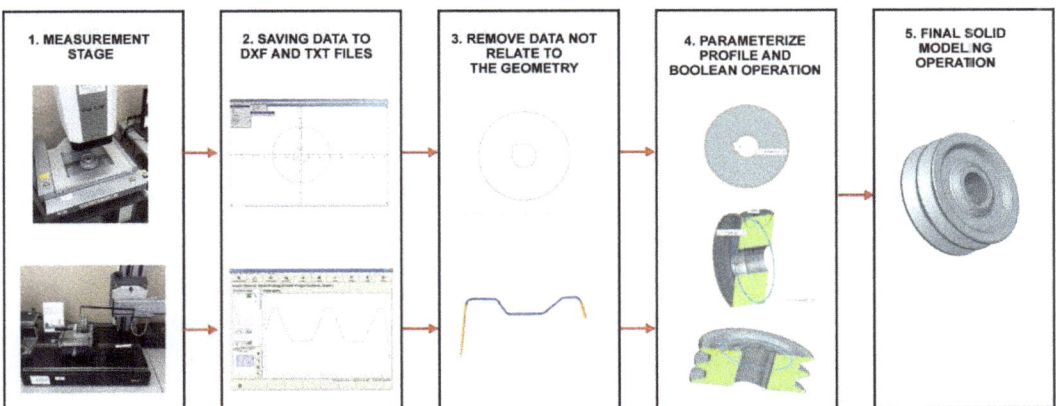

Figure 4. Selected stages of pulley geometry reconstruction into a 3D-CAD model based on 2D profiles acquired during measurement.

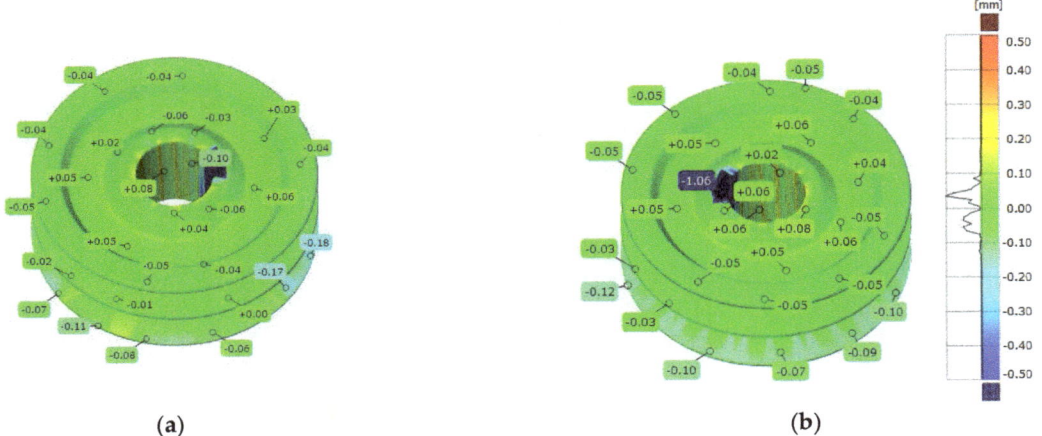

Figure 5. Three-dimensional deviation map representing CAD modeling errors for a pulley model: (**a**) top view; (**b**) bottom view.

Table 1. Statistical parameters representing CAD modeling errors for the pulley model.

Parameters	Pulley Model
Maximum deviation [mm]	0.278
Minimum deviation [mm]	−1.203
Range [mm]	1.481
Mean deviation [mm]	−0.002
Standard deviation [mm]	0.031

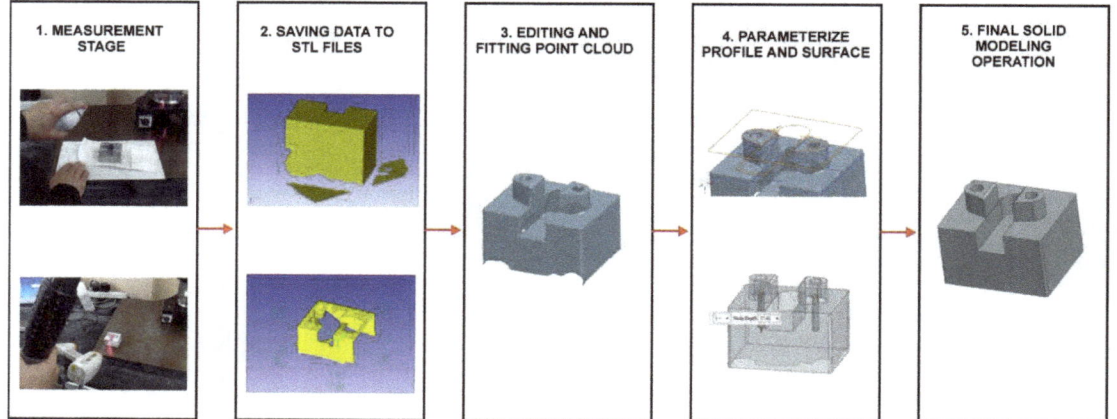

Figure 6. Stages of reconstructing the geometry of a part used for clamping and positioning within a machining process, transformed into a 3D-CAD model based on the obtained 3D point cloud.

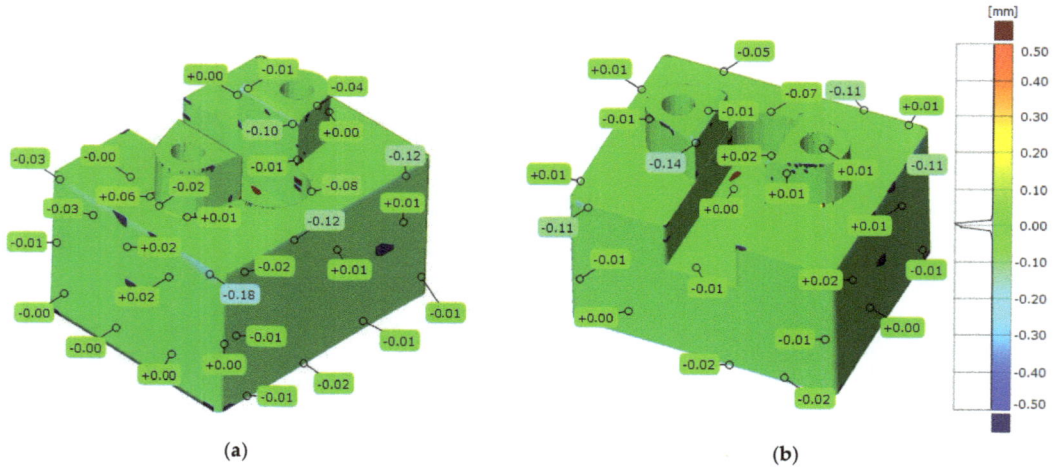

Figure 7. Three-dimensional deviation map representing CAD modeling errors for in model of parts used for clamping and positioning within a machining process: (**a**) back view; (**b**) front view.

Table 2. Statistical parameters representing CAD modeling errors for the model of parts used for clamping and positioning within a machining process.

Parameters	Model for Clamping and Positioning Part
Maximum deviation [mm]	0.161
Minimum deviation [mm]	−0.251
Range [mm]	0.411
Mean deviation [mm]	0.000
Standard deviation [mm]	0.009

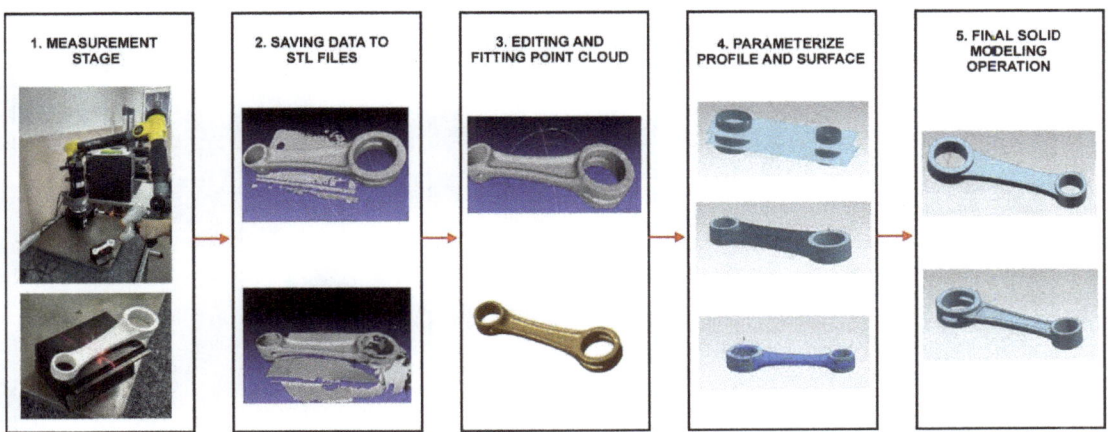

Figure 8. Stages of reconstructing the geometry of the connecting rod into a 3D-CAD model based on the obtained 3D point cloud.

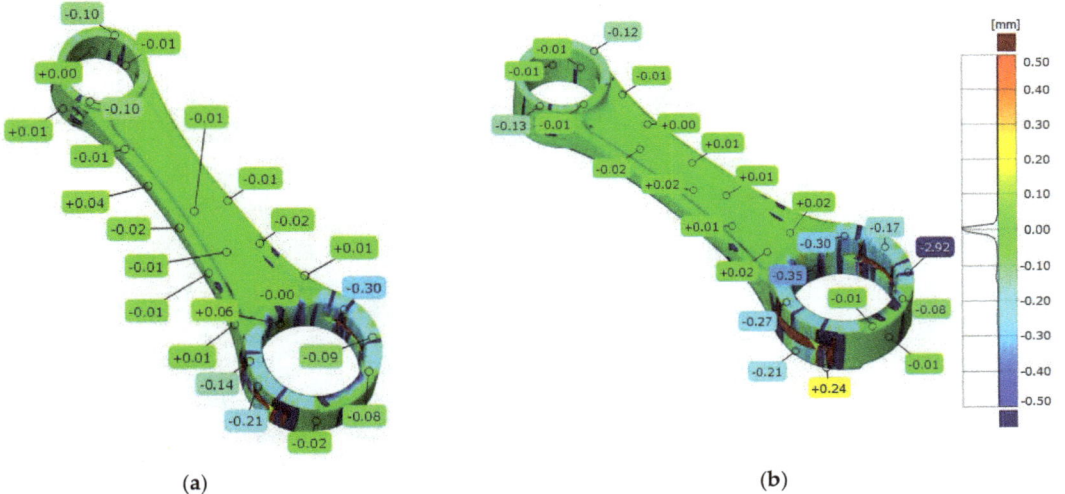

Figure 9. Three-dimensional deviation map representing CAD modeling errors for a connecting rod model: (**a**) top side view; (**b**) bottom side view.

Table 3. Statistical parameters representing CAD modeling errors for the connecting rod model.

Parameters	Connecting Rod Model
Maximum deviation [mm]	0.223
Minimum deviation [mm]	−0.349
Range [mm]	0.571
Mean deviation [mm]	−0.003
Standard deviation [mm]	0.026

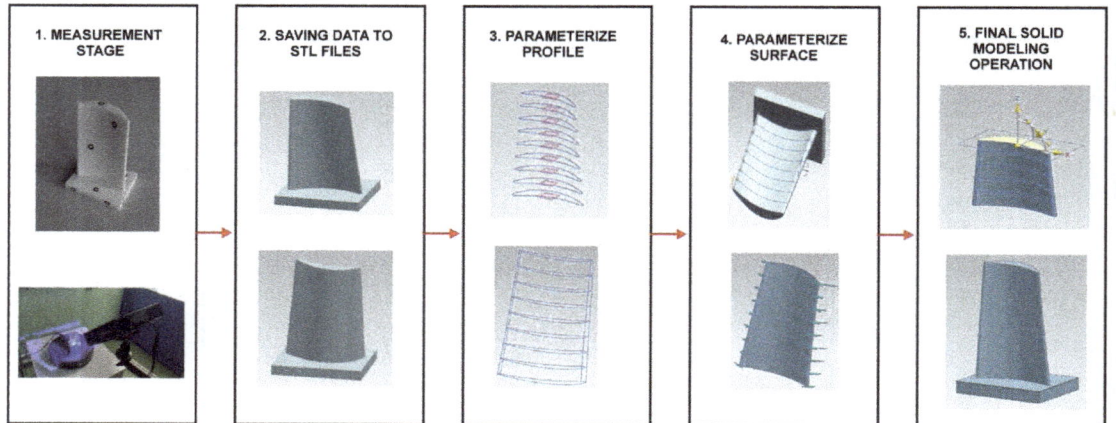

Figure 10. Stages of reconstructing the geometry of the turbine blade model into a 3D-CAD model based on the obtained 3D point cloud.

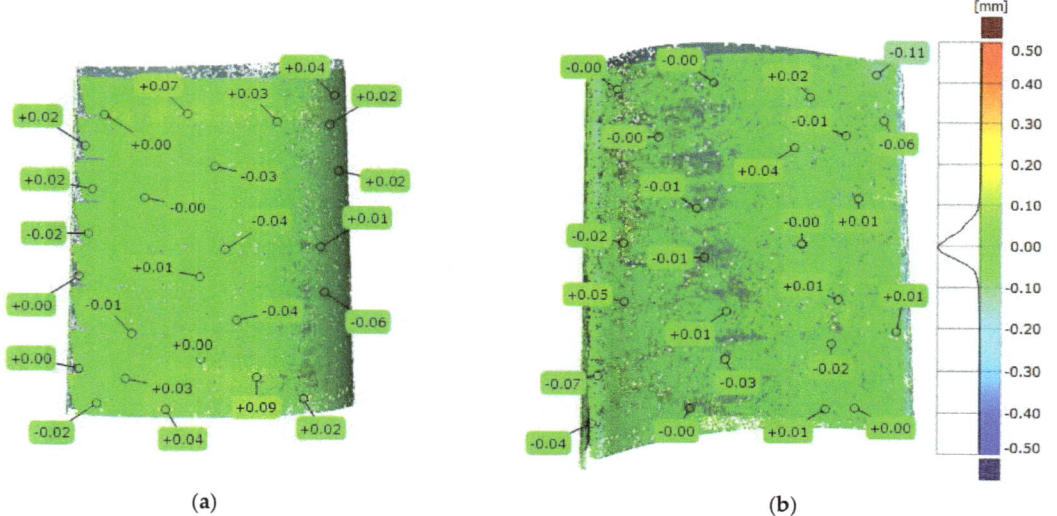

Figure 11. Three-dimensional deviation map representing CAD modeling errors for a turbine blade model: (**a**) convex side view; (**b**) concave side view.

Table 4. Statistical parameters representing CAD modeling errors for the turbine blade model.

Parameters	Turbine Blade Model
Maximum deviation [mm]	0.686
Minimum deviation [mm]	−0.344
Range [mm]	1.030
Mean deviation [mm]	0.000
Standard deviation [mm]	0.045

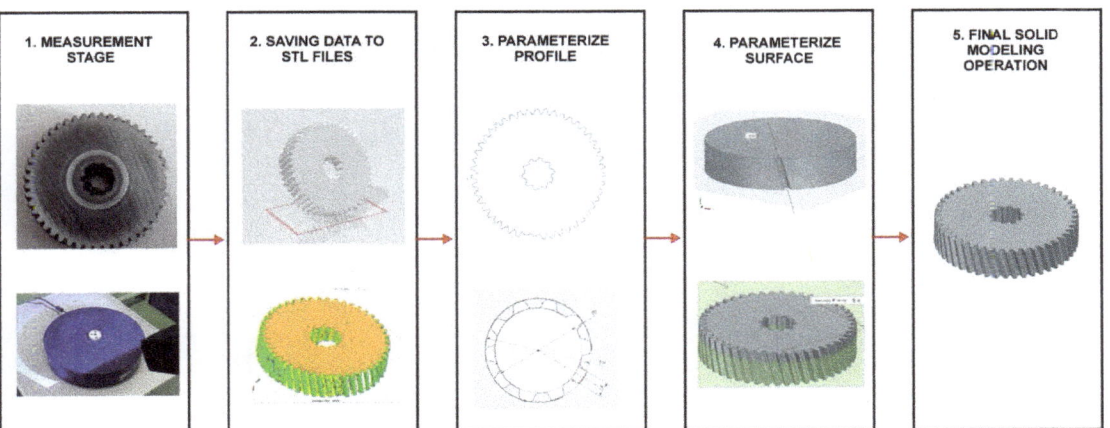

Figure 12. Stages of reconstructing the geometry of the helical gear model into a 3D-CAD model based on the obtained 3D point cloud.

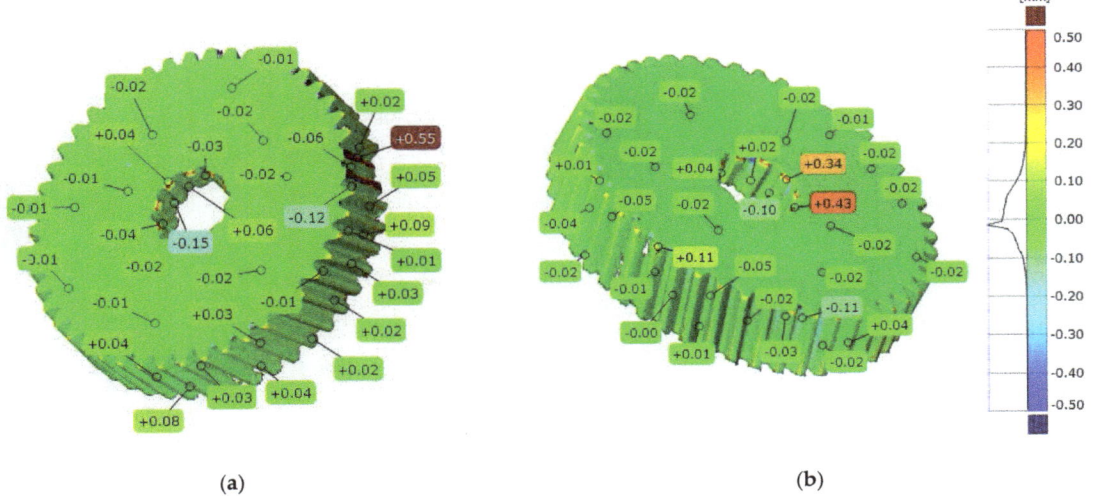

Figure 13. Three-dimensional deviation map representing CAD modeling errors for a helical gear model: (**a**) top view; (**b**) bottom view.

Table 5. Statistical parameters representing CAD modeling errors for the helical gear model.

Parameters	Helical Gear Model
Maximum deviation [mm]	0.693
Minimum deviation [mm]	−0.967
Range [mm]	1.660
Mean deviation [mm]	−0.025
Standard deviation [mm]	0.098

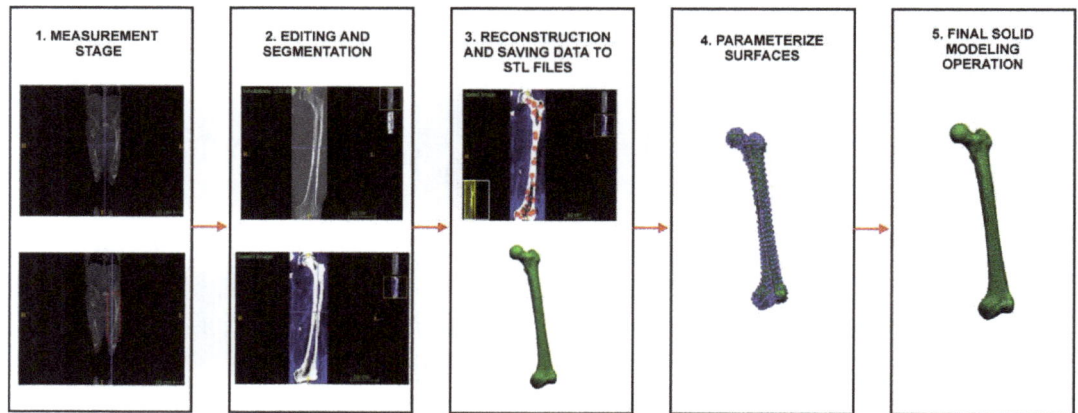

Figure 14. Stages of reconstructing the geometry of the femur model into a 3D-CAD model based on the obtained 2D images.

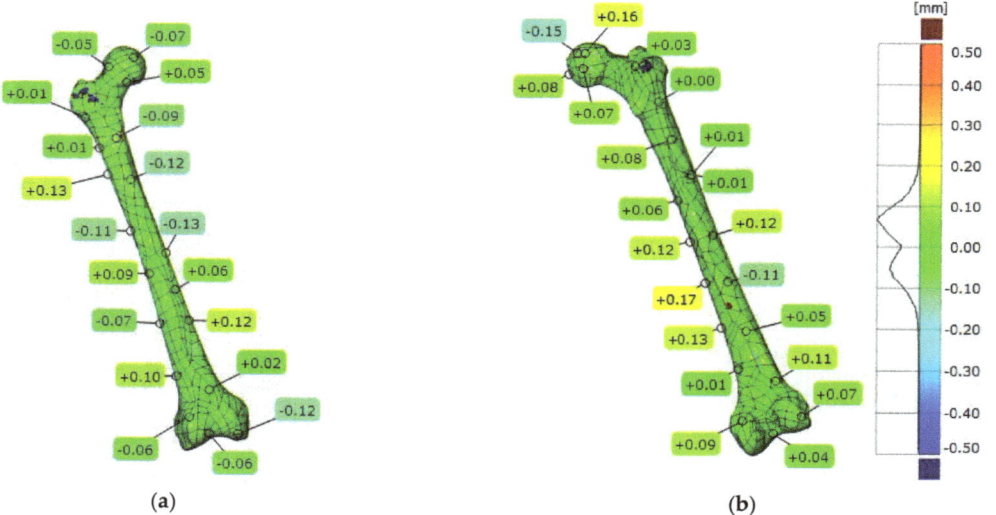

Figure 15. Three-dimensional deviation map representing CAD modeling errors for a femur model: (**a**) front view; (**b**) back view.

Table 6. Statistical parameters representing CAD modeling errors for the femur model.

Parameters	Femur Model
Maximum deviation [mm]	2.984
Minimum deviation [mm]	−0.705
Range [mm]	3.689
Mean deviation [mm]	0.001
Standard deviation [mm]	0.090

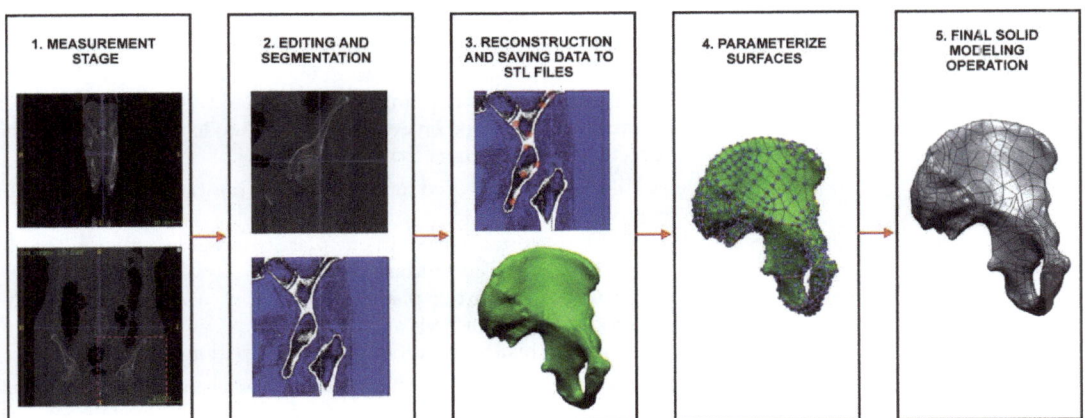

Figure 16. Stages of reconstructing the geometry of the pelvic part model into a 3D-CAD model based on the obtained 2D images.

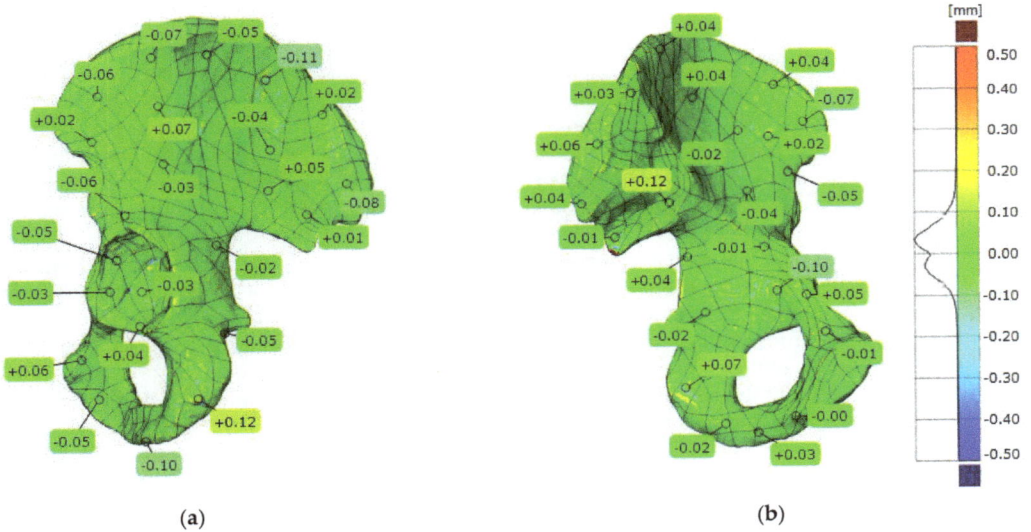

Figure 17. Three-dimensional deviation map representing CAD modeling errors for the pelvic part model: (**a**) back view; (**b**) front view.

Table 7. Statistical parameters representing CAD modeling errors for the pelvic part model.

Parameters	Pelvic Part Model
Maximum deviation [mm]	2.356
Minimum deviation [mm]	−0.651
Range [mm]	3.007
Mean deviation [mm]	0.005
Standard deviation [mm]	0.051

4. Discussion

The RE process is increasingly used in many technological fields like automotive [15], aviation [18], and medicine [48,49]. It can be identified as one of the techniques for designing machine parts closely associated with computer-aided engineering systems. Analyzing the accuracy of the development of the final reconstructed 3D-CAD model is necessary for evaluating the RE process [12,13]. Many factors affect the accuracy of the 3D-CAD model, including measurement errors, data processing errors, and CAD modeling errors [17,18]. The authors of the current study focused on evaluating CAD modeling errors. The model selection procedure focused on geometries characterized by:

(a) basic geometries, such as a model used for clamping and positioning parts to perform the machining process;
(b) the generation of cross-sectional curves in one plane and guide curves in the other plane, such as for a helical gear and turbine blade;
(c) repeatability of features in one or two planes, such as on a pulley;
(d) basic geometries and freeform surfaces, such as on a connecting rod;
(e) freeform surfaces, such as on a femur model and pelvic part model.

The quality of the acquired data was affected by, among other things, the resolution of the measurement, form deviation, and the degree of wear of the digitized object. In the case of measurements with the MarSurf XC20 and iNEXIVE optical microscope systems, the highest possible resolution was used when measuring the pulley. The microscope used had a resolution of 0.02 mm, while the MarSurf XC20 system had a resolution of 0.001 mm. The measurement resolution was kept at least ten times smaller than the dimensional and form tolerances used to define the pulley geometry, to ensure accurate measurements [50]. Therefore, any errors in the obtained measurement results were primarily due to the pulley's manufacturing process and any damage caused during this. In the stage of CAD modeling based on acquired 2D and 3D point cloud data, the most significant impact on the accuracy of obtaining the final 3D-CAD model is the stage of fitting parameterized 2D curves or 3D surfaces to the measurement data, which depends on the quality of the measurement data obtained. When fitting the data to the optical microscope, some points deviated from the correct trend of the measured profile. Therefore, they were not taken into account in the curve fitting process. In the case of data acquired with the MarSurf XC20, data that deviated from the trend were also noticed, but they appeared less significant than with the optical microscope. Therefore, they were not considered blunder errors; they were just data that, in addition to shape detrending, may have contained irregularities from surface roughness. The *Fit Circle* and *Fit Line* options were used to elaborate the parameterized profiles. The average fitting errors were obtained from the data acquired with the optical microscope, which were the highest. For the circle fit, they averaged 0.06 mm; for the line fit, they averaged 0.05 mm. For MarSurf XC20, they were 0.03 mm for the circle and 0.02 mm for the line, respectively. In averaging the matching results, the data mapping of the splineway needed to be considered. Matching the lines to this part of the geometry was difficult due to damage to this part of the model. Therefore, the obtained fitting values significantly differed from the average deviation values. Considering the research described in Figure 18, the factors influencing accuracy at the stages of geometric measurement, measurement data processing, and, finally, the CAD modeling process were identified.

Two methods were used in the CAD modeling based on 3D point clouds: one simplified the modeling process by creating 2D profiles based on the 3D point cloud, and the other developed a 3D-CAD model by fitting traditional geometric figures (e.g., cylinder, flat surface) and freeform surfaces. Considering the data obtained with the laser scanner, an irregular form of a three-dimensional point cloud was observed. It was formed by manually merging the acquired data from different measurement directions. The maximum fitting error of the point cloud was 0.006 mm for the model used for clamping and positioning parts in the machining process and 0.01 mm for the connecting rod. The highest measurement resolution of the laser scanner, which was 0.01 mm, was used to minimize measurement errors. Despite this, an incomplete representation of the geometry of the models was obtained on selected sharp edges, which was combined with the limitations of the laser head itself.

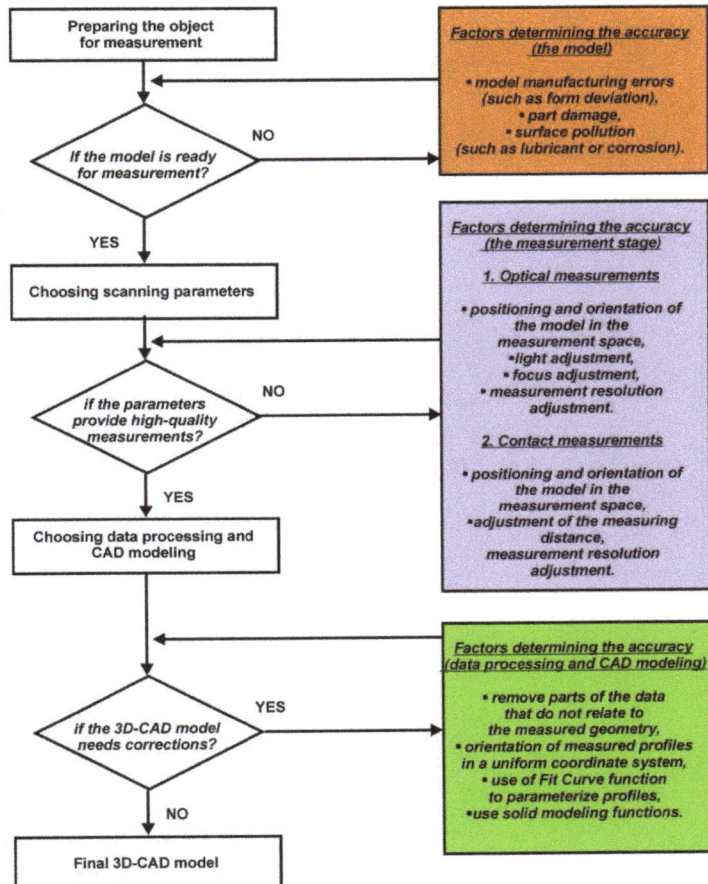

Figure 18. Factors determining the accuracy of geometric reconstruction based on acquired 2D profiles.

Thus, most negative deviations were obtained from models scanned using this method. Most of them were within the ±0.05 mm deviation range. In the case of the model used for clamping and positioning parts for performing the machining process, the highest average values of the deviations of the fit of the line and circle for the parameterized profiles were below −0.1 mm. Thus, they did not exceed the deviation limits for the model's manufacture. The dimensional and form tolerances of the model were within deviations of ±0.1 mm. The model was designed for the company's domestic production needs. In the case of the connecting rod, the results of matching the flat surface and cylindrical surface to the three-dimensional point cloud were also below −0.1 mm in some places. The fitting deviations were much higher for some sections of the connecting rod, mainly due to the wear of the model's surface in this area. The degree and tolerance method fitted the profile with a spline curve for a section of the connecting rod geometry. Based on the generation of a three-degree curve and an assumed tolerance of 0.01 mm, an average fitting error of 0.005 mm was obtained. Thus, the errors of the entire reconstruction process were mainly within the manufacturing tolerances of the connecting rod. Unfortunately, the errors created in the operation process significantly affected the increase in the values of negative deviations in the big end bore. In the case of the wrist pin diameter, the deviations were much smaller and, in most areas, did not exceed the values of manufacturing deviations [51,52]. The deviation of the hole axis spacing was −0.02 mm; the value obtained was within the range of manufacturing deviations, which is ±0.05 mm. Considering the research described in Figure 19, the factors influencing accuracy at the stages of geometric measurement, measurement data processing, and, finally, the CAD modeling process were identified.

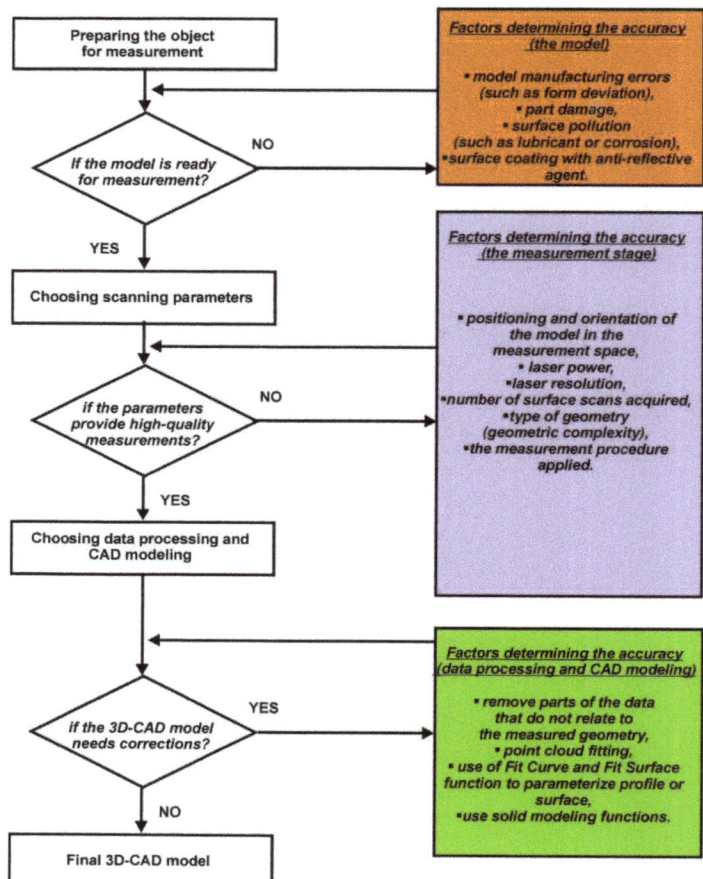

Figure 19. Factors determining the accuracy of geometric reconstruction based on the acquired 3D point cloud using the laser head.

In the case of data obtained from the structured light scanner, a more homogeneous point cloud was obtained. Thus, the error of fitting the point clouds for the turbine blade was 0.003 mm, and for the helical gear was 0.004 mm. This was due to the automation of the entire measurement process. The models of the turbine blade and helical gear were measured with a resolution of 0.01 mm to minimize the impact of measurement errors. The established resolution value was ten times smaller than the tolerances, which defined the accuracy of the model's geometry [53–55]. For the turbine blade geometry, section curves were generated. Spline curves were created on the obtained points. Each profile consisted of four elements of this type, continuously connected. The profile's leading edge, attack edge, and upper and lower parts were modeled separately. The *Fit Spline* command created approximated curves based on the imported points. Based on the generation of a three-degree curve and an assumed tolerance of 0.01 mm, an average fit error of 0.005 mm was obtained. The option to generate a section curve was also used for the helical gear. Similar settings to the *Fit Spline* option were applied to the turbine blade. However, higher average fit errors of about 0.1 mm were obtained based on the settings used. The highest modeling errors occurred within the spline area and the fragment of tooth geometry. These occurred because those areas were damaged. For the development of the side surface of the tooth, the *Fit Surface* option was used. The option chosen was *Fit Freeform Surface*. Based on the selected option, the accuracy of the modeling of the side surface of the tooth was obtained, which was within the range of maximum deviations of ±0.09 mm. Considering the research described in Figure 20, the factors influencing accuracy at the stages of geometric measurement, measurement data processing, and, finally, the CAD modeling process were identified.

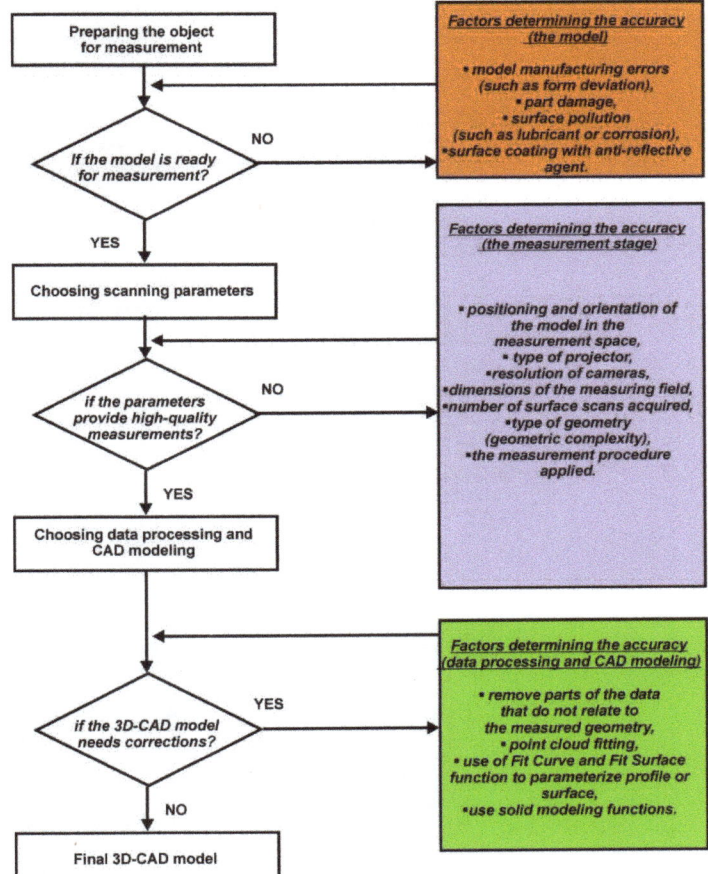

Figure 20. Factors determining the accuracy of geometric reconstruction based on the acquired 3D point cloud using the structured light system.

In the case of models of anatomical structures, it is impossible to relate the results obtained to the accuracy of nominal models (since such do not exist). However, several conclusions can be made about the factors affecting the accuracy of the reconstruction process. Among the most significant are errors in the measurement process, which largely depend on the quality of the spatial resolution of the DICOM data [56,57]. In addition, the accuracy of the obtained geometry is also influenced by the segmentation method used [30,58]. Additionally, it is crucial to know the CAD modeling errors. For models of anatomical structures of the hip joint, the method used was to generate an automatic freeform surface based on curves previously projected onto the 3D-STL model. For non-standard geometries such as anatomical structures, no other 3D-CAD modeling method was possible. To fully parametrize the models, in the case of the femur model, 1060 edges were required to be generated, on which 530 surface patches were spanned. For the pelvic part, 1248 edges were generated, on which 624 surface patches were spanned. The generated parameters achieved CAD modeling accuracy of ±0.2 mm for the femur model and ±0.1 mm for the pelvic part. As with any modeling method, it is possible to develop 3D-CAD models more accurately. This is especially possible for the femur. However, covering the 3D-STL model with a larger number of surface patches significantly increases the 3D-CAD model generation time. Considering the research described in Figure 21, the factors influencing accuracy at the stages of geometric measurement, measurement data processing, and, finally, the CAD modeling process were identified.

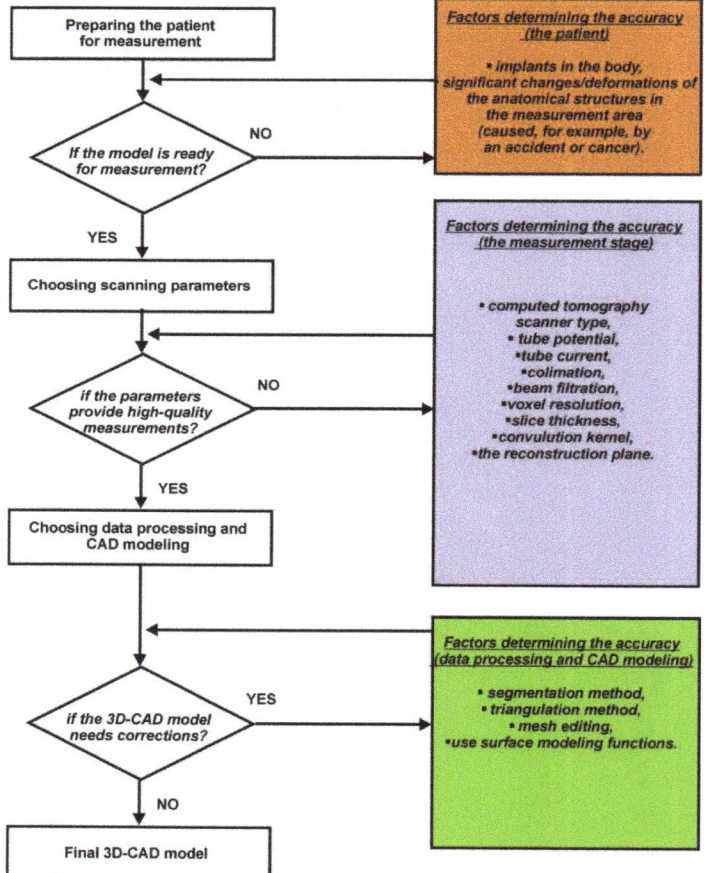

Figure 21. Factors determining the accuracy of geometric reconstruction based on DICOM data acquired using the CT scanner.

5. Conclusions

Reverse engineering is becoming increasingly crucial in reconstructing the geometry of models for which we usually do not have technical documentation. The most significant problem concerning the reconstruction of geometry is related to the occurrence of errors that influence the accuracy of the development of the final 3D-CAD model. The lack of developed procedures and estimated errors at the stage of geometric reconstruction carries the risk that selected dimensions and, most importantly, functional parts of the reconstructed model may be outside the tolerance limits. Therefore, the procedures developed in the article, including the selected resolution of measurement systems, constitute CAD modeling methods to minimize reconstruction errors, allowing the development of copies of model geometries within the tolerance limits of their manufacture. The selection of the system and measurement parameters, the accuracy of fitting together the acquired measurement data, and the parameterization methods used have a major influence on the deviation values obtained. However, all co-authors confirm that it is necessary to test the adopted assumptions further to optimize the presented procedures and to test their functional properties on already manufactured models whose digital documentation was created in the reconstruction process.

Author Contributions: Conceptualization, P.T.; methodology, P.T., W.B., K.C., K.D. and A.F.; software, P.T., W.B., K.C., K.D., A.F. and J.M.; validation, P.T. and J.M.; formal analysis, P.T.; investigation, P.T., W.B., K.C., K.D. and A.F.; writing—original draft preparation, W.B., K.C., K.D. and A.F.; writing—review and editing, P.T.; visualization, P.T.; supervision, P.T. All authors have read and agreed to the published version of the manuscript.

Funding: This research received no external funding.

Data Availability Statement: Data are contained within the article.

Conflicts of Interest: The authors declare no conflicts of interest.

References

1. Neamţu, C.; Hurgoiu, D.; Popescu, S.; Dragomir, M.; Osanna, H. Training in coordinate measurement using 3D virtual instruments. *Measurement* **2012**, *45*, 2346–2358. [CrossRef]
2. Han, D.Y.L.D.Z.; Juan, W.W.W. CAD model-based intelligent inspection planning for coordinate measuring machines. *Chin. J. Mech. Eng.* **2011**, *24*, 1. [CrossRef]
3. He, G.; Huang, X.; Ma, W.; Sang, Y.; Yu, G. CAD-based measurement planning strategy of complex surface for five axes on machine verification. *Int. J. Adv. Manuf. Technol.* **2017**, *91*, 2101–2111. [CrossRef]
4. Wang, X.; Xian, J.; Yang, Y.; Zhang, Y.; Fu, X.; Kang, M. Use of coordinate measuring machine to measure circular aperture complex optical surface. *Measurement* **2017**, *100*, 1–6. [CrossRef]
5. Gapinski, B.; Wieczorowski, M.; Marciniak-Podsadna, L.; Dybala, B.; Ziolkowski, G. Comparison of different method of measurement geometry using CMM, optical scanner and computed tomography 3D. *Procedia Eng.* **2014**, *69*, 255–262. [CrossRef]
6. Roithmeier, R. *Measuring Strategies in Tactile Coordinate Metrology*; Carl Zeiss AG: Jena, Germany, 2014.
7. Li, F.; Hiley, J.; Syed, T.M.; Hitchens, C.; Garcia Lopez-Astilleros, M. A region segmentation method to measure multiple features using a tactile scanning probe. *Int. J. Comput. Integr. Manuf.* **2019**, *32*, 569–579. [CrossRef]
8. Turek, P.; Budzik, G.; Przeszłowski, Ł. Assessing the Radiological Density and Accuracy of Mandible Polymer Anatomical Structures Manufactured Using 3D Printing Technologies. *Polymers* **2020**, *12*, 2444. [CrossRef]
9. Kruth, J.P.; Bartscher, M.; Carmignato, S.; Schmitt, R.; De Chiffre, L.; Weckenmann, A. Computed tomography for dimensional metrology. *CIRP Ann.* **2011**, *60*, 821–842. [CrossRef]
10. Suzuki, K.; Masukawa, A.; Aoki, S.; Arai, Y.; Ueno, E. A new coordinates system for cranial organs using magnetic resonance imaging. *Acta Oto-Laryngol.* **2010**, *130*, 568–575. [CrossRef]
11. Li, F.; Longstaff, A.P.; Fletcher, S.; Myers, A. *Integrated Tactile and Optical Measuring Systems in Three Dimensional Metrology*; University of Huddersfield: Huddersfield, UK, 2012.
12. Raja, V. Introduction to reverse engineering. In *Reverse Engineering: An Industrial Perspective*; Springer: London, UK, 2008; pp. 1–9. [CrossRef]
13. She, S.; Lotufo, R.; Berger, T.; Wąsowski, A.; Czarnecki, K. Reverse engineering feature models. In Proceedings of the 33rd International Conference on Software Engineering, Honolulu, HI, USA, 21–28 May 2011; pp. 461–470. [CrossRef]
14. Bagci, E. Reverse engineering applications for recovery of broken or worn parts and re-manufacturing: Three case studies. *Adv. Eng. Softw.* **2009**, *40*, 407–418. [CrossRef]
15. Štefan, K.; Janette, B. Reverse engineering in automotive design component. *Industry 4.0* **2022**, *7*, 62–65.
16. Dúbravčík, M.; Kender, Š. Application of reverse engineering techniques in mechanics system services. *Procedia Eng.* **2012**, *48*, 96–104. [CrossRef]
17. Rozesara, M.; Ghazinoori, S.; Manteghi, M.; Tabatabaeian, S.H. A reverse engineering-based model for innovation process in complex product systems: Multiple case studies in the aviation industry. *J. Eng. Technol. Manag.* **2023**, *69*, 101765. [CrossRef]

18. Fedorova, I.G.E.; Filimonova, T.S.; Zhuravlev, E.V.E.; Vasiliev, V.V. Estimation of the possibility of using reverse engineering in the aviation industry. *Comput. Nanotechnol.* **2019**, *6*, 68–73. [CrossRef]
19. Mengoni, M.; Leopardi, A. An exploratory study on the application of reverse engineering in the field of small archaeological artefacts. *Comput. Aided Des. Appl.* **2019**, *16*, 1209–1226. [CrossRef]
20. Selden, R.Z.; Jones, B.M. Reverse engineering a bronze cannon from the La Belle shipwreck. *Hist. Archaeol.* **2021**, *55*, 290–299. [CrossRef]
21. Turek, P. Automating the process of designing and manufacturing polymeric models of anatomical structures of mandible with Industry 4.0 convention. *Polimery* **2019**, *64*, 522–529. [CrossRef]
22. Korunovic, N.; Marinkovic, D.; Trajanovic, M.; Zehn, M.; Mitkovic, M.; Affatato, S. In silico optimization of femoral fixator position and configuration by parametric CAD model. *Materials* **2019**, *12*, 2326. [CrossRef] [PubMed]
23. Ciocca, L.; Mazzoni, S.; Fantini, M.; Persiani, F.; Baldissara, P.; Marchetti, C.; Scotti, R. A CAD/CAM-prototyped anatomical condylar prosthesis connected to a custom-made bone plate to support a fibula free flap. *Med. Biol. Eng. Comput.* **2012**, *50*, 743–749. [CrossRef]
24. Turek, P.; Jońca, K.; Winiarska, M. Evaluation of the accuracy of the resection template and restorations of the bone structures in the mandible area manufactured using the additive technique. *Rep. Mech. Eng.* **2023**, *4*, 39–46. [CrossRef]
25. Turek, P.; Jakubiec, J. Geometrical precision and surface topography of mSLA-produced surgical guides for the knee joint. *J. Eng. Manag. Syst. Eng.* **2023**, *2*, 150–157. [CrossRef]
26. Salmi, M. Additive Manufacturing Processes in Medical Applications. *Materials* **2021**, *14*, 191. [CrossRef] [PubMed]
27. Kumar, A.; Jain, P.K.; Pathak, P.M. Reverse engineering in product manufacturing: An overview. *DAAAM Int. Sci. Book* **2013**, *39*, 665–678. [CrossRef]
28. Barbero, B.R.; Ureta, E.S. Comparative study of different digitization techniques and their accuracy. *Comput. Aided Des.* **2011**, *43*, 188–206. [CrossRef]
29. Milovanović, J.; Stojković, M.; Trifunović, M.; Vitković, N. Review of bone scaffold design concepts and design methods. *Facta Univ. Ser. Mech. Eng.* **2023**, *21*, 151–173. [CrossRef]
30. van Eijnatten, M.; Koivisto, J.; Karhu, K.; Forouzanfar, T.; Wolff, J. The impact of manual threshold selection in medical additive manufacturing. *Int. J. Comput. Assist. Radiol. Surg.* **2017**, *12*, 607–615. [CrossRef]
31. Turek, P. Evaluation of the auto surfacing methods to create a surface body of the mandible model. *Rep. Mech. Eng.* **2022**, *3*, 46–54. [CrossRef]
32. VDI/VDE 2634 Blatt 3. Available online: https://www.vdi.eu/guidelines/vdivde_2634_blatt_3-optische_3_d_messsysteme_bildgebende_systeme_mit_flaechenhafter_antastung/ (accessed on 8 April 2024).
33. American Society of Mechanical Engineers (ASME). *B89. 4.22. Methods for Performance Evaluation of Articulated Arm Coordinate Measuring Machines (CMM)*; American Society of Mechanical Engineers (ASME): New York, NY, USA, 2004.
34. VDI/VDE 2634 Blatt 2. Available online: https://www.vdi.eu/guidelines/vdivde_2634_blatt_2-optische_3_d_messsysteme_bildgebende_systeme_mit_flaechenhafter_antastung/ (accessed on 8 April 2024).
35. D'Amato, R.; Caja, J.; Maresca, P.; Gómez, E. Use of coordinate measuring machine to measure angles by geometric characterization of perpendicular planes. Estimating uncertainty. *Measurement* **2014**, *47*, 598–606. [CrossRef]
36. Budzik, G.; Kubiak, K.; Matysiak, H.; Cygan, R.; Tutak, M. Hybrid method for rapid prototyping of core models of aircraft engine blades. *J. Kones* **2012**, *19*, 77–82. [CrossRef]
37. Kawalec, A.; Magdziak, M. Usability assessment of selected methods of optimization for some measurement task in coordinate measurement technique. *Measurement* **2012**, *45*, 2330–2338. [CrossRef]
38. Saqib, S.; Urbanic, J. An experimental study to determine geometric and dimensional accuracy impact factors for fused deposition modelled parts. In *Enabling Manufacturing Competitiveness and Economic Sustainability*; Springer: Berlin/Heidelberg, Germany, 2012; pp. 293–298. [CrossRef]
39. Brajlih, T.; Tasic, T.; Drstvensek, I.; Valentan, B.; Hadzistevic, M.; Pogacar, V.; Acko, B. Possibilities of using three-dimensional optical scanning in complex geometrical inspection. *Stroj. Vestn. J. Mech. Eng.* **2011**, *57*, 826–833. [CrossRef]
40. Pisula, J.; Dziubek, T.; Przeszłowski, Ł. A comparison of the accuracy of bevel gear teeth obtained by means of selected RP techniques and the removal machining method. *Mach. Dyn. Res.* **2016**, *40*, 147–161. Available online: http://mdr.simr.pw.edu.pl/index.php/MDR/article/view/200/182 (accessed on 20 May 2024).
41. Pisula, J.; Dziubek, T.; Przeszłowski, L.; Budzik, G. Evaluation of Geometrical Parameters of a Spur Gear Manufactured in an Incremental Process from GP1 Steel. In *Industrial Measurements in Machining*; Part of the Lecture Notes in Mechanical Engineering book, series; Królczyk, G.M., Niesłony, P., Królczyk, J., Eds.; Springer: Cham, Switzerland, 2020; Volume 975, pp. 109–127. [CrossRef]
42. Bračun, D.; Škulj, G.; Kadiš, M. Spectral selective and difference imaging laser triangulation measurement system for on line measurement of large hot workpieces in precision open die forging. *Int. J. Adv. Manuf. Technol.* **2017**, *90*, 917–926. [CrossRef]
43. Selami, Y.; Tao, W.; Gao, Q.; Yang, H.; Zhao, H. A scheme for enhancing precision in 3-dimensional positioning for non-contact measurement systems based on laser triangulation. *Sensors* **2018**, *18*, 504. [CrossRef]
44. Liang, X.; Lambrichts, I.; Sun, Y.; Denis, K.; Hassan, B.; Li, L.; Pauwels, R.; Jacobs, R. A comparative evaluation of cone beam computed tomography (CBCT) and multi-slice CT (MSCT). Part II: On 3D model accuracy. *Eur. J. Radiol.* **2010**, *75*, 270–274. [CrossRef]

45. Lee, K.Y.; Cho, J.W.; Chang, N.Y.; Chae, J.M.; Kang, K.H.; Kim, S.C.; Cho, J.H. Accuracy of three-dimensional printing for manufacturing replica teeth. *Korean J. Orthod.* **2015**, *45*, 217–225. [CrossRef] [PubMed]
46. Warnett, J.M.; Titarenko, V.; Kiraci, E.; Attridge, A.; Lionheart, W.R.; Withers, P.J.; Williams, M.A. Towards in-process X-ray CT for dimensional metrology. *Meas. Sci. Technol.* **2016**, *27*, 035401. [CrossRef]
47. Townsend, A.; Racasan, R.; Leach, R.; Senin, N.; Thompson, A.; Ramsey, A.; Blunt, L. An interlaboratory comparison of X-ray computed tomography measurement for texture and dimensional characterisation of additively manufactured parts. *Addit. Manuf.* **2018**, *23*, 422–432. [CrossRef]
48. Pais, A.; Moreira, C.; Belinha, J. The Biomechanical Analysis of Tibial Implants Using Meshless Methods: Stress and Bone Tissue Remodeling Analysis. *Designs* **2024**, *8*, 28. [CrossRef]
49. Mejía Rodríguez, M.; González-Estrada, O.A.; Villegas-Bermúdez, D.F. Finite Element Analysis of Patient-Specific Cranial Implants under Different Design Parameters for Material Selection. *Designs* **2024**, *8*, 31. [CrossRef]
50. ISO 9981:2020; Belt Drives—Pulleys and V-Ribbed Belts for the Automotive Industry—PK Profile: Dimensions. ISO: Geneva, Switzerland, 2020.
51. Sharma, G.V.S.S.; Rao, P.S.; Surendra Babu, B. Process-based tolerance assessment of connecting rod machining process. *J. Ind. Eng. Int.* **2016**, *12*, 211–220. [CrossRef]
52. Jezierski, J.; Kowalik, M.; Siemiątkowski, Z. Assembling operations and tolerance analysis of combustion engine crankshaft system. *Arch. Mech. Eng.* **2006**, *53*, 363–371.
53. Petitcuenot, M.; Pierre, L.; Anselmetti, B. ISO specifications of complex surfaces: Application on aerodynamic profiles. *Procedia CIRP* **2015**, *27*, 16–22. [CrossRef]
54. Garaizar, O.R.; Qiao, L.; Anwer, N.; Mathieu, L. Integration of thermal effects into tolerancing using skin model shapes. *Procedia CIRP* **2016**, *43*, 196–201. [CrossRef]
55. ISO 1328-1:2013; Cylindrical Gears—ISO System of Flank Tolerance Classification—Part 1: Definitions and Allowable Values of Deviations Relevant to Flanks of Gear Teeth. ISO: Geneva, Switzerland, 2013.
56. Romans, L. *Computed Tomography for Technologists: A Comprehensive Text*; Wolters Kluwer: Baltimore, MD, USA, 2011.
57. Alsleem, H.; Davidson, R. Factors affecting contrast-detail performance in computed tomography: A review. *J. Med. Imaging Radiat. Sci.* **2013**, *44*, 62–70. [CrossRef] [PubMed]
58. Huotilainen, E.; Jaanimets, R.; Valášek, J.; Marcián, P.; Salmi, M.; Tuomi, J.; Wolff, J. Inaccuracies in additive manufactured medical skull models caused by the DICOM to STL conversion process. *J. CranioMaxillofacial Surg.* **2014**, *42*, e259–e265. [CrossRef]

Disclaimer/Publisher's Note: The statements, opinions and data contained in all publications are solely those of the individual author(s) and contributor(s) and not of MDPI and/or the editor(s). MDPI and/or the editor(s) disclaim responsibility for any injury to people or property resulting from any ideas, methods, instructions or products referred to in the content.

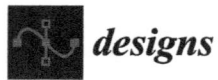 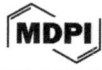

Article

Introduction of Hybrid Additive Manufacturing for Producing Multi-Material Artificial Organs for Education and In Vitro Testing

Konstantinos Chatzipapas [1], Anastasia Nika [2] and Agathoklis A. Krimpenis [3,*]

[1] Core Department, National and Kapodistrian University of Athens, 34400 Psachna, Greece; kchatzipapas@uoa.gr
[2] Industrial Chemistry Laboratory, Department of Chemistry, National and Kapodistrian University of Athens, Zografou, 15771 Athens, Greece; anika@chem.uoa.gr
[3] Mechanical Engineering Department, Hellenic Mediterranean University, Estavromenos, 71410 Heraklion, Greece
* Correspondence: akrimpenis@hmu.gr; Tel.: +30-2810379286

Abstract: The evolution of 3D printing has ushered in accessibility and cost-effectiveness, spanning various industries including biomedical engineering, education, and microfluidics. In biomedical engineering, it encompasses bioprinting tissues, producing prosthetics, porous metal orthopedic implants, and facilitating educational models. Hybrid Additive Manufacturing approaches and, more specifically, the integration of Fused Deposition Modeling (FDM) with bio-inkjet printing offers the advantages of improved accuracy, structural support, and controlled geometry, yet challenges persist in cell survival, interaction, and nutrient delivery within printed structures. The goal of this study was to develop and present a low-cost way to produce physical phantoms of human organs that could be used for research and training, bridging the gap between the use of highly detailed computational phantoms and real-life clinical applications. To this purpose, this study utilized anonymized clinical Computed Tomography (CT) data to create a liver physical model using the Creality Ender-3 printer. Polylactic Acid (PLA), Polyvinyl Alcohol (PVA), and light-bodied silicone (Polysiloxane) materials were employed for printing the liver including its veins and arteries. In brief, PLA was used to create a mold of a liver to be filled with biocompatible light-bodied silicone. Molds of the veins and arteries were printed using PVA and then inserted in the liver model to create empty channel. In addition, the PVA was then washed out by the final product using warm water. Despite minor imperfections due to the printer's limitations, the final product imitates the computational model accurately enough. Precision adjustments in the design phase compensated for this variation. The proposed novel low-cost 3D printing methodology successfully produced an anatomically accurate liver physical model, presenting promising applications in medical education, research, and surgical planning. Notably, its implications extend to medical training, personalized medicine, and organ transplantation. The technology's potential includes injection training for medical professionals, personalized anthropomorphic phantoms for radiation therapy, and the future prospect of creating functional living organs for organ transplantation, albeit requiring significant interdisciplinary collaboration and financial investment. This technique, while showcasing immense potential in biomedical applications, requires further advancements and interdisciplinary cooperation for its optimal utilization in revolutionizing medical science and benefiting patient healthcare.

Keywords: additive manufacturing; personalized medicine; bioprinting; medical education

Citation: Chatzipapas, K.; Nika, A.; Krimpenis, A.A. Introduction of Hybrid Additive Manufacturing for Producing Multi-Material Artificial Organs for Education and In Vitro Testing. *Designs* **2024**, *8*, 51. https://doi.org/10.3390/designs8030051

Academic Editor: Richard Drevet

Received: 23 March 2024
Revised: 23 May 2024
Accepted: 27 May 2024
Published: 28 May 2024

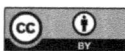

Copyright: © 2024 by the authors. Licensee MDPI, Basel, Switzerland. This article is an open access article distributed under the terms and conditions of the Creative Commons Attribution (CC BY) license (https://creativecommons.org/licenses/by/4.0/).

1. Introduction

Additive manufacturing, with its wide-ranging applications across biomedical engineering, electronics, automotive sectors, education, and microfluidics, has evolved significantly. Initially characterized by high entry costs, recent advancements in printing processes and materials have rendered 3D printing more accessible and cost-effective [1]. The applications of 3D printing in biomedical engineering span from bioprinting tissues imitating natural structures to manufacturing affordable and custom-fit prosthetics [2]. Additionally, the technology facilitates the creation of porous metal orthopedic implants, promoting better integration with natural bones and aiding pharmaceutical testing [3,4]. In educational settings, 3D printing bridges the gap between theoretical concepts and physical manifestations, providing students with hands-on experiences for rapid prototyping. This technology enhances STEM education (Science, Technology, Engineering, and Mathematics) by enabling students to create models, scientific equipment, and replicas of historical artifacts [5].

Recent advances in 3D printing necessitate the development of biomaterials compatible with printing processes. These materials, especially for biomedical applications, require biocompatibility and structural integrity. They aim to create scaffolds for tissue engineering, drug screening, and regenerative medicine [6]. Notable materials include natural polymers like chitosan, sodium alginate, and synthetic polymers [7,8].

Biodegradable bioinks, primarily hydrogels, dominate 3D bioprinting due to their compatibility with living cells, mechanical stability, and high-resolution printing capabilities. Control over powder size and particle flow enhances ceramic-based ink properties [9–14]. Bioink printability depends on various factors, including viscosity, surface tension, and nozzle characteristics. Materials like hydrogels, collagen, alginate, gelatine, PCL, and PLA are widely used for additive manufacturing. These materials vary in biocompatibility, mechanical strength, and biodegradability, catering to diverse applications such as tissue engineering and drug delivery [15–22].

Non-planar 3D printing techniques transcend traditional flat printing surfaces, enabling complex multi-layered structures. Methods include volumetric printing, continuous liquid interface production (CLIP), curved surface printing (CSP), freeform printing, and multi-material printing [23–26]. The technology finds applications in aerospace, healthcare, and consumer products, enabling the production of intricate biomedical implants and complex engine parts [27–29]. However, software limitations in conventional printers hinder the full utilization of 3D capabilities. Various algorithms and software, like Curvislicer and GCodeBending, aim to address this challenge [30–34].

Hybrid 3D printing combines various 3D printing methods to produce intricate, high-accuracy parts. Examples include Fused Deposition Modeling (FDM) with Stereolithography (SLA) or Digital Light Processing (DLP), and Selective Laser Sintering (SLS) with binder jetting [35,36].

Various hybrid 3D printing methods have emerged for biological materials:
- Bio-Inkjet Printing: Deposition of bioink containing cells onto a substrate, cured to form living tissue;
- Electrospinning: Electric field production of nanofiber scaffolds supporting living cells;
- Microfluidic Printing: Droplet deposition of bioink with cells through a microfluidic device;
- Stereolithography with Cell Encapsulation: Encapsulating cells in a cured hydrogel for tissue formation.

Challenges persist in enhancing cell survival rates, ensuring proper cell interactions, and facilitating nutrient delivery within printed structures. Researchers explore temperature-controlled bio-inkjet printing, precise cell placement, and microfluidic channels for improved viability and functionality [37–40].

There is a lot of discussion regarding the implementation of physical phantoms to study cell survival in organs and tissues after an irradiation procedure [41,42]. Nevertheless, the cost for such applications needs a significant budget to be included in every laboratory, as well as a multidisciplinary approach combining many different types of expertise. Additionally, there is a need for physical phantoms for extensive practice with surgical approaches to optimize procedures, limiting the use of real tissues. Likewise, a recent surgical review highlighted the importance of understanding tissue mechanics [43].

More specifically, recent studies have comprehensively explored the use of 3D printing for phantom fabrication, including discussions on material selection [44–46]. A key finding is the limited availability of materials that can accurately mimic the full spectrum of tissue properties [44]. However, the growing accessibility, affordability, and versatility of additive manufacturing techniques point towards its increased adoption in the medical field [46]. With the ever-expanding array of tissue-mimicking materials (TMMs) presented in research and the ongoing surge in investigations, a pressing need exists to focus on the properties of these phantom materials across various imaging and therapeutic applications.

While digital or "computational" anthropomorphic phantoms offer a cost-effective alternative [47], physical phantoms remain the preferred choice for institution-specific acquisition and procedural protocols, which can vary depending on equipment manufacturers, models, and intended uses. The material selection, or the specific TMMs used within these physical phantoms, is crucial for their successful application [48].

This study aims to present a proof-of-concept for a low-cost implementation on combining the FDM technique with inkjet to produce soft-tissue structures, such as a small version of the human liver, using real clinical data (i.e., a CT dataset), following suggestions by the literature [43–46]. Three different materials were utilized to fit the purpose of each structure, namely Polylactic Acid (PLA), Polyvinyl Alcohol (PVA), and light bodied, biocompatible silicone (Polysiloxane), which could incorporate living cells in a future extended implementation.

The following section (Section 2) includes a description of the materials and methods implemented, providing information on the materials and the techniques implemented to develop the whole procedure. Section 3 follows, providing the final printed products of this study and analysis of results. Section 4 provides a comprehensive analytical discussion of the results of this study and possible implementations, and Section 5 draws the final conclusions to summarize the whole study.

2. Materials and Methods

Combining FDM with bio-inkjet printing involves creating a supportive FDM scaffold for bio-inkjet-deposited living cells. The utilization of Ultra-Violet (UV) light for curing forms the living tissue, allowing greater control over geometry and architecture. Its advantages include improved accuracy and structural support, enabling the creation of complex structures. Challenges of this approach encompass enhancing cell survival, promoting proper cell interactions, and ensuring efficient nutrient delivery within the printed structures [49–52].

To start with the formation of the physical phantom, clinical data are needed. For this study, anonymized (for ethical purpose) clinical Computed Tomography (CT) data, featuring a segmented liver including veins and arteries, was utilized. To make the physical phantom more accessible for the laboratory's equipment, as well as to accelerate the additive manufacturing procedure, the liver model was scaled down to 50% of its original size, as this is only a feasibility study. The 3D printing process was conducted using the Creality Ender-3 printer, as this is a widely used, low-cost, and accessible piece of equipment.

Three types of material were employed to assure accessibility, convenience, and biocompatibility, as presented in Table 1. More specifically, they are

- PLA: Used for printing the liver mold to ensure mechanical integrity. Additionally, this material is flexible in the way that it is printed, ensuring that no special conditions are needed;
- PVA: Employed as the mold for veins and arteries, allowing easy removal by washing with hot water. This was crucial as the delicate veins' geometry could not be extracted from a PLA mold without damage;
- Polysiloxane: Medical-grade silicone used to fill the PLA molds. This silicone is harmless to living organisms, and its density is close to the density of organ tissue (~1.1 g/cm^3). For this reason, this material could also be a base in future applications to accommodate living cell populations.

Table 1. Printing and material parameters used during the hybrid additive manufacturing procedure.

Material	Nozzle Temperature (°C)	Bed Temperature (°C)	Water Temperature While Dissolving	Filament Diameter	Wall Thickness	Infill	Layer High
PLA	205	60	-	1.75 mm	0.8 mm	0%	0.28 mm
PVA	220	60	40–60 °C (with stirring)	1.75 mm	0.8 mm	0%	0.28 mm
Polysiloxane	25	60	-	-	-	-	-

Figure 1 depicts a 3D model of the liver used, showcasing the veins in blue and arteries in red. The liver and its intricate network of veins and arteries were derived from anonymized CT data and were previously segmented. The TotalSegmentator tool [53] was considered for the segmentation procedure. The TotalSegmentator is able to segment a big portion of the human body, delineating 117 distinct organs and regions. TotalSegmentator is an AI model, developed and trained by the department of Research and Analysis at University Hospital Basel, on the Zenodo database [54], to be able to recognize human organs in any provided CT data. However, precise clinical implementation may necessitate evaluation and refinement by experienced clinicians.

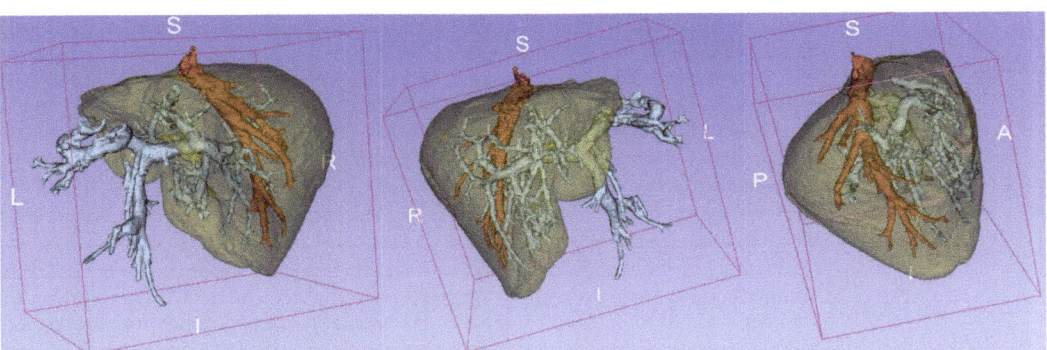

Figure 1. 3D representation of the liver model. Colors differentiate arteries (red) from veins (blue) and the liver (yellow). Letters indicate the anatomical orientation of the organ in the human body: S is for Superior, I for Inferior, L for Left, R for Right, P for Posterior and A for Anterior.

Utilizing 3D-Slicer v.5.6.2 software, the segmented data from DICOM files was exported into STL (Stereo-Lithography) file format, which is a commonly used file format in any CAD software. 3D-Slicer is a free, open-source software for the visualization, processing, segmentation, registration, and analysis of medical, biomedical, and other 3D images and meshes; and planning and navigating image-guided procedures. Based on a large supporting community of users and developers, 3D-Slicer can solve advanced image computing challenges with a focus on clinical and biomedical applications. It allows one to build and deploy custom solutions for research and commercial products.

The produced STL files of the model were then transformed into G-code files using slicers. G-code is a programming language for CNC (Computer Numerical Control) machines. G-code stands for "Geometric Code" and is used to tell a machine what to do or how to do something, translating the path that needs to be followed. UltiMaker Cura v5.6.0 was employed to generate the initial G-code, which was later converted into a non-planar version for this study. For the non-planar implementation, the CurviSlicer (March 2020 build) was employed. The CurviSlicer is a recently developed tool that is able to receive STL files and generate the G-code, including non-planar movement. Nevertheless, the code was not able to run directly with the printer. The next step was to obtain this G-code file and compare it to another file that can be used by the printer, to manually apply modifications in the initial and final part of the G-code, making it recognizable by the printer. In this implementation, a simple G-code file was generated using the Cura software and then used as reference for manual corrections on the non-planar G-code file generated by CurviSlicer. The header part of the file needed to be copied by the Cura G-code file, to make the G-code compatible with the 3D printer. Additionally, the end part of the G-code file produced through CurviSlicer needed to be copied by the Cura G-code file, to help the printer conclude the procedure without problems.

The 3D printing process utilized in this study involved the use of a specialized material known as condensation Polysiloxane, specifically Protolast PF [55]. This material is characterized by its light-based consistency and finds extensive application as a precision impression material in the field of dentistry. It must be stated that this type of silicone could be integrated with living cells, if such an implementation is a target. In our case, as this study is only proof-of-concept, no such step was followed.

We now delve into the methodology in greater detail. The procedure commenced with the precise printing of veins and arteries using PVA. Subsequently, these printed vascular structures were incorporated into the corresponding positions in the liver mold to create areas that would stop the diffusion of the light-bodied silicone. These areas could act as channels that could be filled with liquids to simulate blood circulation. The liver mold was printed in a second step using PLA to ensure the integrity of the mold, as it was completely empty on the inside. The walls of this piece were 0.8 mm, as this thickness was enough for both its integrity and easy removal after being filled with silicone.

It needs to be stated that the injection of the silicone was performed manually by the researchers, during the 3D printing process, using corresponding syringes, that are used in dentistry for this type of silicone, which is both a flexible and durable material. At this stage, the objective was to demonstrate that the integration of these different operations is feasible, and a valid part could be achieved, thus proving the success of the proposed method. To further extend the hybrid procedure, the syringes could be merged with the printer using an extra motor, as well as advanced hardware and software. Nevertheless, additive manufacturing is about prototyping and as such different methods can be applied, meaning automated and semi-automated. Regardless, in many industrial or lab applications it is common ground to perform combinatory processing and manufacturing by implementing robotic arms, thus precisely simulating operations performed by trained personnel who can operate simultaneously or serially with other processes, thus performing Hybrid Manufacturing on the produced part, as it is carried out in the same build space and with the purpose of creating a single part.

After filling the liver mold with the PVA arteries and veins, as well as with the Polysiloxane, an intricate washing process was undertaken to remove the PVA material entirely, leaving behind the final silicone liver including the channels. This process resulted in the creation of a quite detailed and lifelike model: a replica of a liver characterized not only by its external appearance but also by the presence of accurately reproduced arteries and veins. The intricacies of this hybrid additive manufacturing technique are visually demonstrated in Figure 2a–c, showcasing the molds that were created through this innovative process, using both the PLA and the PVA materials.

It is worth noting that the printing of the liver involved the utilization of a non-planar edited G-code. Despite the complexity introduced by this non-planar approach, the final product did not exhibit noticeable differences compared to the model printed with the standard technique. This is due to the complexity and the different levels of the surface of liver geometry. This means that it is not a simple aero-foil, but a more complex shape. For such a case, it was more convenient to use the standard technique for the mold and implement a non-planar approach for the infill of the model, which is the procedure that was finally selected in this study.

3. Results

The FDM-printed mold, crafted using the 3D printing technique, closely resembles the original design depicted in the STL file. However, owing to the limitations of the 3D printer's resolution and precision, some minor roughness and imperfections are discernible along the edges of the printed mold. These slight discrepancies, attributed to the inherent constraints of a low-quality 3D printer, marginally affect the fidelity of the final output when compared to its digital design. Updating the hardware and software of our system could greatly improve the quality of the product.

Subsequently, the final printed product, following the injection of the gel polymer into the FDM-printed mold and subsequent extraction, exhibits a considerable reduction in size compared to the initial FDM mold. This dimensional variation is an anticipated outcome owing to the presence of the polymer shell, which contributes to a fractional decrease in the overall size of the produced item. However, this disparity in dimensions can be effectively compensated for, by factoring in the thickness of the shell during the design phase. By incorporating adjustments to accommodate the shell's effect on the final product's size, such as modifying the initial STL file dimensions, precise calibration can be achieved, minimizing discrepancies between the digital design and the physical outcome. It needs to be mentioned that the size difference between the 3D printed product and the STL file was less than 10% in all dimensions (i.e., x, y, and z axes, or non-orthogonal axes). The calculated volume also differed by less than 8% when measured in the STL file (~156 mL) and as water volume (~145 mL) inside the PLA liver mold.

Moreover, to further enhance the surfacing and extraction of the final product from the mold, the utilization of a thin layer of Vaseline could augment the surface quality of the final product, which is shown in Figure 3. This additional step aids in optimizing the release of the printed product, ensuring a smoother surface finish, and facilitating a more efficient extraction process. Incorporating such refinements into the production process significantly contributes to achieving a final output that aligns closely with the intricacies of the initial digital design, bridging the gap between the STL file's precision and the physical manifestation of the printed product.

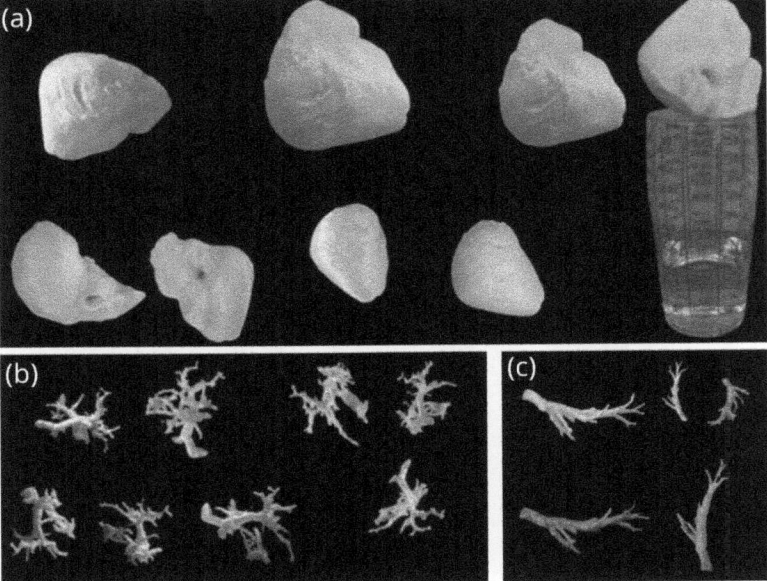

Figure 2. (**a**) 3D-printed liver mold (145 mL of internal volume); (**b**) 3D-printed liver vein mold; (**c**) 3D printed liver artery mold.

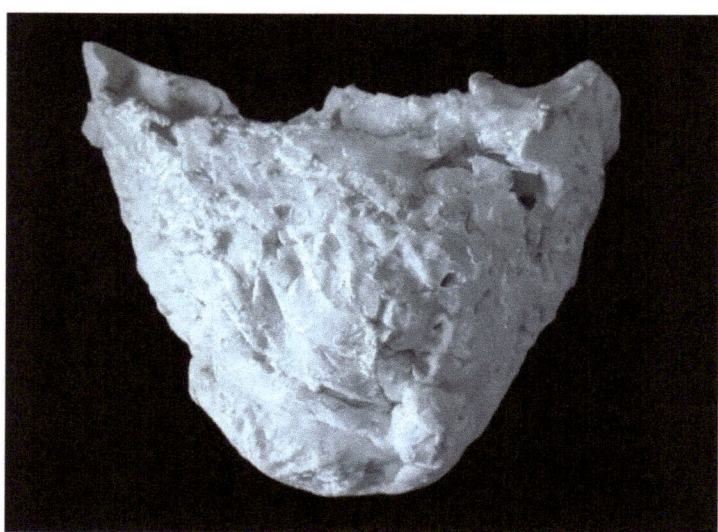

Figure 3. 3D-printed final product.

4. Discussion

In summary, this study showcases a novel low-cost additive manufacturing methodology, combining advanced materials and intricate techniques to produce anatomically accurate models. Through the meticulous integration of silicone veins and arteries into a PLA mold, the research team successfully created a liver model that not only captures the external features of the organ but also replicates its internal vascular network with precision. This innovative approach holds immense promise for various applications in the fields of medical education, research, and surgical planning.

One of the most significant implications lies in the field of medical education and training. Clinical scientists could utilize this advanced technique for injection training, allowing medical professionals to optimize their skills with highly detailed and realistic in vitro simulations. This also minimizes the use of animals as well as the need for human tissue, offering a more ethical and advanced platform for medical training while preparing future healthcare professionals for complex clinical scenarios. Moreover, innovation should not stop here; this technology could be expanded upon to explore more sophisticated robotic methods for intricate injections, opening doors to previously unattainable medical procedures.

Furthermore, this technique holds immense promise in the realm of personalized medicine. By refining the process and investing in higher-grade materials, it could contribute to the creation of complete, personalized anthropomorphic phantoms. These phantoms, akin to the RTsafe devices [56], could revolutionize radiation therapy quality assurance, ensuring that treatments are precisely calibrated and tailored to individual patients. The potential benefits for patients' well-being and treatment outcomes are immeasurable.

However, the true marvel of this technology lies in its potential for organ transplantation. With further advancements and investment in cutting-edge materials, this technique could be integrated with living cells, pushing the boundaries of medical science. Functional living organs could be artificially created by the exploitation of such a low-cost technique, offering hope to countless patients on transplant waiting lists. Such an endeavor, though, demands an interdisciplinary collaboration of epic proportions and a substantial financial commitment. The fusion of expertise from various fields, including biology, materials science, and engineering, is essential to navigate the complexities of producing living organs in a controlled environment.

It is crucial to acknowledge the challenges and avenues for future research in this groundbreaking study. Rigorous testing—including pressure assessments, radiation scanning, and dose measurements—is imperative to ensure the safety and efficacy of the developed product. While the initial indications from the existing literature are promising, comprehensive experimentation and validation are necessary steps in this pioneering journey. As the research community delves deeper into this innovative technique, the potential to transform the landscape of medical education, personalized medicine, and organ transplantation becomes increasingly tangible. The ongoing dedication to exploration and refinement will undoubtedly pave the way for a future where the boundaries of medical science are pushed further than ever before, bringing hope and healing to millions around the globe.

Moreover, while this study successfully demonstrates the feasibility of hybrid 3D printing using biocompatible materials, it is imperative to note that the assessment of cell cultures and the viability of cells throughout the complete printing procedure remains an area requiring further investigation. The interaction between printed structures and living cells is a crucial aspect in biomedical applications, necessitating in-depth analyses to ensure optimal cell survival, proliferation, and functionality post-printing.

Future research endeavors should focus on comprehensive studies involving cell cultures to evaluate the biocompatibility and cytocompatibility of the printed structures. Assessing cell behavior, including adhesion, proliferation, and differentiation, throughout the printing process and post-printing stages is crucial for the development of functional tissue constructs or biomedical devices. Furthermore, exploring innovative bioinks and refining printing parameters to enhance cell viability within the printed constructs is fundamental.

Assessing such approaches will enable the scientific community to study the survivability of cells and tissues, even when such population of cells is irradiated. This way, radiation therapy procedures could be highly improved. Addressing these aspects will not only advance our understanding of the interaction between printed materials and cells but also pave the way for the utilization of hybrid additive manufacturing techniques in various biomedical applications, ranging from tissue engineering to drug delivery systems. Drug delivery studies on such phantoms will improve the understanding of Physiologically Based Pharmacokinetic Modeling (PBPK) that will allow for the optimization of therapeutic procedures.

5. Conclusions

In conclusion, this study presents a promising proof-of-concept for the hybrid 3D printing of biocompatible materials, highlighting the successful integration of two distinct steps: FDM printing utilizing PLA and PVA, and inkjet printing employing gel polymers. While the implemented procedure was not automated, the groundwork laid in this research provides a foundational framework for potential automation in the future [57]. Achieving full automation would necessitate a multidimensional approach encompassing advancements in hardware, software evolution, and cross-disciplinary collaborations across fields such as physics, mechanics, biology, and software development. The envisioned automated process holds immense potential, offering efficiency and scalability in the fabrication of biocompatible structures. Overall, this study underscores the feasibility and potential avenues for the development of an automated hybrid 3D printing procedure, marking a significant stride towards innovative applications in biocompatible material fabrication. This study showcases a groundbreaking methodology in 3D printing, successfully integrating advanced materials and intricate techniques to produce highly detailed and anatomically accurate organ models. The potential applications include medical education, research, and surgical planning, emphasizing the promise and utility of this innovative approach.

Author Contributions: Conceptualization, A.A.K.; methodology, A.A.K., K.C. and A.N.; software, K.C.; validation, A.A.K. and K.C.; formal analysis, A.A.K.; investigation, K.C. and A.N.; resources, A.A.K. and K.C.; data curation, K.C.; writing—original draft preparation, K.C., A.A.K. and A.N.; writing—review and editing, K.C., A.A.K. and A.N.; visualization, K.C., A.A.K. and A.N.; supervision, A.A.K.; project administration, A.A.K.; funding acquisition, A.A.K. and K.C. All authors have read and agreed to the published version of the manuscript.

Funding: This research received no external funding.

Data Availability Statement: The data presented in this study are available on request from the corresponding author. The data are not publicly available due to ethical restrictions.

Conflicts of Interest: The authors declare no conflicts of interest.

References

1. Liu, J.; Sun, L.; Xu, W.; Wang, Q.; Yu, S.; Sun, J. Current advances and future perspectives of 3D printing natural-derived biopolymers. *Carbohydr. Polym.* **2019**, *207*, 297–316. [CrossRef] [PubMed]
2. Rengier, F.; Mehndiratta, A.; von Tengg-Kobligk, H.; Zechmann, C.M.; Unterhinninghofen, R.; Kauczor, H.U.; Giesel, F.L. 3D printing based on imaging data: Review of medical applications. *Int. J. Comput. Assist. Radiol. Surg.* **2010**, *5*, 335–341. [CrossRef] [PubMed]
3. You, Y.; Niu, Y.; Sun, F.; Huang, S.; Ding, P.; Wang, X.; Zhang, X.; Zhang, J. Three-dimensional printing and 3D slicer powerful tools in understanding and treating neurosurgical diseases. *Front. Surg.* **2022**, *9*, 1030081. [CrossRef] [PubMed]
4. Cui, W.; Zhou, Y.; Chang, J. Electrospun nanofibrous materials for tissue engineering and drug delivery. *Sci. Technol. Adv. Mater.* **2010**, *11*, 014108. [CrossRef] [PubMed]
5. Ford, S.; Minshall, T. Invited review article: Where and how 3D printing is used in teaching and education. *Addit. Manuf.* **2019**, *25*, 131–150. [CrossRef]
6. Suntornnond, R.; An, J.; Chua, C.K. Bioprinting of Thermoresponsive Hydrogels for Next Generation Tissue Engineering: A Review. *Macromol. Mater. Eng.* **2017**, *302*, 1600266. [CrossRef]
7. Li, H.; Liu, S.; Li, L. Rheological study on 3D printability of alginate hydrogel and effect of graphene oxide. *Int. J. Bioprint.* **2016**, *2*, 54–66. [CrossRef]
8. Ng, W.L.; Yeong, W.Y.; Naing, M.W. Polyelectrolyte gelatin-chitosan hydrogel optimized for 3D bioprinting in skin tissue engineering. *Int. J. Bioprint.* **2016**, *2*, 53–62. [CrossRef]
9. Arifin, N.; Sudin, I.; Ngadiman, N.H.A.; Ishak, M.S.A. A Comprehensive Review of Biopolymer Fabrication in Additive Manufacturing Processing for 3D-Tissue-Engineering Scaffolds. *Polymers* **2022**, *14*, 2119. [CrossRef]
10. Chung, J.J.; Im, H.; Kim, S.H.; Park, J.W.; Jung, Y. Toward Biomimetic Scaffolds for Tissue Engineering: 3D Printing Techniques in Regenerative Medicine. *Front. Bioeng. Biotechnol.* **2020**, *8*, 586406. [CrossRef]
11. Hart, L.R.; Harries, J.L.; Greenland, B.W.; Colquhoun, H.M.; Hayes, W. Molecular design of a discrete chain-folding polyimide for controlled inkjet deposition of supramolecular polymers. *Polym. Chem.* **2015**, *6*, 7342–7352. [CrossRef]
12. Hart, L.R.; Harries, J.L.; Greenland, B.W.; Colquhoun, H.M.; Hayes, W. Supramolecular Approach to New Inkjet Printing Inks. *ACS Appl. Mater. Interfaces* **2015**, *7*, 8906–8914. [CrossRef]
13. Tolbert, J.W.; Hammerstone, D.E.; Yuchimiuk, N.; Seppala, J.E.; Chow, L.W. Solvent-Cast 3D Printing of Biodegradable Polymer Scaffolds. *Macromol. Mater. Eng.* **2021**, *306*, 2100442. [CrossRef]
14. Trachtenberg, J.E.; Mountziaris, P.M.; Miller, J.S.; Wettergreen, M.; Kasper, F.K.; Mikos, A.G. Open-source three-dimensional printing of biodegradable polymer scaffolds for tissue engineering. *J. Biomed. Mater. Res. Part A* **2014**, *102*, 4326–4335. [CrossRef] [PubMed]
15. Fatimi, A.; Okoro, O.V.; Podstawczyk, D.; Siminska-Stanny, J.; Shavandi, A. Natural Hydrogel-Based Bio-Inks for 3D Bioprinting in Tissue Engineering: A Review. *Gels* **2022**, *8*, 179. [CrossRef] [PubMed]
16. Li, J.; Wu, C.; Chu, P.K.; Gelinsky, M. 3D printing of hydrogels: Rational design strategies and emerging biomedical applications. *Mater. Sci. Eng. R Rep.* **2020**, *140*, 100543. [CrossRef]
17. Mancha Sánchez, E.; Gómez-Blanco, J.C.; López Nieto, E.; Casado, J.G.; Macías-García, A.; Díaz Díez, M.A.; Carrasco-Amador, J.P.; Torrejón Martín, D.; Sánchez-Margallo, F.M.; Pagador, J.B. Hydrogels for Bioprinting: A Systematic Review of Hydrogels Synthesis, Bioprinting Parameters, and Bioprinted Structures Behavior. *Front. Bioeng. Biotechnol.* **2020**, *8*, 776. [CrossRef] [PubMed]
18. Taneja, H.; Salodkar, S.M.; Singh Parmar, A.; Chaudhary, S. Hydrogel based 3D printing: Bio ink for tissue engineering. *J. Mol. Liq.* **2022**, *367*, 120390. [CrossRef]
19. Unagolla, J.M.; Jayasuriya, A.C. Hydrogel-based 3D bioprinting: A comprehensive review on cell-laden hydrogels, bioink formulations, and future perspectives. *Appl. Mater. Today* **2020**, *18*, 100479. [CrossRef]
20. Fazeli, N.; Arefian, E.; Irani, S.; Ardeshirylajimi, A.; Seyedjafari, E. 3D-Printed PCL Scaffolds Coated with Nanobioceramics Enhance Osteogenic Differentiation of Stem Cells. *ACS Omega* **2021**, *6*, 35284–35296. [CrossRef]
21. Liu, S.; Sun, L.; Zhang, H.; Hu, Q.; Wang, Y.; Ramalingam, M. High-resolution combinatorial 3D printing of gelatin-based biomimetic triple-layered conduits for nerve tissue engineering. *Int. J. Biol. Macromol.* **2021**, *166*, 1280–1291. [CrossRef]

22. Radhakrishnan, S.; Nagarajan, S.; Belaid, H.; Farha, C.; Iatsunskyi, I.; Coy, E.; Soussan, L.; Huon, V.; Bares, J.; Belkacemi, K.; et al. Fabrication of 3D printed antimicrobial polycaprolactone scaffolds for tissue engineering applications. *Mater. Sci. Eng. C* **2021**, *118*, 111525. [CrossRef]
23. Düzgün, D.E.; Nadolny, K. Continuous liquid interface production (CLIP) method for rapid prototyping. *J. Mech. Energy Eng.* **2018**, *2*, 5–12. [CrossRef]
24. Nisja, G.A.; Cao, A.; Gao, C. Short review of nonplanar fused deposition modeling printing. *Mater. Des. Process. Commun.* **2021**, *3*, e221. [CrossRef]
25. Rogers, J.A. Techniques and applications for non-planar lithography. *MRS Online Proc. Libr.* **2002**, *739*, 121–128. [CrossRef]
26. Tumbleston, J.R.; Shirvanyants, D.; Ermoshkin, N.; Janusziewicz, R.; Johnson, A.R.; Kelly, D.; Chen, K.; Pinschmidt, R.; Rolland, J.P.; Ermoshkin, A.; et al. Continuous liquid interface production of 3D objects. *Science* **2015**, *347*, 1349–1352. [CrossRef] [PubMed]
27. Farahani, R.D.; Chizari, K.; Therriault, D. Three-dimensional printing of freeform helical microstructures: A review. *Nanoscale* **2014**, *6*, 10470–10485. [CrossRef]
28. O'Connell, J. Non-Planar 3D Printing: All You Need to Know. Available online: https://all3dp.com/2/non-planar-3d-printing-simply-explained/ (accessed on 21 March 2024).
29. Zhang, H.; Liu, D.; Huang, T.; Hu, Q.; Lammer, H. 3D Printing Method of Spatial Curved Surface by Continuous Natural Fiber Reinforced Composite. *IOP Conf. Ser. Mater. Sci. Eng.* **2020**, *782*, 022059. [CrossRef]
30. Ahlers, D.; Wasserfall, F.; Hendrich, N.; Zhang, J. 3D Printing of Nonplanar Layers for Smooth Surface Generation. In Proceedings of the 2019 IEEE 15th International Conference on Automation Science and Engineering (CASE), Vancouver, BC, Canada, 22–26 August 2019; pp. 1737–1743.
31. CNCKitchen. GCodeBending. Available online: https://github.com/CNCKitchen/GCodeBending (accessed on 21 March 2024).
32. Etienne, J.; Ray, N.; Panozzo, D.; Hornus, S.; Wang, C.C.L.; Martínez, J.; McMains, S.; Alexa, M.; Wyvill, B.; Lefebvre, S. CurviSlicer: Slightly curved slicing for 3-axis printers. *ACM Trans. Graph.* **2019**, *38*, 81. [CrossRef]
33. Gleadall, A. FullControl GCode Designer: Open-source software for unconstrained design in additive manufacturing. *Addit. Manuf.* **2021**, *46*, 102109. [CrossRef]
34. Loepmeier, H. Nozzleboss. Available online: https://github.com/Heinz-Loepmeier/nozzleboss (accessed on 21 March 2024).
35. Gibson, I.; Rosen, D.; Stucker, B. *Additive Manufacturing Technologies: 3D Printing, Rapid Prototyping, and Direct Digital Manufacturing*; Springer: New York, NY, USA, 2014; pp. 451–474.
36. Srivatsan, T.S.; Sudarshan, T.S. *Additive Manufacturing: Innovations, Advances, and Applications*; CRC Press: Boca Raton, FL, USA, 2015; pp. 390–420.
37. Chen, E.P.; Toksoy, Z.; Davis, B.A.; Geibel, J.P. 3D Bioprinting of Vascularized Tissues for in vitro and in vivo Applications. *Front. Bioeng. Biotechnol.* **2021**, *9*, 664188. [CrossRef] [PubMed]
38. Dey, M.; Ozbolat, I.T. 3D bioprinting of cells, tissues and organs. *Sci. Rep.* **2020**, *10*, 14023. [CrossRef] [PubMed]
39. Ghidini, T. Regenerative medicine and 3D bioprinting for human space exploration and planet colonisation. *J. Taorac. Dis.* **2018**, *10*, S2363–S2375. [CrossRef] [PubMed]
40. Hinton, T.J.; Jallerat, Q.; Palchesko, R.N.; Park, J.H.; Grodzicki, M.S.; Shue, H.J.; Ramadan, M.H.; Hudson, A.R.; Feinberg, A.W. Three-dimensional printing of complex biological structures by freeform reversible embedding of suspended hydrogels. *Sci. Adv.* **2015**, *1*, e1500758. [CrossRef] [PubMed]
41. Chatzipapas, K.; Dordevic, M.; Zivkovic, S.; Tran, N.H.; Lampe, N.; Sakata, D.; Petrovic, I.; Ristic-Fira, A.; Shin, W.-G.; Zein, S.; et al. Geant4-DNA simulation of human cancer cells irradiation with helium ion beams. *Phys. Medica* **2023**, *112*, 102513. [CrossRef] [PubMed]
42. Chatzipapas, K.P.; Papadimitroulas, P.; Emfietzoglou, D.; Kalospyros, S.A.; Hada, M.; Georgakilas, A.G.; Kagadis, G.C. Ionizing Radiation and Complex DNA Damage: Quantifying the Radiobiological Damage Using Monte Carlo Simulations. *Cancers* **2020**, *12*, 799. [CrossRef] [PubMed]
43. Li, P.; Yang, Z.; Jiang, S. Tissue mimicking materials in image-guided needle-based interventions: A review. *Mater. Sci. Eng. C* **2018**, *93*, 1116–1131. [CrossRef] [PubMed]
44. Filippou, V.; Tsoumpas, C. Recent advances on the development of phantoms using 3D printing for imaging with CT, MRI, PET, SPECT, and ultrasound. *Med. Phys.* **2018**, *45*, e740–e760. [CrossRef]
45. Glick, S.J.; Ikejimba, L.C. Advances in digital and physical anthropomorphic breast phantoms for X-ray imaging. *Med. Phys.* **2018**, *45*, e870–e885. [CrossRef]
46. Tino, R.; Yeo, A.; Leary, M.; Brandt, M.; Kron, T. A systematic review on 3D-printed imaging and dosimetry phantoms in radiation therapy. *Technol. Cancer Res. Treat.* **2019**, *18*, 1533033819870208. [CrossRef]
47. Xu, X.G. An exponential growth of computational phantom research in radiation protection, imaging, and radiotherapy: A review of the fifty-year history. *Phys. Med. Biol.* **2014**, *59*, R233. [CrossRef] [PubMed]
48. McGarry, C.K.; Grattan, L.J.; Ivory, A.M.; Leek, F.; Liney, G.P.; Liu, Y.; Miloro, P.; Rai, R.; Robinson, A.P.; Shih, A.J.; et al. Tissue mimicking materials for imaging and therapy phantoms: A review. *Phys. Med. Biol.* **2020**, *65*, 23TR01. [CrossRef] [PubMed]
49. Jamieson, C.; Keenan, P.; Kirkwood, D.A.; Oji, S.; Webster, C.; Russell, K.A.; Koch, T.G. A Review of Recent Advances in 3D Bioprinting With an Eye on Future Regenerative Therapies in Veterinary Medicine. *Front. Vet. Sci.* **2021**, *7*, 584193. [CrossRef] [PubMed]

50. Pai, R.R.; Anupama Sekar, J.; Ajit, S.; Velayudhan, S.; Kasoju, N.; Anil Kumar, P.R. 5—Three-dimensional bioprinting of tissues and organs. In *Biomedical Product and Materials Evaluation*; Woodhead Publishing Series in Biomaterials; Mohanan, P.V., Ed.; Woodhead Publishing: Sawston, UK, 2022; pp. 135–150. [CrossRef]
51. Salaoru, I.; Maswoud, S.; Paul, S. Inkjet Printing of Functional Electronic Memory Cells: A Step Forward to Green Electronics. *Micromachines* **2019**, *10*, 417. [CrossRef] [PubMed]
52. Yan, X.; Bethers, B.; Chen, H.; Xiao, S.; Lin, S.; Tran, B.; Jiang, L.; Yang, Y. Recent Advancements in Biomimetic 3D Printing Materials With Enhanced Mechanical Properties. *Front. Mater.* **2021**, *8*, 518886. [CrossRef]
53. Wasserthal, J.; Breit, H.-C.; Meyer, M.T.; Pradella, M.; Hinck, D.; Sauter, A.W.; Heye, T.; Boll, D.T.; Cyriac, J.; Yang, S.; et al. TotalSegmentator: Robust Segmentation of 104 Anatomic Structures in CT Images. *Radiol. Artif. Intell.* **2023**, *5*, e230024. [CrossRef]
54. Wasserthal, J. Dataset with segmentations of 117 important anatomical structures in 1228 CT images (2.0.1). Available online: https://zenodo.org/records/10047292 (accessed on 27 March 2024). [CrossRef]
55. Dental-Co. Available online: https://dental-co.gr/product/protolast-pf-150ml/ (accessed on 21 March 2024).
56. RTsafe. RTsafe. Available online: https://rt-safe.com/ (accessed on 21 March 2024).
57. Langer, L.; Schmitt, M.; Schlick, G.; Schilp, J. Development of an Automated Process Chain for Hybrid Additive Manufacturing using Laser Powder Bed Fusion. *Procedia CIRP* **2022**, *112*, 358–363. [CrossRef]

Disclaimer/Publisher's Note: The statements, opinions and data contained in all publications are solely those of the individual author(s) and contributor(s) and not of MDPI and/or the editor(s). MDPI and/or the editor(s) disclaim responsibility for any injury to people or property resulting from any ideas, methods, instructions or products referred to in the content.

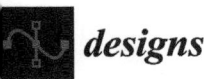

Article

Biomechanics of a Novel 3D Mandibular Osteotomy Design

Carlos Aurelio Andreucci [1], Elza M. M. Fonseca [2,*] and Renato N. Jorge [1]

1. Mechanical Engineering Department, Faculty of Engineering, University of Porto, Rua Dr. Roberto Frias, 712, 4200-465 Porto, Portugal; candreucci@hotmail.com (C.A.A.); rnatal@fe.up.pt (R.N.J.)
2. Mechanical Engineering Department, School of Engineering, Polytechnic Institute of Porto, R. Dr. António Bernardino de Almeida 431, 4249-015 Porto, Portugal
* Correspondence: elz@isep.ipp.pt

Abstract: Elective mandibular surgical osteotomies are commonly used to correct craniofacial discrepancies. Since the modifications proposed by Obwegeser, Dal Pont, and Hunsuck, no effective variations have been proposed to improve the biomechanical results of these mandibular osteotomies. With technological developments and the use of three-dimensional images from CT scans of patients, much has been done to plan and predict outcomes with greater precision and control. To date, 3D imaging and additive manufacturing technologies have not been used to their full potential to create innovative mandibular osteotomies. The use of 3D digital images obtained from CT scans as DICOM files, which were then converted to STL files, proved to be an efficient method of developing an innovative mandibular ramus beveled osteotomy technique. The new mandibular osteotomy is designed to reduce the likelihood of vasculo-nervous damage to the mandible, reduce the time and ease of surgery, and reduce post-operative complications. The proposed osteotomy does not affect traditional osteotomies. Anatomical structures such as the inferior alveolar nerve and intraoral surgical access were preserved and maintained, respectively. The results obtained from the digital images were validated on an additively manufactured 3D synthetic bone model.

Keywords: orthognathic surgery; mandibular osteotomy; 3D design; DICOM

Citation: Andreucci, C.A.; Fonseca, E.M.M.; Jorge, R.N. Biomechanics of a Novel 3D Mandibular Osteotomy Design. *Designs* **2024**, *8*, 57. https://doi.org/10.3390/designs8030057

Academic Editor: Richard Drevet

Received: 25 May 2024
Revised: 8 June 2024
Accepted: 11 June 2024
Published: 13 June 2024

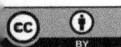

Copyright: © 2024 by the authors. Licensee MDPI, Basel, Switzerland. This article is an open access article distributed under the terms and conditions of the Creative Commons Attribution (CC BY) license (https://creativecommons.org/licenses/by/4.0/).

1. Introduction

This study describes the feasibility of developing a novel mandibular osteotomy through 3D digital planning, 3D model validation, and patient-matched surgical guide fabrication.

Muscle biomechanics is the study of the internal and external forces that act on the human body to produce movement. It examines how muscles, bones, tendons, and ligaments work together to produce function. Muscles can only pull and come in antagonistic pairs. When one muscle in a pair contracts, the other relaxes, and vice versa. The function of muscles depends on their intrinsic properties and extrinsic arrangement [1].

Contraction refers to the generation of tension within a muscle fiber through actin and myosin cross-bridge cycling. The sarcoplasm of a muscle can lengthens, shorten, or remain the same length under tension. The names of the contractions are based on how the length of the sarcoplasm changes during this tension [2].

Isokinetic contractions occur at a constant rate. Isotonic contractions involve constant tension as the muscle changes length and can be either concentric (shortening the muscle) or eccentric (lengthening the muscle). Isometric contractions involve no change in muscle length [2,3].

The mandible has seven main muscles: the buccinator, which assists in chewing and originates from the alveolar process of the mandible; the mylohyoid, which is the primary muscle of the mouth floor; the superior pharyngeal constrictor, which attaches to the mylohyoid and plays a crucial role in swallowing [3].

The motor fibers of the mandibular branch of the trigeminal nerve (CN V3) innervate all masticatory muscles, while the main arterial supply comes from branches of the maxillary artery. Muscle is essential for developing bone strength, providing mechanical protection, and preserving or repairing skeletal tissue [1].

Bone undergoes adaptive processes in response to habitual loading, regulating its structure based on various components of its loading regime and mechanical environment [1,4,5].

The interaction between stress and strain provides insight into the mechanical behavior of the properties of bone material as it deforms under load [1].

Tooth loss affects the fine proprioceptive control of jaw function and influences the precision of occlusal load application. This is due to the removal of intra-dental and periodontal mechanoreception. Osseoperception, on the other hand, depends on central influences from corollary discharge from cortico-motor commands to jaw muscles and contributions from peripheral mechanoreceptors in orofacial and temporomandibular tissues [3,6].

The plasticity of neuromotor mechanisms is recognized in the processing of central influences to accommodate the loss of dental and periodontal inputs [6].

Proprioceptive signals from mechanoreceptors in the joints, muscles, tendons, and skin are crucial for the neural control of movement. The absence of proprioceptive afferents can affect muscle tone control and bone formation, disrupt postural reflexes, and severely impair the spatial and temporal aspects of voluntary movement. There is initial evidence suggesting that proprioceptive training induces cortical reorganization, which reinforces the notion that proprioceptive training is a viable method for improving sensorimotor function [7].

When performing an osteotomy on the mandible, the muscles separated by the posterior and anterior fractured bone segments exert a vectorial force with direction and directionality [3,8].

Pathological fractures can be classified as either favorable or unfavorable to fracture reduction and immobilization treatment. A fracture is considered favorable if the muscle vector force brings the fractured bone segments closer together and unfavorable if it separates the fragments [8].

During elective osteotomy for maxillofacial correction with mandibular osteotomy, it is essential to monitor muscle action. This is necessary not only to maintain stability after immobilization of the surgical fracture but also to ensure a controlled outcome during the period of bone healing and repair [9].

Based on the biomechanics, physiology, and anatomy of the mandible, the ideal mandibular osteotomy for treating craniofacial discrepancies can be determined. The ramus and angle of the mandible bilaterally have been the most commonly used region for osteotomy in elective mandibular surgery throughout history [7–9].

The masseter, temporalis, medial, and lateral pterygoid muscles are directly associated with the posterior mandibular fragment in a bilateral sagittal split osteotomy. They exert unnecessary force that can cause unfavorable displacement of the sagittal split osteotomy [3,5].

The other muscles—the mylohyoid, buccinator, and superior pharyngeal constrictor—are directly related to the displacement of the anterior segment of the mandibular osteotomy performed at the angle of the mandible [9].

This work presents an innovative osteotomy technique developed using three-dimensional (3D) technologies, digital imaging, and additive manufacturing of a human mandible obtained from a computed tomography scan. The technique aims to preserve the inferior alveolar vasculo-nervous bundle and the dento-alveolar boundaries while maintaining the integrity of the teeth. To achieve this, the position of the mandibular canal was assessed using the obtained image.

The 3D osteotomy line was determined to preserve anatomical structures and efficiently approximate and preserve surgically fractured segments in an innovative biomechanical approach. The digital mandible was sectioned according to the proposed parameters (Figure 1). The black area in the image shows where the surgical guide will be supported to perform the osteotomy. This makes it possible to determine the direction, angle, and depth of the cut to be made with the piezoelectric cutting instrument.

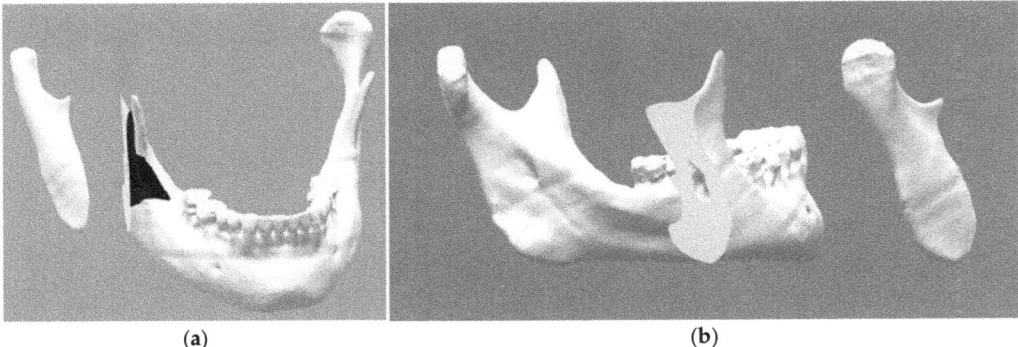

Figure 1. Three-dimensional digital images: (**a**) the black area shows where the surgical guide will be supported to perform the osteotomy; (**b**) the surface obtained with the oblique cut of the mandibular ramus.

To validate the results, a 3D model of the mandible was printed using a material with a density like that of human bone. The described osteotomy was then performed, allowing for a comparison between the results of the digital osteotomy and the laboratory experiment, thus validating the results.

2. Materials and Methods

2.1. Materials

A Digital Imaging and Communications in Medicine (DICOM) image of a mandible converted into the stereolithography (STL) file format was obtained from a patient. The 3D image was segmented into three parts simulating the proposed bilateral bone section in the mandible using software available in Windows, 3D Builder (Windows 10 version), making it easy for users of this operating system to reproduce the method. The position of the surgical guide was delineated using 3D paint, which is also available in the same software (Figure 2).

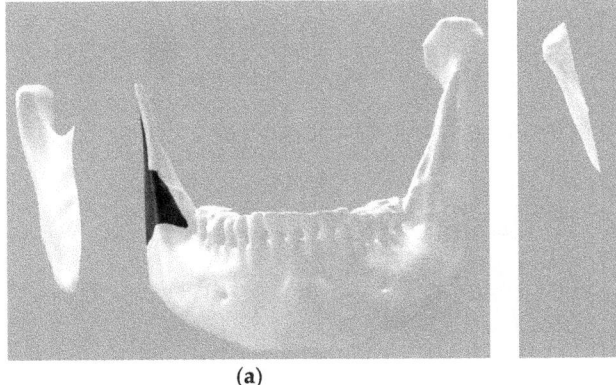
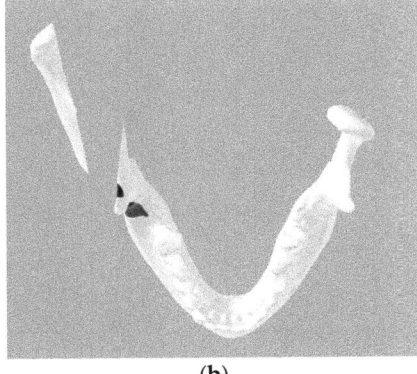

Figure 2. Three-dimensional digital image: (**a**) frontal view; (**b**) top view.

Digital bone cutting was performed using the 3D Builder software tool to cut the digital models for 3D printing. It is possible to make three-dimensional cuts to visualize the anatomical structures to be preserved. Through trial and error, a visual analysis of the mandibular canal was made with each digital cut at different angles. On average, 50 trial cuts were needed to find the ideal osteotomy.

A model was printed using additive manufacturing in nylon (0.8 g/cm^3) with a tensile modulus of 1.7 GPa, simulating the density of mandibular bone. The model was used to validate the osteotomy by cutting the bone using the author's proposed handcrafted polymethylmethacrylate guide.

The model was subjected to cuts using a surgical motor (Tech Drill) and a 2 mm carbide cylindrical drill.

2.2. Methods

To determine the ideal bilateral mandibular osteotomy, the first parameter analyzed was the position of the foramen oval, where the mandibular nerve bundle enters the medial side or lingula of the mandibular ramus/angle. Using the posterior wall of the foramen oval as the boundary for the bone section, after marking the osteotomy line with the 3D Builder software, a digital bone section was made where it was possible to determine the preservation of the mandibular canal (Figure 3).

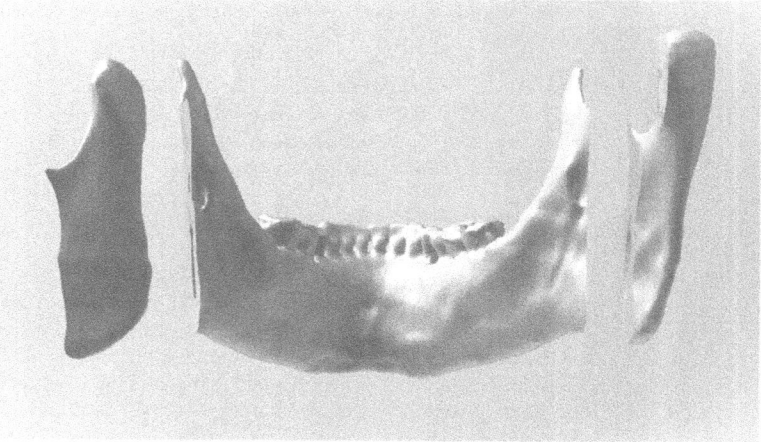

Figure 3. Three-dimensional image that displays the mandibular dental arch.

In this figure, the 3D image displays the contact surface of the osteotomized right posterior mandibular segment, which involves the temporomandibular joint condyle. In the anterior segment, which involves the mandibular dental arch, the preservation of the mandibular canals in bilateral osteotomies is visible. The left posterior segment is visible on the right side of the picture, parallel to the incision.

The 3D mandible was printed before and after the digital cuts were made. The mandible with the bone cuts was used to make the surgical guide in vitro with methyl methacrylate (Figure 4), with the direction and angle of the cut to be made being precisely adjusted. This guide was used as a directional and angular support for the tungsten carbide drill used to perform the osteotomy. It was also possible to limit the depth of the cut, increasing the safety of the procedure in vivo.

The same bicortical bone cut was made on the mandible model from the glenoid fossa (Figure 5); the cut was made obliquely to facilitate the cutting angle with the surgeon's field of view through the intraoral surgical approach and straight to the determined limit of the inferior posterior wall plus 1 mm from the foramen oval. In vivo, this bicortical cut should be made with a piezoelectric cutting instrument to preserve internal anatomical structures, especially the internal maxillary artery and the inferior alveolar vascular–nervous bundle.

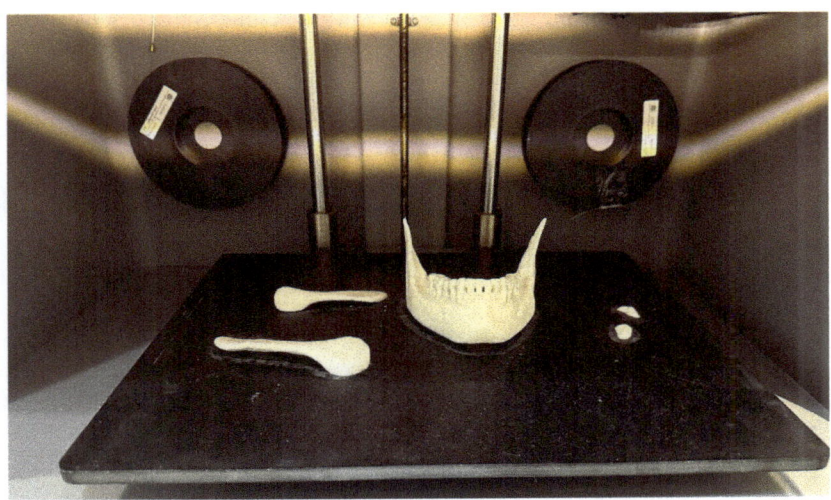

Figure 4. Three-dimensional mandible printed after the digital osteotomy.

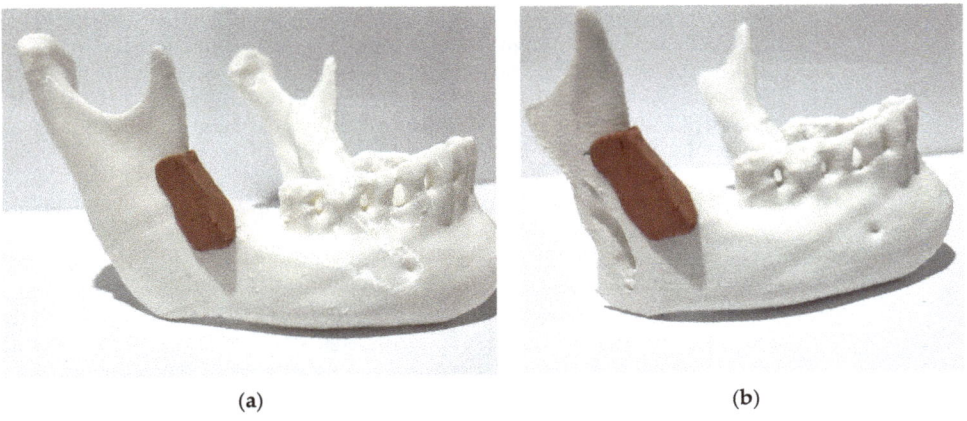

Figure 5. Positioning of the surgical guide: (**a**) before osteotomy; (**b**) after osteotomy.

3. Results

The osteotomies made in the digital images were validated after 3D printing the models in synthetic bone (nylon) with a density of 0.8 g/cm^3. The models were analyzed to ensure that the mandibular foramen and canal were preserved. The bone contact surface between the posterior and anterior segments was also validated and measured using a manual caliper with a maximum contact surface that was 20 mm wide and 57 mm high. These values provide a safety margin for mandibular retraction and advancement procedures within these limits.

The bone cut made on the synthetic bone model was accurate due to the correct angulation obtained using the surgical guide for the cut, as well as the location from the top of the mandibular notch to the final point at the edge of the mandible (Figure 5a).

The primary objective of the proposed method was to create a novel mandibular osteotomy, determined by 3D digital images and validated on a 3D printed model, which would preserve anatomical regions and, most importantly, optimize muscle action in the approximation of the osteotomized segments. This objective was successfully achieved by analyzing the final result of the osteotomized segments (Figure 5b).

The temporalis muscle will retract and elevate the anterior segment (with the mandibular dental arch), and the masseter muscle will approximate the posterior segment (mandibular ramus), maintaining contact between the osteotomized bone segments. The retention of the coronoid process (Figure 5b) in the anterior segment represents a significant biomechanical distinction when compared to the conventional techniques that are currently employed (bilateral sagittal split osteotomy).

The cut can be made with a 2 mm tungsten carbide bur, a surgical saw, or a straight piezoelectric cutting instrument. The piezoelectric device is best for the in vivo procedure, as it protects soft tissues, such as vessels and nerves.

The cutting angles applied in the osteotomy varied due to individual anatomical characteristics. This factor highlights the importance of 3D digital and laboratory technology in creating innovative guided bilateral mandibular osteotomy (GBMO).

4. Discussion

In recent years, the advantages of 3D planning and guided surgery have become apparent in maxillofacial surgery. It can be challenging for a surgeon to accurately reproduce the exact positioning of the cutting and drilling guides on the flat mandibular angles defined by the engineer, which can affect the reliability of guided bilateral sagittal split osteotomy [10].

Reference screws placed on the skeleton before the acquisition of medical computed tomographic data can serve as a fixed landmark for use during surgery and by engineers during the design phase. The results suggest that the use of reference screws is an efficient method for accurately positioning guides during guided bilateral sagittal split osteotomy [10].

Computer-aided design/computer-aided manufacturing (CAD/CAM) technologies have become increasingly popular in orthognathic surgery, especially for complex cases. These technologies are used to create cutting and drilling guides, which require virtual surgical planning and 3D modeling before they can be printed in materials such as titanium, polyamide, or resin [11].

It has been reported that a personalized titanium device can be used to support bilateral sagittal split osteotomy (BSSO) with or without genioplasty combined with individual implants for repositioning and fixation. This one-piece guide for both sides of the BSSO allows for less invasive drill placement and greater accuracy during cutting and drilling [12].

The use of this technique limited the amount of tissue detachment required and provided the necessary strength for precise bone cutting and drilling. Additionally, it facilitated the accurate fixation of preformed plates to achieve occlusion as planned virtually [11].

Since the introduction of the sagittal cut of the mandible for osteotomy of craniofacial discrepancies in 1957, few major innovations have been proposed. The only changes made have been to the angle, size, and height of the osteotomies [13].

There have been no significant innovations since that time. Suggestions for improving established techniques are mostly based on professional experience and adapting surgical procedures to individual patient needs [14].

This article presents a novel bilateral mandibular osteotomy (GBMO) that simplifies the previously performed procedure. This is accomplished using imaging technology, 3D printing, surgical guides, and bone-cutting guides.

The procedure involves a single oblique transversal cut that is guided surgically by a prefabricated model after previous surgery on models. The lingual surface of the mandibular ramus is not exposed.

The proposal is based on a digitally made cut in a 3D image, from which the surgical guide model is created. This innovative technique is used for bilateral mandibular osteotomy to advance and retract the mandible. The innovation lies in the novel design technique, rather than in the use of 3D digital models and surgical guides, which have already been extensively described in the literature.

In addition, the biomechanical advantages of the proposed technique are described by analyzing the region of the bone cut and the consequent muscular action in the posterior and anterior segments of the osteotomized mandible.

In the osteotomized posterior segment, we find the insertions of the masseter, medial pterygoid, and lateral pterygoid muscles.

The lateral pterygoid muscle is responsible for depressing the mandible, as well as assisting with protrusion and lateral movement. The depression of the mandible is largely due to gravity [15].

The medial pterygoid is a rectangular muscle with a superficial and deep head. The superficial head originates from the maxillary tuberosity of the lower jaw. The tendon fibers of the medial pterygoid insert into the angle of the mandible. The muscle assists in the elevation and protrusion of the mandible [16].

In this innovative osteotomy (GBMO), the temporalis muscle, which inserts into the mandibular coronoid process, is inserted into the osteotomized anterior segment where the mandibular dental arch is located. The anterior and mid fibers are responsible for elevating the mandible, while the posterior fibers retract it [17].

As a result, the action of the temporalis muscle lifting the mandible posteriorly helps to bring the segmented bony boundaries closer together, which is exactly the opposite of what happens with conventional bilateral sagittal cut techniques [15–17].

The biomechanical advantages of muscle actions in fracture stabilization, reduction, and osteotomy are well documented in the literature [8,9].

A favorable osteotomy can eliminate the need for plates and screws for bone fixation, with excellent short- and medium-term benefits for the patient and surgeon [14].

The difference between the technique proposed here and the vertical mandibular incision that was previously proposed and is still used [18,19] is the oblique transversal angle, which allows the procedure to be performed intraorally, and the fact that the angle of the incision is not vertical but defined according to the patient's anatomy after all of the planning with digital and 3D-printed models (Figure 1).

The access to the intraoral surgical field for performing this innovative osteotomy is the same as that used for the IVRO technique or the non-oblique vertical osteotomy, requiring only minor modifications relative and inherent to the specific anatomy of each patient, like any regular intraoral surgery [20].

The method described here can also be used to train surgeons in maxillofacial surgery residencies to perform other conventional techniques, such as the bilateral sagittal split, the bilateral horizontal cut, the intraoral and/or extraoral vertical cut, and the extraoral inverted "L" osteotomy [14,21].

The limitations of the proposed technique include the need for prior training of the surgeon or the need for a technician in the team to analyze the 3D images and perform the digital bone section accurately according to predefined standards. It also adds another step in the laboratory to create a surgical guide, which should be done by a trained technician or the surgeon.

In addition, during the planning process, the surgical section must be tested on the 3D model to be printed to validate the digital planning, adding another step to the process.

The use of surgical guides as occlusal splints and or as bone-cutting guides in both the maxilla and mandible has already been shown in the literature to have advantages in terms of time savings and precision during surgery [22–35].

The most frequent complications of routinely performed mandibular osteotomies include injury to the vascular–nerve bundle of the inferior alveolar nerve, short- and medium-term mandibular position recurrences, temporomandibular joint pain and dysfunction, and infections [36,37].

The proposed technique (GBMO) aims to reduce surgical complications by minimizing the risk of injury inherent to the sagittal split procedure (Figure 6) [38,39]. During sagittal split osteotomy surgery, the mandible needs to be fractured around the inferior alveolar nerve, which unavoidably increases the risk of injury.

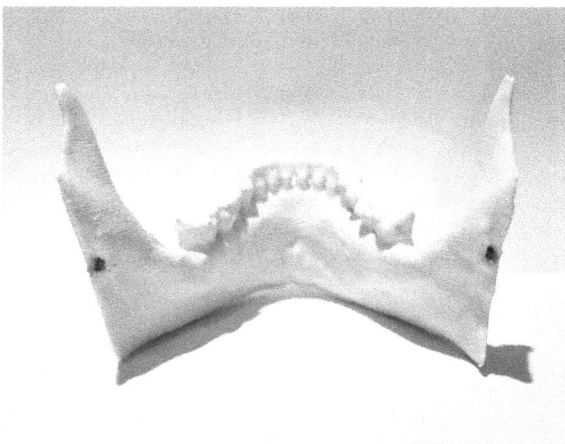

Figure 6. Preservation of the bilateral insertion of the inferior alveolar nerve into the mandible.

In the bilateral sagittal split osteotomy, the bone cut is finalized using bone separators. However, the location and shape of the fracture in the internal region of the mandibular ramus are not standardized. This lack of standardization can result in a bad split, as mentioned in the literature [37].

The use of the finite element method and analysis of the results could provide important data and predictions, with validation of the results occurring in procedures performed in clinical trials. The implementation of the new osteotomy described here and other proposals using the same innovative method to obtain novel osteotomies based on analyses of anatomical structures and biomechanical neuromuscular forces through digital images and 3D models is the present and future of surgical technique innovation [40].

In addition to the 3D printing of monophasic and multiphase scaffolds, bioprinting and tissue engineering have emerged as innovative technologies that may change the way we view guided tissue engineering [41].

Orthognathic surgery using virtual 3D surgical planning and CAD/CAM technologies is very accurate [42]. Its application in clinical practice has increased the predictability and comfort of surgery, and it will be important for clinicians to make continuous efforts to apply the most advanced technologies that will be developed in the future to patient diagnosis and surgery [43–45].

The proposed method of creating a guide for the surgical bone cut was found to be safe and effective in achieving the desired outcome. The experience of the surgeon is crucial for planning and executing the digital bone section, 3D model, and future surgery.

The osteotomy procedure is proposed to be performed through an intraoral surgical approach, as extraoral approaches are not feasible with the described cutting angle.

Maintaining the insertion of the temporalis muscle in the anterior segment of the dental arch facilitates the approximation of the osteotomized anterior and posterior segments. This technique also offers the safe option of not requiring rigid fixation.

The potential challenges in clinical implementation are related to the technical training of surgeons to learn how to validate the novel osteotomy in the 3D model and to create a feasible angle for implementing the bone cut in the limited space of the mouth opening during intraoral approach surgery.

Future studies should analyze the performance of the proposed osteotomy (GBMO) by different surgeons and compare the results obtained with 3D models. A further cadaver study should then be carried out to validate the results obtained with the models, thus preparing the procedure for a clinical trial.

5. Conclusions

The utilization of digital 3D images acquired from CT scans in the form of DICOM files, which were then converted into STL files, proved to be an efficient method for developing an innovative mandibular osteotomy technique. The use of the 3D Builder software enabled the models to be digitally cut and printed before and after the digital cuts without requiring extensive computer expertise.

The described 3D osteotomy (GBMO) simplifies bilateral mandibular osteotomy by using a single and continuous oblique and transversal incision in the mandible. This preserves the fundamental anatomical regions, including the inferior alveolar nerve and the internal maxillary artery, in a safe and controlled manner.

Future studies will analyze the advantages and limitations of the technique in vivo, as well as its application in training maxillofacial surgeons in this specialty.

Author Contributions: Conceptualization, C.A.A.; methodology, C.A.A.; formal analysis, C.A.A.; investigation, C.A.A.; writing—original draft preparation, C.A.A.; writing—review and editing, E.M.M.F.; visualization, E.M.M.F.; supervision, R.N.J. All authors have read and agreed to the published version of the manuscript.

Funding: This research received no external funding.

Data Availability Statement: Data are contained within the article.

Conflicts of Interest: The authors declare no conflicts of interest.

References

1. Hart, N.H.; Nimphius, S.; Rantalainen, T.; Ireland, A.; Siafarikas, A.; Newton, R.U. Mechanical basis of bone strength: Influence of bone material, bone structure and muscle action. *J. Musculoskel Neuron Interact* **2017**, *17*, 114–139.
2. Gash, M.C.; Kandle, P.F.; Murray, I.V.; Varacallo, M. Physiology, Muscle Contraction. In *StatPearls [Internet]*; StatPearls Publishing: Treasure Island, FL, USA, 2024. Available online: https://www.ncbi.nlm.nih.gov/books/NBK537140/ (accessed on 24 May 2024).
3. Breeland, G.; Aktar, A.; Patel, B.C. Anatomy, Head and Neck, Mandible. In *StatPearls [Internet]*; StatPearls Publishing: Treasure Island, FL, USA, 2024. Available online: https://www.ncbi.nlm.nih.gov/books/NBK532292 (accessed on 24 May 2024).
4. Basit, H.; Tariq, M.A.; Siccardi, M.A. Anatomy, Head and Neck, Mastication Muscles. In *StatPearls [Internet]*; StatPearls Publishing: Treasure Island, FL, USA, 2024. Available online: https://www.ncbi.nlm.nih.gov/books/NBK541027/ (accessed on 24 May 2024).
5. Bakke, M. Mandibular elevator muscles: Physiology, action, and effect of dental occlusion. *Scand. J. Dent. Res.* **1993**, *101*, 314–331. [CrossRef]
6. Klineberg, I.; Murray, G. Osseoperception: Sensory function and proprioception. *Adv. Dent. Res.* **1999**, *13*, 120–129. [CrossRef]
7. Aman, J.E.; Elangovan, N.; Yeh, I.L.; Konczak, J. The effectiveness of proprioceptive training for improving motor function: A systematic review. *Front. Hum. Neurosci.* **2015**, *8*, 1075. [CrossRef]
8. Panesar, K.; Susarla, S.M. Mandibular Fractures: Diagnosis and Management. *Semin. Plast. Surg.* **2021**, *35*, 238–249. [CrossRef]
9. Van den Bempt, M.; Vinayahalingam, S.; Han, M.D.; Bergé, S.J.; Xi, T. The role of muscular traction in the occurrence of skeletal relapse after advancement bilateral sagittal split osteotomy (BSSO): A systematic review. *Orthod. Craniofac. Res.* **2022**, *25*, 1–13. [CrossRef]
10. Philippe, B. Accuracy of position of cutting and drilling guide for sagittal split guided surgery: A proof of concept study. *Br. J. Oral Maxillofac. Surg.* **2020**, *58*, 940–946. [CrossRef]
11. Savoldelli, C.; Vandersteen, C.; Dassonville, O.; Santini, J. Dental occlusal-surface-supported titanium guide to assist cutting and drilling in mandibular bilateral sagittal split osteotomy. *J. Stomat. Oral Maxillofac. Surg.* **2018**, *119*, 75–78. [CrossRef]
12. Van den Bempt, M.; Liebregts, J.; Maal, T.; Bergé, S.; Xi, T. Toward a higher accuracy in orthognathic surgery by using intraoperative computer navigation, 3D surgical guides, and/or customized osteosynthesis plates: A systematic review. *J. Cranio-Maxillofac. Surg.* **2018**, *46*, 2108–2119. [CrossRef]
13. Trauner, R.; Obwegeser, H. Zur Operationstechnik bei der Progenia und anderen Unterkieferanomalien. *Dtsch. Zahn. Mund. Kieferhlkd.* **1955**, *23*, 11–25.
14. Andreucci, C.A. Sixty Years of Innovation in Biomechanical Orthognatic Surgery: The State of the Art and Future Directions. *Osteology* **2024**, *4*, 11–32. [CrossRef]
15. Roberts, W.E.; Goodacre, C.J. The Temporomandibular Joint: A Critical Review of Life-Support Functions, Development, Articular Surfaces, Biomechanics and Degeneration. *J. Prosthodont.* **2020**, *29*, 772–779. [CrossRef]
16. Li, G.W.; Liu, C.K.; Liu, P.; Deng, T.G.; Li, J.L.; Hu, K.J. Anatomical study of rat trigeminal motor nucleus-lateral pterygoid muscle projection pathway. *Zhonghua Kou Qiang Yi Xue Za Zhi* **2020**, *55*, 259–263.

17. Arsenina, O.I.; Komarova, A.V.; Popova, N.V.; Popova, A.V.; Egorova, D.O. Primenenie elastokorrektora dlya ustraneniya diskoordinatsii raboty zhevatel'nykh myshts u patsientov s disfunktsiei visochno-nizhnechelyustnogo sustava [Elimination of discoordination of the masticatory muscles work in patients with muscular-articular dysfunction of the temporomandibular joint by using «elastocorrector» appliance]. *Stomatologiia* **2020**, *99*, 61–65. [CrossRef]
18. Obwegeser, H.L. Orthognathic surgery and a tale of how three procedures came to be: A letter to the next generations of surgeons. *Clin. Plast. Surg.* **2007**, *34*, 331–355. [CrossRef]
19. Caldwell, J.B.; Letterman, G.S. Vertical osteotomy in the mandibular rami for correction of prognathism. *J. Oral. Surg.* **1954**, *12*, 185–202.
20. Peleg, O.; Mahmoud, R.; Shuster, A.; Arbel, S.; Kleinman, S.; Mijiritsky, E.; Ianculovici, C. Vertical Ramus Osteotomy, Is It Still a Valid Tool in Orthognathic Surgery? *Int. J. Environ. Res. Public Health* **2022**, *19*, 10171. [CrossRef]
21. Aziz, S.R.; Greenberg, A.M.; Escobar, V.; Schwimmer, A. Mandibular Osteotomies. In *Craniomaxillofacial Reconstructive and Corrective Bone Surgery*; Greenberg, A., Schmelzeisen, R., Eds.; Springer: New York, NY, USA, 2019. [CrossRef]
22. Chakravarthy, C.; Sunder, S.; Malyala, S.K.; Tahmeen, A. 3D Printed Surgical Guides in Orthognathic Surgery—A Pathway to Positive Surgical Outcomes. In *Proceedings of the International Conference on ISMAC in Computational Vision and Bio-Engineering 2018 (ISMAC-CVB), ISMAC 2018, Pandian, India, 16–17 May 2018*; Pandian, D., Fernando, X., Baig, Z., Shi, F., Eds.; Lecture Notes in Computational Vision and Biomechanics; Springer: Cham, Switzerland, 2019; Volume 30. [CrossRef]
23. Xiao, Y.; Sun, X.; Wang, L.; Zhang, Y.; Chen, K.; Wu, G. The Application of 3D Printing Technology for Simultaneous Orthognathic Surgery and Mandibular Contour Osteoplasty in the Treatment of Craniofacial Deformities. *Aesth. Plast. Surg.* **2017**, *41*, 1413–1424. [CrossRef]
24. Wang, L.; Tian, D.; Sun, X.; Xiao, Y.; Chen, L.; Wu, G. The Precise Repositioning Instrument for Genioplasty and a Three-Dimensional Printing Technique for Treatment of Complex Facial Asymmetry. *Aesth. Plast. Surg.* **2017**, *41*, 919–929. [CrossRef]
25. Rubio-Palau, J.; Prieto-Gundin, A.; Cazalla, A.A.; Serrano, M.B.; Fructuoso, G.G.; Ferrandis, F.P.; Baró, A.R. Three-dimensional planning in craniomaxillofacial surgery. *Ann. Maxillofac. Surg.* **2016**, *6*, 281–286. [CrossRef]
26. Jong, W.C.; Namkug, K. Clinical Application of Three-Dimensional Printing Technology in Craniofacial Plastic Surgery. *Arch. Plast. Surg.* **2015**, *42*, 267–277. [CrossRef]
27. Lin, H.H.; Lonic, D.; Lo, L. 3D printing in orthognathic surgery—A literature review. *J. Formos. Med. Assoc.* **2018**, *117*, 547–558. [CrossRef]
28. Yushkevich, P.A.; Piven, J.; Hazlett, H.C.; Smith, R.G.; Ho, S.; Gee, J.C.; Gerig, G. User-guided 3D active contour segmentation of anatomical structures: Significantly improved efficiency and reliability. *NeuroImage* **2016**, *31*, 1116–1128. [CrossRef]
29. Wrzosek, M.K.; Peacock, Z.S.; Laviv, A.; Goldwaser, B.R.; Ortiz, R.; Resnick, C.M.; Troulis, M.J.; Kaban, L.B. Comparison of time required for traditional versus virtual orthognathic surgery treatment planning. *Int. J. Oral Maxillofac. Surg.* **2016**, *45*, 1065–1069. [CrossRef]
30. Tetsworth, K.; Block, S.; Glatt, V. Putting 3D modelling and 3D printing into practice: Virtual surgery and preoperative planning to reconstruct complex post-traumatic skeletal deformities and defects. *J. Soc. Int. Chir. Orthop. Traumatol.* **2017**, *3*, 16. [CrossRef]
31. Steinhuber, T.; Brunold, S.; Gärtner, C.; Offermanns, V.; Ulmer, H.; Ploder, O. Is Virtual Surgical Planning in Orthognathic Surgery Faster Than Conventional Planning? A Time and Workflow Analysis of an Office-Based Workflow for Single- and Double-Jaw Surgery. *J. Oral Maxillofac. Surg.* **2018**, *76*, 397–407. [CrossRef]
32. Resnick, C.M.; Inverso, G.; Wrzosek, M.; Padwa, B.L.; Kaban, L.B.; Peacock, Z.S. Is There a Difference in Cost between Standard and Virtual Surgical Planning for Orthognathic Surgery? *J. Oral Maxillofac. Surg.* **2016**, *74*, 1827–1833. [CrossRef]
33. Plooij, J.M.; Maal, T.J.J.; Haers, P.; Borstlap, W.A.; Kuijpers-Jagtman, A.M.; Berge, S.J. Digital three-dimensional image fusion processes for planning and evaluating orthodontics and orthognathic surgery. A systematic review. *Int. J. Oral Maxillofac. Surg.* **2011**, *40*, 341–352. [CrossRef]
34. Franz, L.; Isola, M.; Bagatto, D.; Tuniz, F.; Robiony, M. A novel approach to skull-base and orbital osteotomies through virtual planning and navigation. *Laryngoscope* **2019**, *129*, 823–831. [CrossRef] [PubMed]
35. Brüllmann, D.; Schulze, R.K.W. Spatial resolution in CBCT machines for dental/maxillofacial applications—What do we know today? *Dentomaxillofac. Radiol.* **2015**, *44*, 20140204. [CrossRef] [PubMed]
36. Movahed, R.; Ivory, J.W.; Delatour, F. Complications Associated with Maxillomandibular Advancement. In *Management of Obstructive Sleep Apnea*; Kim, K.B., Movahed, R., Malhotra, R.K., Stanley, J.J., Eds.; Springer: Cham, Switzerland, 2021. [CrossRef]
37. Steenen, S.A.; Becking, A.G. Bad splits in bilateral sagittal split osteotomy: Systematic review of fracture patterns. *Int. J. Oral Maxillofac. Surg.* **2016**, *45*, 887–897. [CrossRef] [PubMed]
38. Andreucci, C.A.; Fonseca, E.M.M.; Jorge, R.N. 3D Printing as an Efficient Way to Prototype and Develop Dental Implants. *BioMedInformatics* **2022**, *2*, 671–679. [CrossRef]
39. Fernandes, M.G.; Alves, J.L.; Fonseca, E.M.M. Diaphyseal femoral fracture: 3D biomodel and intramedullary nail created by additive manufacturing. *Int. J. Mater. Eng.* **2016**, *7*, 130–142. [CrossRef]
40. Sioustis, I.-A.; Axinte, M.; Prelipceanu, M.; Martu, A.; Kappenberg-Nitescu, D.-C.; Teslaru, S.; Luchian, I.; Solomon, S.M.; Cimpoesu, N.; Martu, S. Finite Element Analysis of Mandibular Anterior Teeth with Healthy, but Reduced Periodontium. *Appl. Sci.* **2021**, *11*, 3824. [CrossRef]

1. Sufaru, I.-G.; Macovei, G.; Stoleriu, S.; Martu, M.-A.; Luchian, I.; Kappenberg-Nitescu, D.-C.; Solomon, S.M. 3D Printed and Bioprinted Membranes and Scaffolds for the Periodontal Tissue Regeneration: A Narrative Review. *Membranes* **2022**, *12*, 902. [CrossRef] [PubMed]
2. Ha, S.H.; Youn, S.M.; Kim, C.Y.; Jeong, C.G.; Choi, J.Y. Surgical Accuracy of 3D Virtual Surgery and CAD/CAM-Assisted Orthognathic Surgery for Skeletal Class III Patients. *J. Craniofac. Surg.* **2023**, *34*, 96–102. [CrossRef] [PubMed]
3. Kim, M.K.; Ham, M.J.; Kim, W.R.; Kim, H.G.; Kwon, K.J.; Kim, S.G.; Park, Y.W. Investigating the accuracy of mandibulectomy and reconstructive surgery using 3D customized implants and surgical guides in a rabbit model. *Maxillofac. Plast. Reconstr. Surg.* **2023**, *45*, 8. [CrossRef] [PubMed]
4. Si, J.; Zhang, C.; Tian, M.; Jiang, T.; Zhang, L.; Yu, H.; Shi, J.; Wang, X. Intraoral Condylectomy with 3D-Printed Cutting Guide versus with Surgical Navigation: An Accuracy and Effectiveness Comparison. *J. Clin. Med.* **2023**, *12*, 3816. [CrossRef]
5. Kim, S.H.; Lee, S.M.; Park, J.H.; Yang, S.; Kim, J.W. Effectiveness of individualized 3D titanium-printed Orthognathic osteotomy guides and custom plates. *BMC Oral Health* **2023**, *23*, 255. [CrossRef]

Disclaimer/Publisher's Note: The statements, opinions and data contained in all publications are solely those of the individual author(s) and contributor(s) and not of MDPI and/or the editor(s). MDPI and/or the editor(s) disclaim responsibility for any injury to people or property resulting from any ideas, methods, instructions or products referred to in the content.

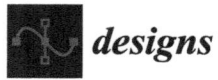

Article

Design and Implementation of a Low-Power Device for Non-Invasive Blood Glucose

Luis Miguel Pires [1,2,*] and José Martins [2,3,*]

[1] Department of Electronical Engineering, Telecommunications and Computers (DEETC), Instituto Superior de Engenharia de Lisboa (ISEL), 1959-007 Lisbon, Portugal
[2] Technologies and Engineering School (EET), Instituto Politécnico da Lusofonia (IPLuso), 1700-098 Lisbon, Portugal
[3] Department of Systems and Informatics (DSI), Setúbal School of Technology, Instituto Politécnico de Setúbal (IPS), 2914-508 Setúbal, Portugal
* Correspondence: luis.pires@ipluso.pt (L.M.P.); p3451@ipluso.pt (J.M.)

Abstract: Glucose is a simple sugar molecule. The chemical formula of this sugar molecule is $C_6H_{12}O_6$. This means that the glucose molecule contains six carbon atoms (C), twelve hydrogen atoms (H), and six oxygen atoms (O). In human blood, the molecule glucose circulates as blood sugar. Normally, after eating or drinking, our bodies break down the sugars in food and use them to obtain energy for our cells. To execute this process, our pancreas produces insulin. Insulin "pulls" sugar from the blood and puts it into the cells for use. If someone has diabetes, their pancreas cannot produce enough insulin. As a result, the level of glucose in their blood rises. This can lead to many potential complications, including blindness, disease, nerve damage, amputation, stroke, heart attack, damage to blood vessels, etc. In this study, a non-invasive and therefore easily usable method for monitoring blood glucose was developed. With the experiment carried out, it was possible to measure glucose levels continuously, thus eliminating the disadvantages of invasive systems. Near-IR sensors (optical sensors) were used to estimate the concentration of glucose in blood; these sensors have a wavelength of 940 nm. The sensor was placed on a small black parallelepiped-shaped box on the tip of the finger and the output of the optical sensor was then connected to a microcontroller at the analogue input. Another sensor used, but only to provide more medical information, was the heartbeat sensor, inserted into an armband (along with the microprocessor). After processing and linear regression analysis, the glucose level was predicted, and data were sent via the Bluetooth network to a developed APP. The results of the implemented device were compared with available invasive methods (commercial products). The hardware consisted of a microcontroller, a near-IR optical sensor, a heartbeat sensor, and a Bluetooth module. Another objective of this experiment using low-cost and low-power hardware was to not carry out complex processing of data from the sensors. Our practical laboratory experiment resulted in an error of 2.86 per cent when compared to a commercial product, with a hardware cost of EUR 8 and a consumption of 50 mA.

Keywords: blood glucose monitoring; embedded systems; heartbeat sensor; near-IR sensors

Citation: Pires, L.M.; Martins, J. Design and Implementation of a Low-Power Device for Non-Invasive Blood Glucose. *Designs* **2024**, *8*, 63. https://doi.org/10.3390/designs8040063

Academic Editors: Richard Drevet and Hicham Benhayoune

Received: 16 May 2024
Revised: 14 June 2024
Accepted: 18 June 2024
Published: 24 June 2024

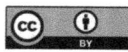

Copyright: © 2024 by the authors. Licensee MDPI, Basel, Switzerland. This article is an open access article distributed under the terms and conditions of the Creative Commons Attribution (CC BY) license (https://creativecommons.org/licenses/by/4.0/).

1. Introduction

Carbohydrates are molecules of enormous biological importance that have empirical formulas such as $C_n(H_2O)_n$ or $C_n(H_2O)_{n-1}$. These formulas suggest they are "hydrates of carbon" and that is why early chemists gave them the general name carbohydrates. We commonly call carbohydrates sugars, and they are also known as saccharides. They are organic compounds represented by the formulas above. Since these compounds are synthesized through photosynthesis in plants, they are mostly components specific to plant foods. However, they are also the building blocks of many vital tissues in animals. Glucose is the most important carbohydrate group; it is called simple sugar (monosaccharide) and is abundant in foods. Another area where determining glucose values is very important is the health sector. Measurements to determine blood glucose levels are important in the treatment of patients with diabetes and hyperglycemia [1]. Diabetes Mellitus type I has a strong genetic component and is a very common hereditary disease today. It causes blindness, heart attack, kidney failure, amputation, and in later stages, death. The rapidly increasing number of patients makes it necessary to control and constantly monitor diabetes. Monitoring diabetes is also extremely important in terms of reducing the progression of the disease and healthcare costs [2]. Non-invasive techniques for blood glucose monitoring have attracted significant research interest due to their high sensitivity and better patient compliance, unlike invasive ones. Typical non-invasive biosensors based on different approaches include iontophoretic extraction of glucose from the skin, surface plasmon resonance, Raman spectroscopy, visible or near-infrared (NIR) spectroscopy, polarimetry, photo-acoustic probes, and fluorescence methods. These methods may be alternative options for continuous glucose measurement [3]. Some studies have already been carried out on this subject, either describing or comparing the several technologies at our disposal [3–5] and choosing and testing NIR spectroscopy [6–8].

Other developing technologies like flexible sensors based on carbon nanotube paper film (CNTF) and stress-induced square frustum structures (SSFSs) [9] have shown very promising results in research and potential to be applied in the medical field, but it is important to note that while these technologies have shown significant potential in a research context, the transition to commercial application is still ongoing and often this transition involves additional challenges and considerations, including scalability, cost-effectiveness, and regulatory approval. For now, this technology is still not ready for commercial applications.

Other technologies like durable superhydrophobic surfaces [10] are already in a different stage of development but still give rise to concerns related to poor durability and short service life [11]; due to this, to date, the practical applications of superhydrophobic materials have been greatly restricted. Researchers are still focusing on ways to prolong the lifetime of superhydrophobic surfaces with respect to two aspects, namely surface structures and materials [11].

The development and creation of low-cost, non-invasive glucose-measuring equipment would generate interest both among people who suffer from diabetes and among people who do not yet suffer but are in risk groups. One advantage of being non-invasive is that there are people who avoid taking the test using conventional invasive equipment because they do not like the prospect of having their finger pricked (it is uncomfortable and could lead to infection) and others who are very sensitive to the sight of blood, making self-testing with conventional invasive equipment unlikely for a good part of the population. A non-invasive technique would allow the acquisition by everyone of equipment that would be used regularly at home and at work, allowing continuous monitoring and control and thus preventing sudden emergencies in the population already suffering from this disease (if blood glucose remains too high or is steadily rising, the person will speak with their doctor, as they may need to adjust their treatment) or even an increase in the population with this problem. Optical detection of glucose allows for more frequent and better monitoring for people with diabetes.

The environmental aspect cannot be forgotten either; the fact that people stop using (and throw away) meter blood strips and have to periodically change the needles with the conventional equipment is another point in favor of changing to the use of non-invasive equipment.

The International Organization for Standardization [12] in their ISO 15197:2015 [13] recommends some goals for glucose meters and for system accuracy. Firstly, 95% of the glucose results should fall within ± 15 mg/dL of the reference result at glucose concentrations <100 mg/dL and within $\pm 15\%$ at glucose concentrations ≥ 100 mg/dL [13,14]. Secondly, 99% of individual glucose measured values should fall within clinically acceptable zones A and B of the consensus error grid (CEG) for diabetes [13–15]. Under optimal circumstances, many meters meet these accuracy standards.

Also, the Food and Drug Administration (FDA) has given non-binding guidance for commercial equipment; devices should deliver measurements that are within +/−15% of a highly precise lab measurement 95% of the time and within +/−20% of a highly precise lab measurement 99% of the time [16].

Yet, user-related errors are a more significant source of errors than are instrument-related errors [17]. This is also a point in favor of the adoption of a non-invasive method that reduces the number of steps for glucose measurements, thus minimizing errors and essentially leading to better control and monitoring of glucose. In our study, using commercial invasive equipment as a standard and with an error rate for this equipment lower than the ISO recommendation, we minimized typical user-related errors by adopting recommended procedures, such as ensuring that the glucose meter was correctly calibrated (according to the manufacturer's instructions), making sure that the test strips (and control solution) were stored in appropriate conditions (to prevent damage or degradation) and were clean and free of substances that could interfere with the reading, and using the correct amount of blood for the test strip, thus leading to accurate and reliable standard glucose-monitoring values to later be able to compare with our measurements from the non-invasive equipment, and thus being sure to significantly reduce the typical errors associated with measurement of glucose with commercial meters.

Classic commercial equipment is not easy to use. The following are typical user-related errors with the strip: not fully inserting it in the meter, moving it after insertion, and not keeping it at the recommend temperature (as the control solution); these are common errors and lead to errors in readings. Insufficient amount of blood or squeezing the fingertip too much (because the blood is not flowing) are also typical errors and consequently lead to repeated attempts. Users' failure to calibrate the glucose meter regularly is also a common cause of error.

A more recent adopted solution is the continuous glucose monitor (CGM) applied typically by a patch in the arm of the user. They have more stable results than the classic meters but rely on the interstitial fluid that surrounds the body cells (instead of blood). So, they rely on an algorithm to give us a prediction of the blood sugar level. Also, they need calibration. It could take up to an hour and is usually completed on the first day. But reports [18] by users say that the first day is the worst day to calibrate since the data gathered show less accuracy in the sensors in the first 24 h. Adding to this, the reading of the interstitial fluid lags behind the blood glucose by an average of 17 minutes [19]; this is due to the physiological time lag of glucose transport from the vascular to the interstitial space, which makes difficult to predict sudden changes in the glucose level and prevent crisis. And every two weeks, the patch needs to be changed and the calibration process repeated. So, as a good option for the continuing monitoring for the population with diabetes, CGMs do not replace the need and usefulness for a non-invasive low-cost optical solution like ours.

In terms of sensitivity and accuracy, while invasive equipment has traditionally been regarded as more sensitive than non-invasive equipment [20], user-related errors associated with the procedures required for invasive equipment can diminish this advantage or even shift it in favor of non-invasive devices in real-world usage. User-related errors in invasive glucose monitoring equipment can significantly impact the overall sensitivity and accuracy of these devices. This demonstrates the potential viability of Near-Infrared (NIR) equipment for glucose monitoring, even when considering sensitivity and accuracy.

The aim of our study is to identify a straightforward solution that allows us to demonstrate, through the correlation derived from linear regression between the values measured by conventional invasive equipment (considered the standard) and our non-invasive equipment, that our Near-Infrared (NIR) equipment provides a superior alternative. This is particularly significant for individuals who are not yet at risk but seek to monitor their glucose levels, as well as for those in high-risk groups.

The equation derived from the linear regression analysis will establish the correlation between the two sets of readings. A program will be developed and installed on a microprocessor, which will take the readings from the NIR sensors as input and use the correlation from the linear regression analysis to output the corresponding glucose values.

2. Research and System Design

This section explains the elements that make up the architecture of this project: microcontroller (Arduino Uno), optical sensors, heartbeat sensor, and wireless communication via the Bluetooth network. The firmware flowchart and its explanation are also presented, as well as the experimental tests and all the results obtained, which prove the functionality of the work as defined.

2.1. Light Spectrum and 940 nm Infrared Spectrum

Within the vast electromagnetic spectrum, beyond the boundaries of human vision, lies the enigmatic realm of infrared radiation. Among its myriad wavelengths, the 940 nm infrared spectrum stands out for its diverse applications across various fields, from telecommunications to healthcare [21,22]. In this work, we embark on a journey to explore the intricacies of the 940 nm IR spectrum (see Figure 1), shedding light on its properties, practical uses, and significance in contemporary science and technology.

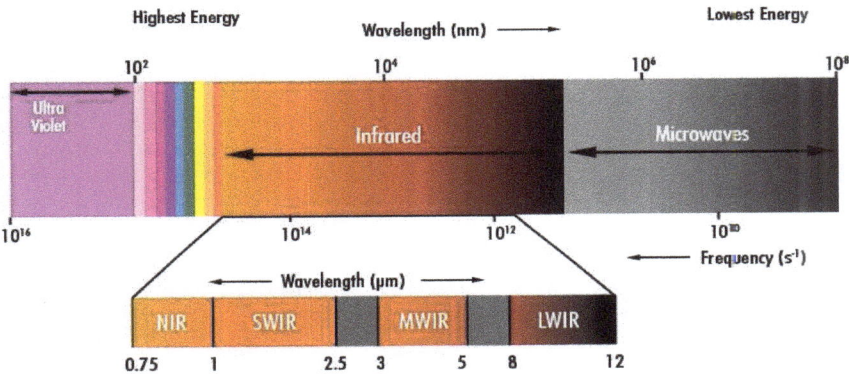

Figure 1. Light spectrum [23].

The electromagnetic spectrum encompasses a broad range of wavelengths (the wavelength is the distance between repetitions of a wave), including those of visible light and beyond. Situated adjacent to the visible spectrum, the infrared region comprises wavelengths longer than those of visible light. Within this domain, the 940 nm wavelength occupies a special place, offering unique characteristics that make it indispensable for numerous applications [21,22]. The versatility of the 940 nm infrared spectrum lends itself to a wide array of applications, each harnessing its distinct properties to achieve specific objectives. Let us delve into some key domains where the 940 nm IR spectrum plays a pivotal role.

Telecommunications and Data Transmission: The 940 nm wavelength serves as a cornerstone for optical communication systems, enabling high-speed data transmission over fiber optic networks. Its ability to travel through optical fibers with minimal attenuation ensures efficient and reliable communication over short/medium distances (e.g., LAN). Vertical Cavity Surface Emitting Lasers (VCSELs), for example, operate at 940 nm.

Sensing and Imaging Technologies: In fields such as surveillance, medical diagnostics, and environmental monitoring, the 940 nm infrared spectrum is instrumental in enhancing sensing and imaging capabilities. Night vision cameras, for instance, utilize 940 nm IR illuminators to capture clear images in low-light conditions, while medical devices leverage near-infrared spectroscopy (NIRS) for non-invasive tissue analysis.

Biomedical and Healthcare Applications: Researchers and healthcare practitioners harness the 940 nm infrared spectrum for various biomedical applications, including diagnostics and therapeutic interventions. Near-infrared light, at 940 nm wavelength, exhibits excellent tissue penetration properties, making it suitable for deep tissue imaging and photo biomodulation therapy [21,22].

Security and Defense Systems: In the realm of security and defense, infrared technology, including the 940 nm spectrum, plays a critical role in surveillance and threat detection. Infrared surveillance cameras equipped with 940 nm IR illuminators enable covert monitoring and perimeter protection, enhancing security measures in both civilian and military contexts.

In summary, the 940 nm infrared spectrum represents a captivating convergence of science, technology, and innovation, offering insight into the invisible forces that shape our world. Its applications, ranging from facilitating high-speed communication to advancing medical diagnostics and enhancing security, are as diverse as they are profound. As we continue to unlock the potential of the 940 nm IR spectrum, it stands as a testament to human ingenuity and our relentless pursuit to explore the unseen [22].

2.2. System Design

This section explains the elements that make up the architecture of this project: microcontroller (ATmega328), optical sensors (near IR), heartbeat sensor, and wireless communication via the Bluetooth network.

Figure 2 shows the project's block diagram, which consists of a microcontroller (ATmega328), the main component, as it receives information from the optical near-IR sensor and the heartbeat sensor, the two sensors used in the project. The Arduino is powered by 5 VDC so that it can work, receive data from the sensor, and send it via the Bluetooth module. The Bluetooth module communicates these data with the application.

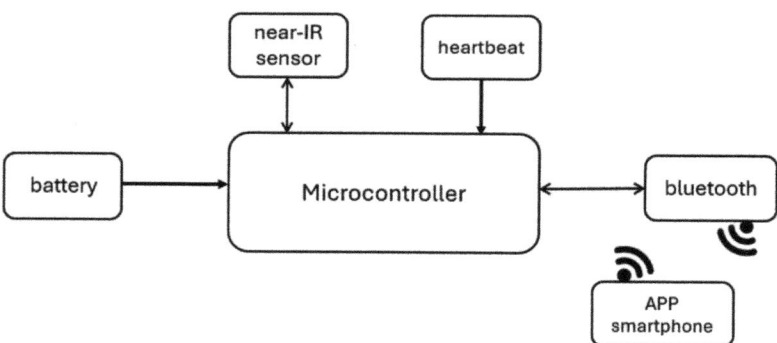

Figure 2. System architecture.

The development board used for this project is Arduino Uno [24], with the ATMega328 microcontroller [25]. The ATMega328 is a low-power chip, so it only needs 1.8–5.5 VDC to work, which is one of the main advantages of implementing it on Arduino boards, making power consumption extremely low [25]. This microcontroller has an Analog-to-Digital Converter (ADC) with ten-bit resolution. With this ADC it is possible to measure analogue signals and convert them into digital values for processing. Some of the features of the ADC in the ATMega328 are:

- Ten-bit resolution: Converts analog signals into digital ones, allowing through this resolution the production of 2^{10} (1024) possible values for each conversion.
- Input voltage range: Possibility of measuring input voltages in the 0 V to 5 V range.
- Input channels: This ADC offers six input channels, labelled ADC0 to ADC5, each of which can be individually selected for conversion.

- Sample rate: The ADC's maximum sample rate is 15,000 samples per second.

In addition to these features, the ADC uses the process of successive approximations to carry out the conversion. This process consists of a binary search algorithm to determine the digital representation of the analog input signal. In this process, the ADC compares the analog input voltage with a reference voltage and determines whether this voltage is higher or lower than the reference voltage. This process is repeated until the digital representation of the input voltage is determined within the desired resolution, which, in the case of this microcontroller, is 10 bits. The process of successive approximations is an efficient ADC conversion method for producing precise results with relatively low power consumption. However, there are other methods that are faster and more effective, such as flash conversion, which can provide a conversion time in just one clock cycle. Unfortunately, flash converters consume more power and need many comparators, making them impractical for precisions greater than eight bits. So, on an Arduino Uno, which has a clock of 16 MHz, if we use a prescaler of 128, the ADC will work with a clock of 16 MHz/128 = 125 kHz.

Sensors are devices which, using energy from the medium being measured, provide the output with a processable signal that is a function of a measurement variable. A sensor is classified as a device which, when subjected to the action of a non-electrical physical quantity, produces a characteristic of an electrical nature. Although the concept is broader, the concept of sensor and transducer is often confused. Transducers are devices that convert a signal of one physical form into another of a different physical form; in short, they convert one type of energy into another. The physical quantities associated with transducers are mechanical, thermal, magnetic, electrical, optical, and chemical. There are three classes of sensors: passive, active, and digital sensors. Passive (analogue) sensors are those whose variation in the property to be measured is reflected in variations in impedance. Active (analog) sensors are those whose energy is directly used by the process to be measured. Digital sensors are those that measure discrete quantities such as logic states and devices with a frequency output.

Non-invasive methods can generally be categorized as thermal, electrical, optical, and nanotechnology. Much current research concentrates on optical methods, mid- and near-infrared spectroscopy in particular [26–28].

Near-infrared spectroscopy (NIRS) is a form of vibrational spectroscopy in which electromagnetic radiation causes vibrations such as stretching and bending of bonds in a chemical species [6]. Each molecule consists of several different bonds that absorb radiation in different specific characteristic spectra. The absorption of radiation by a molecule leads to an increase in the energy level from an electronic ground state to a higher electronic excited state. The absorption of infrared radiation makes the transition from the energy level to the electron excited state. The NIR spectrum consists of harmonics and combined absorption bands of fundamental vibrations of C-H, O-H, N-H and S-H bonds [29]. In more detail:

C-H Bonds (Carbon–Hydrogen): C-H bonds are present everywhere in organic molecules. They appear as distinctive bands in NIR spectra between 2050 nm and 2180 nm.

O-H Bonds (Water): Water molecules exhibit strong absorption in the NIR range. Their absorption bands are broad and dominant. The main absorption bands from liquid water are located around 1450 nm and 1940 nm.

N-H Bonds (Protein): Protein content is challenging to spot at lower concentrations, but it manifests as two distinctive bands. These bands occur at 2050 nm and 2180 nm.

S-H Bonds (Thiols): S-H bonds represent the presence of thiols, which are sulfur-containing organic compounds. Thiols are commonly found in proteins, amino acids, and other biological molecules. The absorption bands associated with S-H bonds typically occur around 2500 nm in the NIR spectrum.

There are essentially three bands: the second or upper harmonic band (750–1400 nm), the first harmonic band (1400–2000 nm), and the combined harmonic band (2000–2500 nm). In more detail:

Second (Upper) Harmonic Band (750–1400 nm): This band corresponds to the second harmonic of fundamental vibrations.

- Key Features:
    - Overtone Absorptions: In this range, we observe overtone absorptions related to fundamental vibrations of various chemical bonds.
    - C-H Bonds: The second harmonic band includes overtones (multiples of the fundamental frequency) of C-H bonds, which are prevalent in organic compounds.
    - Protein and Lipid Content: Researchers often use this band to assess protein and lipid content in samples.

When analyzing food products or biological tissues, the second harmonic band provides valuable information about their composition.

First Harmonic Band (1400–2000 nm): The first harmonic band corresponds to the fundamental vibrations of specific bonds.

- Key Features:
    - O-H Bonds (Water): Water molecules exhibit strong absorption in this range. Monitoring water content is crucial for various applications.
    - Protein Bands: The first harmonic band includes absorption features related to protein content (e.g., amide bonds).
    - Starch and Sugar Bands: Starch and sugar content also contribute to the absorption in this region.

By analyzing the first harmonic band, researchers can assess hydration levels, protein concentrations, and carbohydrate content.

Combined Harmonic Band (2000–2500 nm): This band combines both fundamental vibrations and overtones.

- Key Features:
    - C-H, N-H, and O-H Bonds: The combined harmonic band includes absorption features related to C-H, N-H, and O-H bonds.
    - Thiols (S-H Bonds): Thiols (sulfur-containing compounds) also contribute to absorption in this range.

When studying biological samples or assessing chemical reactions, the combined harmonic band offers valuable insights into various functional groups.

As reported in [28], this region has a series of optical windows characterized by low absorption of water, hemoglobin, and lipids. This allows NIR radiation to penetrate areas with a higher concentration of blood beneath the skin while remaining non-destructive. Most importantly, the NIR method is relatively low-cost, as the necessary materials, such as 940 nm Near-IR emitter and receiver LEDs, can be purchased affordably. Additionally, NIR can penetrate deeper into the skin compared to mid-range IR radiation, making it the optimal choice.

The frequency of 940 nm was chosen for this experiment because, even though glucose has light absorption peaks at other wavelengths belonging to the NIR range (e.g., 970 nm, 1197 nm, and others), it is this wavelength that has the lowest signal attenuation by other biological components, such as red blood cells, water, and platelets. There are other possible choices related with higher peak absorptions of glucose in other regions, like the first harmonic or the combined region being traded for the area of the second harmonic, by the crucial fact that the second allows deeper penetration in the biological tissue. Also, for lower wavelengths, the absorption of deoxyhemoglobin, oxyhemoglobin, and melanin increases, while for larger wavelengths, water absorption has an increasing impact.

In addition, there is no need for prior sample preparation with this method and it provides rapid results.

However, shorter NIR wavelengths cause a high level of scattering in the tissue. Other disadvantages include poor sensitivity to low blood glucose concentrations, which makes accurate detection difficult, and interference from compounds with similar absorption characteristics to glucose.

The key to a successful non-invasive optical measurement of glucose is the collection of an optical spectrum with a very high signal-to-noise ratio in a spectral region containing significant glucose. Optical sensors exploit different interaction properties of light with glucose molecules in a concentration-dependent manner. Infrared (IR) provides an optical window through which it passes subcutaneously, independent of the epidermis and skin pigmentation.

The optical sensor detects transmitted infrared radiation and converts it into electrical signals. Arduino Uno is connected to the near-IR emitter and collects the data from the near-IR receiver via the 10-bit analog–digital converter (ADC) that is part of the microcontroller's architecture, with an accuracy per bit of 4.8 mV, after which the glucose level was calculated using a linear regression based on the measured values (this point is developed in Section 3).

$$blood_{glucose_{level}} = -0.03 \times ADC_{level} + 22145 \quad (1)$$

The near-IR emitter and receiver have been integrated into a black housing to reduce the noise that can be caused by ambient light. A set of two emitter LEDs and receiver photodiode were arranged opposite each other, with a small space in the middle to allow the finger to be placed. Among the various places where we could place our NIR sensor and obtain our measurements are the lips, tongue, earlobes, or fingertips, all of which are rich in blood vessels. The fingertip ended up being chosen for practical reasons relating to the construction of the black box that houses the NIR sensor. In Figure 3, we can see the image of an IR LED of 940 nm (TSAL6200) as well as the photodiode used as the optical receiver (BPV22NF) with peak sensitivity at 940 nm, both from Vishay, used in our experiment.

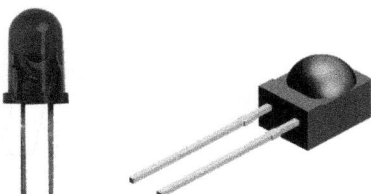

Figure 3. NIR emitter LED (**left**) and optical receiver (**right**).

Another sensor used in the experiment, the MAX30102 (Figures 4 and 5), is not relevant for measuring glucose levels, but is used to provide the user with more information, such as a heartbeat (and thus relating the measured individuals with a healthier, or not, lifestyle). The MAX30102 is an integrated pulse oximeter and heart rate sensor IC, from Analog Devices. It combines two LEDs (IR and red LEDs), a photodetector, optimized optics, and low-noise analog signal processing to detect pulse oximetry (Saturation of Peripheral Oxygen, SpO$_2$) and heart rate signals.

In our experiment, we use the version of the MAX30102 with 5 pins.

The board has two voltage regulators, 3.3 VDC to power the LEDs and 1.8 VDC to power the IC of the MAX30102. Communication with the Arduino Uno is via I2C. One of the most important features of the MAX30102 is its low power consumption; the MAX30102 consumes less than 600 µA during measurement (in standby mode only 0.7 µA). The IR LED wavelength is of 880 nm (Figure 6).

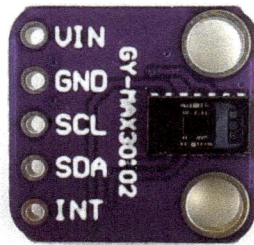

Figure 4. MAX30102 board (5-pin version).

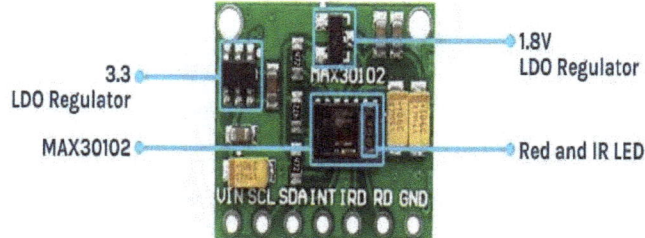

Figure 5. MAX30102 board (7-pin version).

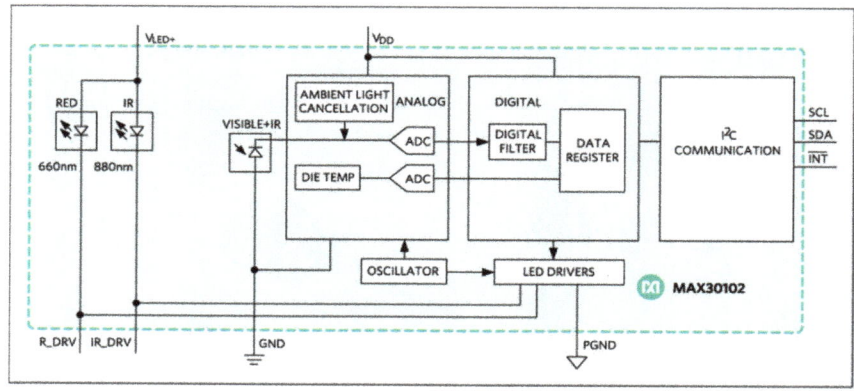

Figure 6. MAX30102 block diagram.

Our body comprises veins and arteries, with veins visually represented by blue lines (see Figure 7) and arteries by red lines. In the veins, blood travels through the body's tissues toward the heart, whereas in the arteries, blood flows from the heart toward the rest of the body. Structurally, arteries are blood vessels with thick, resistant walls through which blood flows at high pressure. In contrast, veins have thinner walls and blood flows through them at lower pressure. The blood flowing through the arteries is rich in oxygen and is referred to as oxyhemoglobin (a complex formed by the binding of oxygen (O_2) to hemoglobin). Arteries absorb more infrared light compared to other tissues. Conversely, the blood flowing through the veins is low in oxygen, known as deoxyhemoglobin (the form of hemoglobin that has released its bound oxygen). Deoxyhemoglobin has a particular affinity for red light, contributing to the purplish-blue appearance of deoxygenated blood. As light passes through our tissues, deoxyhemoglobin selectively absorbs red wavelengths, allowing other colors to pass through.

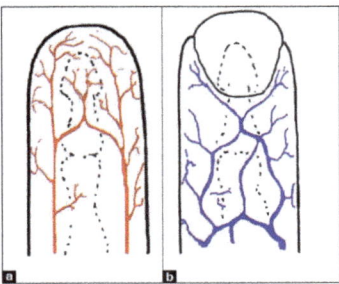

Figure 7. Blood circulation example: arteries (**a**) and veins (**b**).

By comparing the absorption levels of oxyhemoglobin and deoxyhemoglobin, the sensor will calculate the SpO_2 percentage.

The blood that runs through the arteries is rich in oxygen. The more oxygenated the blood, the more hemoglobin it contains, so the blood is redder and consequently absorbs more infrared light. In short, the more oxygenated the blood, the greater the amount of infrared light absorbed. As was said previously, the sensor IR and red LEDs are used to generate the light that penetrates the skin and red-colored tissues. The infrared LED penetrates the skin and is predominantly absorbed by the arteries, while the red LED penetrates even further away and is predominantly absorbed by the veins. When the light passes through the skin, it encounters reflection from the flowing blood in the blood vessels. The sensor employs a photodiode (along with a photonic filter for ambient light cancellation) to measure the amount of light reflected by the blood. The photodiode receives the light-reflected signals and converts them into analog data. These data are then converted into digital data by the ADC (electrical scheme in Figure 8). As the heart pumps, the reflected light (that which is not absorbed) is altered, generating a wave reading on the photodetector, which then generates a waveform that correlates the heartbeat rate.

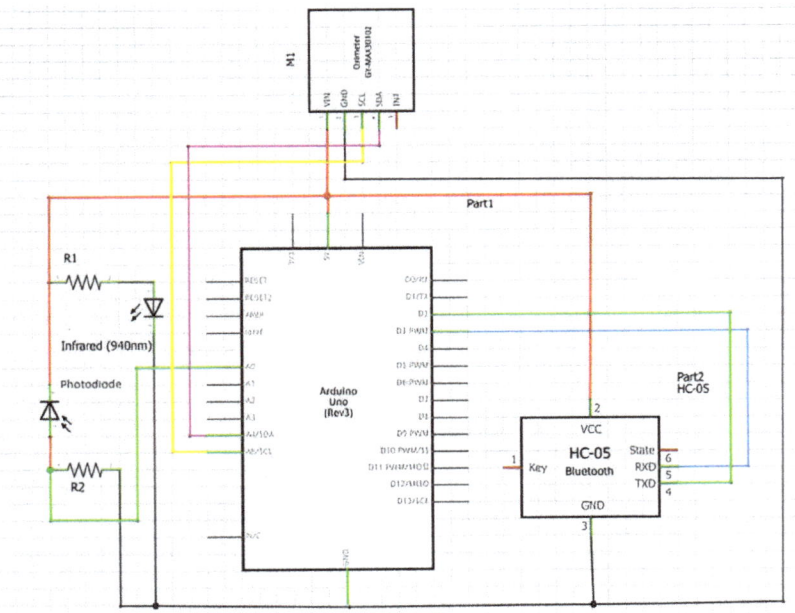

Figure 8. Electrical scheme of experiment.

The Bluetooth module used in this work is the HC-05. It has a range of up to ten meters without obstacles and can be configured in two modes, Master and Slave.

This work uses two programming languages, C/C++ and block programming. The C/C++ programming language is used to develop the firmware for the Arduino Uno. Block programming (APP Inventor) is used to program the application (APP) resident on the smartphone.

2.3. Algorithm Design

Figure 9 shows the flowchart of the firmware developed for the microcontroller and the algorithm developed.

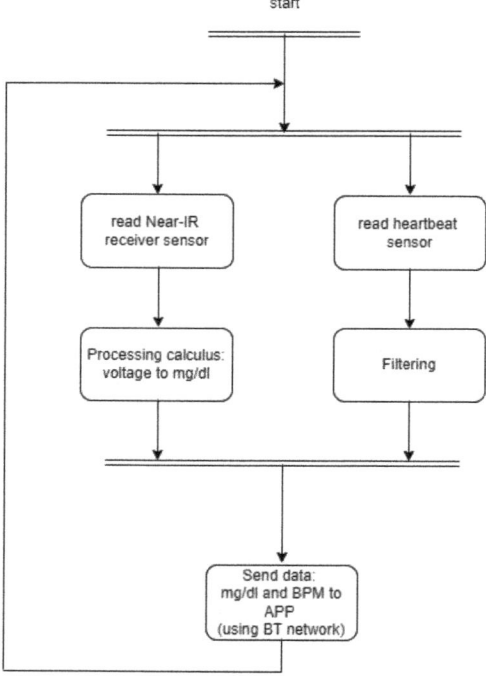

Figure 9. Firmware flowchart.

Declare integer variable i
Declare float variable value and initialize to 0
Declare integer variable numReadings and initialize to 3000
Declare integer variable r
Declare float variable rs
Declare float variable gluc
Loop infinitely:
  Read analog value from pin 0 into r
  Calculate rs:
    rs = (r * (5.0 / 1023.0)) * 1000
  For i from 0 to numReadings - 1
    Add rs to value
    Wait for 1 ms
  Calculate the average value:
    value = value / numReadings
  Calculate gluc:

gluc = (−0.03 * value) + 221.45
Send gluc via Bluetooth serial interface

3. Results and Discussion

In this work, tests were conducted on the optical sensors (Near IR emitter LED and Near IR receiver photodiode), measuring the voltage at the receiver Near IR photodiode, so that the values could be acquired by the microcontroller's ADC on the Arduino Uno board. As previously mentioned, this ADC has a resolution of 10 bits. To implement a process for reading glucose levels, measurements were taken and compared with commercial meters, specifically the OneTouch Select Plus. The OneTouch Select Plus is a conventional device that requires applying blood to a test strip. It associates the custom interval limit, either before or after a meal, with the result, based on whether a corresponding meal marker has been added.

One Touch Select Plus Meter meets international standards of EN ISO 15197:2015 [13]. For system accuracy, the standard requires the following:

- First criterion: 95% of the glucose results must fall within ±15 mg/dL of the reference result at glucose concentrations <100 mg/dL and within ±15% at glucose concentrations ≥100 mg/dL [13,14].
- Second criterion: 99% of individual glucose measured values shall fall within clinically acceptable zones A and B of the Consensus Error Grid (CEG) for diabetes [13–15].

It should be noted that the manufacturer carried out a set of tests that meet these requirements and this can be seen in [30].

The standard also adds that for measurement repeatability and intermediate measurement precision, the standard deviation (SD) should be ≤4.1 mg/dL for glucose levels <100 mg/dL and the coefficient of variation (CV) should be ≤4.2% for glucose concentrations ≥100 mg/dL.

Between the several choices of tests that detect diabetes (e.g., glucose tolerance test (GTT), random blood sugar test, fast blood sugar test), the fast blood sugar test, also known by Fasting Plasma Glucose test (FPG), is typically the best option based on its ability to provide a stable baseline (not influenced by recent meals or physical activity). This stability allows for accurate assessment of glucose metabolism. Fasting means not having anything to eat or drink (except water) for at least 8 h before the test. This test is usually performed first thing in the morning, before breakfast. Diabetes is diagnosed at a fasting blood glucose of greater than or equal to 126 mg/dL [31]. To have an idea of what type of results we should expect (interval limits):

- Normal: less than 100 mg/dL;
- Prediabetes: between 100 and 125 mg/dL;
- Diabetes: 126 mg/dL or higher.

For a different type of population group, such as children or pregnant women, other levels than these should be considered.

In our experiment and to achieve a range of values that is robust and wide enough to be able to establish the connection between the infrared optical receiver voltage supplied to the Arduino and the glucose values, we used the values of 10 different persons aged 18 to 24 whose physical condition was considered healthy. These 10 people measured their glucose values on the commercial conventional equipment (One Touch Select Plus meter) and then in our experiment.

The recorded values were obtained before and after meals, and their average is presented in Table 1. We specifically used six values in Table 1 because some of them were equal. By reducing the number of values to six, we aimed to achieve better linearization for implementing Equation (1) in the firmware development process. This approach allows us to establish a correlation between ADC levels and blood glucose levels with more samples, ultimately reducing the processing load on the microcontroller and minimizing energy consumption.

Table 1. Values measured (in mV) and commercial meter.

Values Obtained by IR (mV)	OneTouch Select Plus Meter (mg/dL)
4354.98	89
4174	92
3841.71	103
3499.6	110
3465.3	116
3200	125

In programming terms, the implementation required linear regression to derive the expression in Equation (1). Linear regression is an essential tool for estimating the expected value of a dependent variable (y). By analyzing real measured values, we can graphically approximate a linear line that best fits the data points. In our project, linear regression helped us estimate glucose values in mg/dL based on the mV readings obtained from the sensor.

Additionally, we considered Lambert's law, which states that the intensity of light decreases exponentially as the thickness of the absorbing medium increases linearly. When infrared radiation passes through the finger and reaches the infrared receiver, it undergoes attenuation due to the presence of blood glucose molecules. Depending on the glucose concentration, the IR light received by the photodetector can be higher (indicating low glucose levels) or lower (indicating higher glucose levels). Figure 10 illustrates this phenomenon.

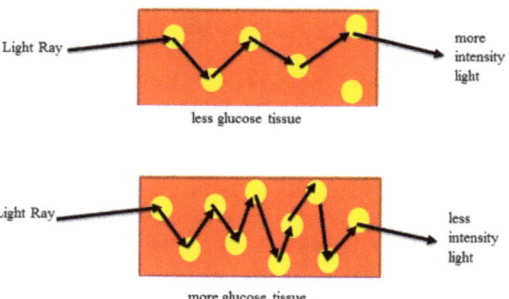

Figure 10. Influence of light propagation in glucose molecules.

For reference, an integrated image of our glucose meter is shown in Figure 11.

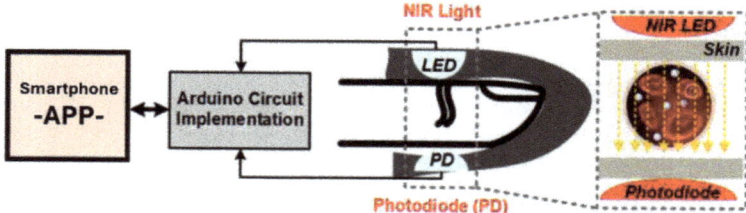

Figure 11. Experimental diagram of the glucose meter.

Based on the results in Table 1, we implemented linear regression using Geogebra, as illustrated in Figure 12. The expression from Equation (1) was then incorporated into the C/C++ programming language for the Arduino Uno microcontroller. In Table 2, we compare the average values measured by the Arduino with the glucose level values obtained from the One Touch Select Plus commercial meter.

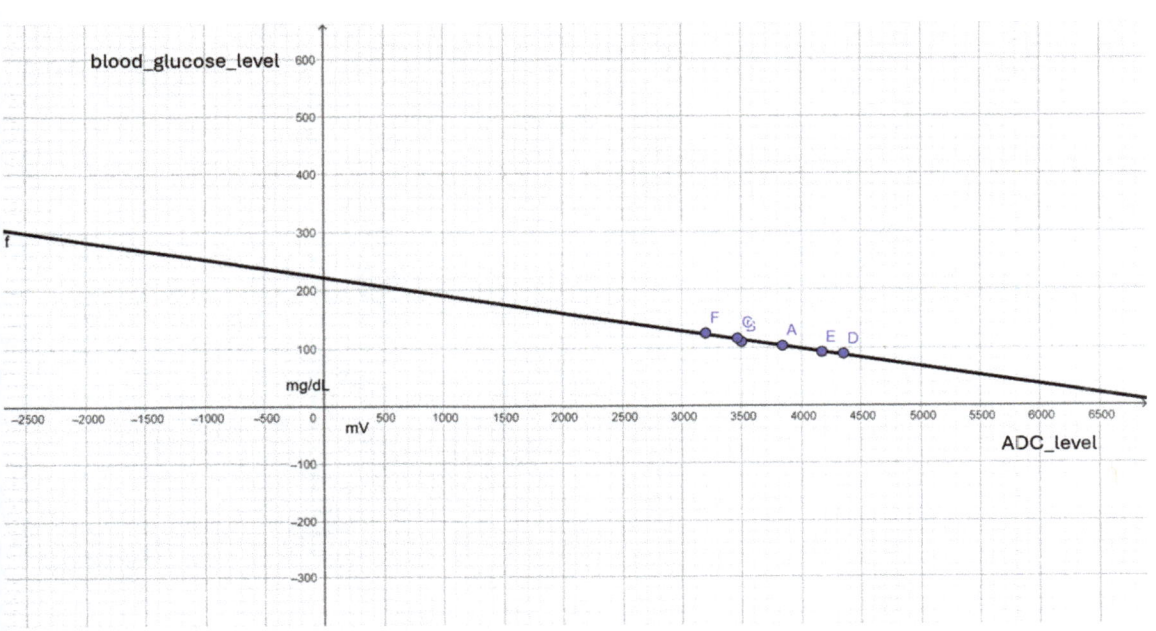

Figure 12. Point cloud and linear regression to expression in (1).

Table 2. Comparing the measured values to those obtained from a commercial meter.

OneTouch Select Plus Meter (mg/dL)	Values Calculated Using the Expression (mg/dL)	Error (%)
89	90.8	2.02
92	96.23	4.59
103	106.19	3.09
110	116.46	5.87
116	117.49	1.23
125	125.45	0.35

For the heartbeat sensor, the results shown in Table 3 were obtained.

Table 3. Measured heart rate values.

Values Obtained Heart Rate (BPM)	Average Value (BPM)
56.79	57
56.87	57
54.79	55
54.88	55
56.79	57
56.79	57

Figures 13 and 14 depict our experiment during the testing phase, along with the application developed and the corresponding experimental results.

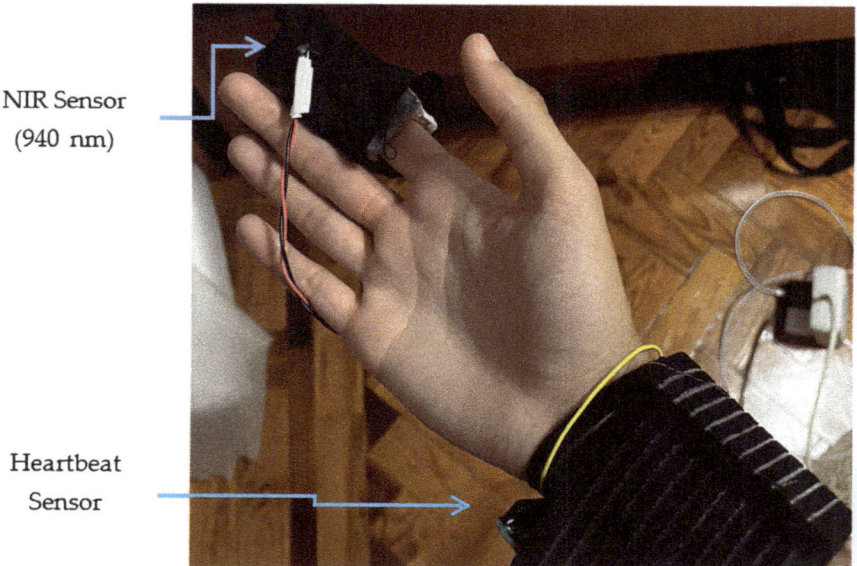

Figure 13. Visual design of the experimental prototype.

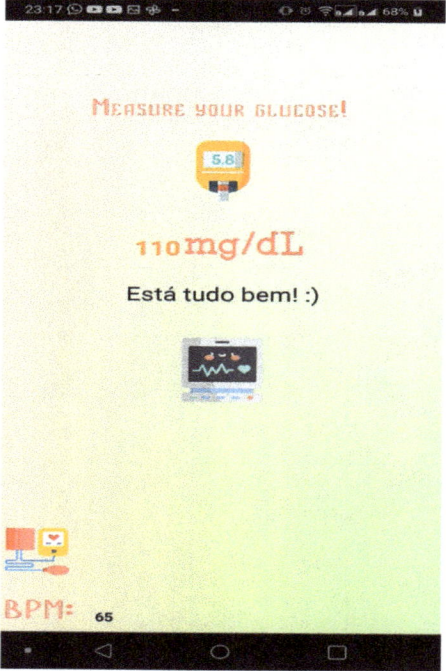

Figure 14. Appearance of the app.

4. Conclusions

The adoption by the population of a crucial piece of equipment for their health depends on two main premises: reliability and affordability. Reliability ensures that the equipment performs consistently and accurately, providing the user with confidence in the results it provides. This is especially important for health-related equipment. On the other hand, affordability ensures that the equipment is accessible to as many people as possible. Health is a universal need, and thus, it is important that critical health equipment is priced in a way that allows the population to afford it.

In our academic and experimental work, we provided, by finding a solid and simple solution (regression analysis) for the correlation between the values measured from the pair of photoemitter/receiver and the values of glucose, that the implementation of a simple algorithm/program in an Arduino microprocessor is viable and makes the two initial premises come true. The precision and simplicity of our solution leads therefore to the low-cost solution (and availability) announced in the introduction of this study. Other factors, like the ease of use of such equipment, also play a significant role in its adoption.

Also, in this work, using the method of the linear regression to achieve a correlation between the measured ADC values and glucose, we were able to achieve an average error of 2.86 per cent when compared to commercial glucose meters, which is very promising (because it shows us that are highly correlated), as we were able to develop a system that cost around EUR 8 in terms of hardware and demonstrated low consumption (during use, it consumes around 50 mA).

Invasive glucose meters, which require a blood sample, typically require a series of time-consuming procedures (also increasing user errors), and our equipment will be easy to use and able to provide readings within a few seconds (the total time from placing your finger on the reader to reading by the microprocessor, which has the ADC with a sample rate of 125 kHz, is 8 microseconds).

The possibility of the user and/or doctor being able to visualize the data collected via an app is an added value, because it can share with healthcare providers the data for further analysis, enabling early detection of any potential issues. The app provides features such as real-time tracking, historical data and alerts (high/low level of glucose), and heartbeat.

Extensive testing in different types of populations, such as type I or II diabetics or risk groups, was not in the initial scope of our work. So, the next steps will be to perform more extensive tests looking at different populations (and diabetics). Integrating screenings carried out by the Ministry of Health or by private clinics, with the aim of detecting and preventing this type of disease, would also be an objective, as we would then have access to a sample of the wider population and could compare it with the values obtained by various pieces of commercial equipment used in these screenings.

Author Contributions: Conceptualization, L.M.P. and J.M.; methodology, L.M.P. and J.M.; software, L.M.P. and J.M.; validation, L.M.P. and J.M.; formal analysis, L.M.P. and J.M.; investigation, L.M.P. and J.M.; resources, L.M.P.; data curation, L.M.P. and J.M.; writing—original draft preparation, L.M.P. and J.M.; writing—review and editing, L.M.P. and J.M.; visualization, L.M.P. and J.M.; supervision, L.M.P. and J.M. All authors have read and agreed to the published version of the manuscript.

Funding: This research received no external funding.

Data Availability Statement: Data are contained within the article.

Conflicts of Interest: The authors declare no conflicts of interest.

References

1. Gonzales, W.V.; Mobashsher, A.T.; Abbosh, A. The progress of glucose monitoring—A review of invasive to minimally and non-invasive techniques, devices and sensors. *Sensors* **2019**, *19*, 800. [CrossRef] [PubMed]
2. Cho, O.K.; Kim, Y.O.; Mitsumaki, H.; Kuwa, K. Noninvasive measurement of glucose by metabolic heat conformation method. *Clin. Chem.* **2004**, *50*, 1894–1898. [CrossRef]
3. Lin, T.; Gal, A.; Mayzel, Y.; Horman, K.; Bahartan, K. Non-invasive glucose monitoring: A review of challenges and recent advances. *Curr. Trends Biomed. Eng. Biosci.* **2017**, *6*, 555696. [CrossRef]
4. Di Filippo, D.; Sunstrum, F.N.; Khan, J.U.; Welsh, A.W. Non-Invasive Glucose Sensing Technologies and Products: A Comprehensive Review for Researchers and Clinicians. *Sensors* **2023**, *23*, 9130. [CrossRef]
5. Xue, Y.; Thalmayer, A.S.; Zeising, S.; Fischer, G.; Lübke, M. Commercial and Scientific Solutions for Blood Glucose Monitoring—A Review. *Sensors* **2022**, *22*, 425. [CrossRef]

6. Islam, M.M.; Manjur, S.M. Design and Implementation of a Wearable System for Non-Invasive Glucose Level Monitoring. In Proceedings of the 2019 IEEE International Conference on Biomedical Engineering, Computer and Information Technology for Health (BECITHCON), Dhaka, Bangladesh, 28–30 November 2019.
7. Venkataramanan, S.; Kamble, D.; Bairolu, A.; Singh, A.; Rao, R. A Novel Heart Rate and Non-Invasive Glucose Measuring Device. In Proceedings of the International Conference on Communication and Signal Processing, Chennai, India, 6–8 April 2017.
8. Naresh, M.; Peddakrishna, S. Non-invasive glucose measurement using 950 nm reflective short wave NIR technique. *Res. Biomed. Eng.* **2023**, *39*, 747–757. [CrossRef]
9. Wang, C.; Gong, D.; Feng, P.; Cheng, Y.; Cheng, X.; Jiang, Y.; Zhang, D.; Cai, J. Ultra-Sensitive and Wide Sensing-Range Flexible Pressure Sensors Based on the Carbon Nanotube Film/Stress-Induced Square Frustum Structure. *ACS Appl. Mater. Interfaces* **2023**, *15*, 8546–8554. [CrossRef] [PubMed]
10. Dai, Z.; Lei, M.; Ding, S.; Zhou, Q.; Ji, B.; Wang, M.; Zhou, B. Durable superhydrophobic surface in wearable sensors: From nature to application. *Explor. J.* **2023**, *4*, 20230046. [CrossRef] [PubMed]
11. Quan, Y.-Y.; Chen, Z.; Lai, Y.; Huang, Z.-S.; Li, H. Recent advances in fabricating durable superhydrophobic surfaces: A review in the aspects of structures and materials. *J. Mater. Chem. Front.* **2021**, *5*, 1655–1682. [CrossRef]
12. ISO. Available online: http://www.iso.org (accessed on 10 June 2024).
13. *ISO 15197:2013*; In Vitro Diagnostic Test Systems—Requirements for Blood-Glucose Monitoring Systems for Self-Testing in Managing Diabetes Mellitus. International Organization for Standardization: Geneva, Switzerland, 2013.
14. Pleus, S.; Jendrike, N.; Baumstark, A.; Mende, J.; Wehrstedt, S.; Haug, C.; Freckmann, G. Evaluation of System Accuracy, Precision, Hematocrit Influence, and User Performance of Two Blood Glucose Monitoring Systems Based on ISO 15197:2013/EN ISO 15197:2015. *Diabetes Ther.* **2014**, *15*, 447–459. [CrossRef] [PubMed]
15. Parkes, J.L.; Pardo, S.; Slatin, S.L.; Ginsberg, B.H. A New Consesus Error Grid to Evaluate the Clinical Significance of Inaccuracies in the Measurement of Blood Glucose. *Diabetes Care* **2000**, *23*, 1143–1148. [CrossRef] [PubMed]
16. Food Drug Administration. Available online: https://www.fda.gov/media/87721/download (accessed on 10 June 2024).
17. Lewandrowski, K.; Cheek, R.; Nathan, D.M.; Godine, J.E.; Hurxthal, K.; Eschenbach, K.; Laposata, M. Implementation of capillary blood glucose monitoring in a teaching hospital and determination of program requirements to maintain quality testing. *Am. J. Med.* **1992**, *93*, 419–426. [CrossRef] [PubMed]
18. Diabetes Daily. How Accurate Are Blood Sugar Meters and Continuous Glucose Monitors, Really?—Diabetes Daily. Available online: https://www.diabetesdaily.com/ (accessed on 10 June 2024).
19. Kulcu, E.; Tamada, J.A.; Reach, G.; Potts, R.O.; Lesho, M.J. Physiological Differences Between Interstitial Glucose and Blood Glucose Measured in Human Subjects. *Diabetes Care* **2003**, *26*, 2405–2409. [CrossRef] [PubMed]
20. Lindner, N.; Kuwabara, A.; Holt, T. Non-invasive and minimally invasive glucose monitoring devices: A systematic review and meta-analysis on diagnostic accuracy of hypoglycaemia detection. *Syst. Rev. J.* **2021**, *10*, 145. [CrossRef] [PubMed]
21. Karim, A.; Andersson, J.Y. Infrared detectors: Advances, challenges and new technologies. *IOP Conf. Ser. Mater. Sci. Eng.* **2013**, *51*, 012001. [CrossRef]
22. Shaikh, S.; Nazneen, A.; Ramesh, M. Current Trends in the Application of Thermal Imaging in Medical Condition Analysis. *Int. J. Innov. Technol. Explor. Eng.* **2019**, *8*, 2708–2712.
23. Edmundoptics. Available online: https://www.edmundoptics.com/knowledge-center/application-notes/imaging/what-is-swir/ (accessed on 24 April 2024).
24. Arduino. Available online: http://arduino.cc/en/Main/ArduinoBoardUno (accessed on 8 March 2024).
25. Microchip. Available online: https://www.microchip.com/en-us/product/atmega328 (accessed on 11 April 2024).
26. Reich, G. Near-infrared spectroscopy and imaging: Basic principles and pharmaceutical applications. *Adv. Drug Deliv. Rev.* **2005**, *57*, 1109–1143. [CrossRef] [PubMed]
27. Goodarzi, M.; Sharma, S.; Ramon, H.; Saeys, W. Multivariate calibration of NIR spectroscopic sensors for continuous glucose monitoring. *TrAC Trends Anal. Chem.* **2015**, *67*, 147–158. [CrossRef]
28. Yadav, J.; Rani, A.; Singh, V.; Murari, B.M. Prospects and limitations of non-invasive blood glucose monitoring using near-infrared spectroscopy. *Biomed. Signal Process. Control* **2015**, *18*, 214–227. [CrossRef]
29. Agelet, L.E.; Hurburgh, C.R. A Tutorial on Near Infrared Spectroscopy and Its Calibration. *Crit. Rev. Anal. Chem.* **2010**, *40*, 246–260. [CrossRef]
30. One Touch Select Plus. Available online: https://www.onetouch.in/sites/default/files/2024-01/07262803B_Owners_Guide_SPS_IN_LEG_R1_web.pdf (accessed on 10 June 2024).
31. Diabetes Diagnosis & Tests. Available online: https://diabetes.org/about-diabetes/diagnosis (accessed on 21 April 2024).

Disclaimer/Publisher's Note: The statements, opinions and data contained in all publications are solely those of the individual author(s) and contributor(s) and not of MDPI and/or the editor(s). MDPI and/or the editor(s) disclaim responsibility for any injury to people or property resulting from any ideas, methods, instructions or products referred to in the content.

MDPI AG
Grosspeteranlage 5
4052 Basel
Switzerland
Tel.: +41 61 683 77 34

Designs Editorial Office
E-mail: designs@mdpi.com
www.mdpi.com/journal/designs

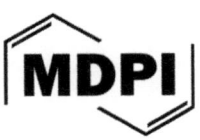

Disclaimer/Publisher's Note: The statements, opinions and data contained in all publications are solely those of the individual author(s) and contributor(s) and not of MDPI and/or the editor(s). MDPI and/or the editor(s) disclaim responsibility for any injury to people or property resulting from any ideas, methods, instructions or products referred to in the content.